THE AUTOIMMUNE CONNECTION

ESSENTIAL INFORMATION FOR WOMEN ON DIAGNOSIS, TREATMENT, AND GETTING ON WITH YOUR LIFE

RITA BARON-FAUST

JILL P. BUYON, M.D.

Contemporary Books

Chicago   New York   San Francisco   Lisbon   London   Madrid   Mexico City
Milan   New Delhi   San Juan   Seoul   Singapore   Sydney   Toronto

616.978 B

Library of Congress Cataloging-in-Publication Data

Baron-Faust, Rita.
    The autoimmune connection : essential information for women on diagnosis,
treatment, and getting on with your life / Rita Baron-Faust and Jill P. Buyon.
        p.   cm.
    Includes bibliographical references.
    ISBN 0-658-02131-1
    1. Autoimmune diseases—Popular works.   2. Women—Diseases—
Popular works.   I. Buyon, Jill P.   II. Title.

RC600 .B37   2002
616.97'8—dc21   2002074147

For my cousin Donna S. Scheib, who always believed.
I miss you.
—RBF

1 2 3 4 5 6 7 8 9 0   AGM/AGM   2 1 0 9 8 7 6 5 4 3

ISBN 0-658-02131-1

Illustrations by Marina Terletsky

McGraw-Hill books are available at special quantity discounts to use as premiums and
sales promotions, or for use in corporate training programs. For more information, please
write to the Director of Special Sales, Professional Publishing, McGraw-Hill, Two Penn
Plaza, New York, NY 10121-2298. Or contact your local bookstore.

This book is printed on acid-free paper.

Contents

Foreword

Rita Baron-Faust and Dr. Jill Buyon have written a groundbreaking overview of a disease category that affects the lives of more than fifty million Americans. *Autoimmunity*—in which the body attacks the very organs it is supposed to protect—is the underlying cause of more than eighty serious, chronic illnesses. Of those afflicted, 75 percent are women. In fact, these diseases represent the third largest cause of chronic illness among women in the United States. Even more alarming, a recent study cites autoimmune diseases as among the top ten leading causes of all deaths among U.S. women ages sixty-five and younger. It's no wonder that autoimmune diseases have been named a major women's health issue and a research priority by the National Institutes of Health's Office of Research on Women's Health.

Yet few women know about autoimmune diseases or the threat they pose until they are faced with a diagnosis. The public, patients, and even the medical community suffer from a lack of information and a plethora of misinformation and myths about these disorders, making early recognition difficult. Tragically, many women are not diagnosed until illness has progressed, and some become very ill before their symptoms are taken seriously.

It can be difficult to diagnose these illnesses. Symptoms of autoimmune diseases vary widely, sometimes even within the same disease, and can affect multiple body systems. Symptoms can be vague and sporadic, sometimes masking the seriousness of a developing illness. Too many physicians are quick to dismiss a woman's symptoms as stress related. An American Autoimmune Related Diseases Association (AARDA) survey found that many patients were labeled as being chronic complainers in the earliest stages of their illnesses. The time wasted costs hundreds of lives and creates untold pain for individuals and families each year.

This book will make great strides toward educating women about an important area affecting their health, well-being, and families. In fact, many women are not aware of their own family history of autoimmune disease, because family members are affected by different diseases (which they may not even recognize as autoimmune disease). Giving women the facts about autoimmunity will provide an assurance that symptoms are not an "all in your head" problem to be pushed aside but rather a problem that needs to be taken seriously—and that can be helped.

Progress is steadily being made in research into understanding the causes of these diseases and developing potential treatments. Early diagnosis and treatment has taken on new urgency, as biological therapies for conditions like rheumatoid arthritis are now able to change the course of an illness that once meant certain disability and disfigurement.

This book will enable more women with autoimmune diseases to find help . . . and hope.

Virginia T. Ladd
President, American Autoimmune Related Diseases Association

Acknowledgments

This was a book literally "years in the making." When I was diagnosed with hypothyroidism in 1971, the word *autoimmune* was never mentioned. I first learned about autoimmune diseases more than twenty years later, at the First Annual Congress on Women's Health in 1992, sponsored by the Society for Women's Health Research. It was there that I met Virginia Ladd, founder and president of the then-fledgling American Autoimmune Related Diseases Association, and began a decade-long friendship.

Throughout my quest to write this book, Virginia continued to encourage me, alerting me to research meetings and inviting me to serve on the AARDA board of directors. I cannot sufficiently express the deep gratitude I feel for her continued support. Virginia, AARDA, and its tireless board members and volunteers have successfully fought to bring autoimmunity to public attention. The existence of this book is testament to their efforts. It was through AARDA that I met Dr. Noel Rose, whom I'd like to especially thank for all of his help in researching this book and helping me to understand the finer points of the immune system. Special appreciation also goes to Dr. Denise Faustman, who enthusiastically gave of her time over the years and generously contributed the afterword for this volume, and to my longtime friend Samuel L. Uretsky, PharmD, for taking the time to review the material on medications.

I am also deeply grateful to the Marine Biological Laboratory at Woods Hole, Massachusetts, (and communications director Pam Clapp Hinkle) which selected me as a Science Writing Fellow in 1997 and afforded me the opportunity to attend an intensive course on the pathogenesis of neuroimmunological diseases. A brilliant cadre of lecturers, led by Drs. Byron Waksman, Celia Brosnan, and Jack Rosenbluth, provided extensive background on the workings of the immune system and the nervous system that increased my knowledge and proved invaluable in researching this book.

I also want to acknowledge two indispensable reference texts that have sat open on my desk for a year and a half: *The Autoimmune Diseases* (1998, Academic Press), edited by Dr. Noel R. Rose and Dr. Ian R. Mackay; and the *Textbook of the Autoimmune Diseases* (2000, Lippincott, Williams & Wilkins), edited by Dr. Robert G. Lahita.

My thanks also go to the following people for the resources and assistance they provided during the research and writing of this book: Arney Rosenblatt of the National Multiple Sclerosis Society; Deb Boelz of the Myasthenia Gravis Foundation; Lynne Sykora Unglo of the Arthritis Foundation; Tammy Cussimanio of the American College of Rheumatology; Joan Young of the Platelet Disorders Support Association; Mark Overbay of the American Diabetes Association; Mary Lou Ballweg of the Endometriosis Association; and Phyllis Greenberger, president of the Society for Women's Health Research.

My agent, Vicky Bijur, understood the concept of this book and recognized its potential from the outset, urging me to keep working on my proposal until we found the right approach and the right editor. Vicky, thanks for not giving up.

My editor at Contemporary Books, Judith McCarthy, "got it" right away. She understood the importance of educating women about autoimmune diseases, recognized that they may suffer from more than one disorder, and understood how these diseases can affect various life stages. Thanks Judith!

My coauthor, Dr. Jill Buyon, is both a dedicated clinician and passionate researcher. When I first approached her more than five years ago with the idea of a book on women and autoimmune diseases, she was immediately enthusiastic. When I became overwhelmed with other work, she spurred me on. Her goal is always excellence; I hope we've achieved that.

Heartfelt thanks go to all the women who shared with me their personal experiences, especially Kathleen Turner, who took the time during her Broadway run in *The Graduate* to sit down and talk with me; Hannah Wallace for sharing her story and the names of other women; Mary Kay Blakely; Lori Silverman (who also helped transcribe interview and conference tapes); Annemarie Durocher; and my old friend Ann Gold, as well as the scores of other women I met at advocacy conferences or spoke to over the phone. I'm in your debt. I hope this book will fill the need so many of you expressed to me over the years.

Loving thanks go to my mother and my son Alexander, who cheer me—and cheer me on.

To my husband, Allen: thanks for putting up with a year and a half of (very) late nights and stress of my juggling a complicated book project and a full-time job. Your love means everthing.

RBF

Above all, I wish to thank each and every one of my patients with SLE who have taught me more about lupus than any textbook, to be humble, caring, and involved. These individuals manage to cope with the ever-present uncertainty of a chronic disease that can lay dormant for months to years only to explode at the most inopportune times.

Working on this book has certainly been a major departure from the basic and clinical research activities that I hold so dear. Despite hours of my obsessive editing and struggling with the right words to communicate to the lay public about extraordinarily complex medical issues, some of which are rapidly evolving, Rita Baron-Faust continued to put up with me. I believe she has managed to capture the depth of autoimmune diseases in an extraordinarily reader-friendly way. I salute her incredible tenacity in putting this omnibus book together and putting up with me. I am confident that this final product will provide an invaluable reference to patients and their families.

On a personal note, I would like to thank my husband, Richard Backer, for being so tolerant of the back of my head; my son, Shane, for keeping me company in the wee hours of the night; my daughter, Chelsea, for her own extraordinary passion for science, relentlessly inquisitive mind, and often uncanny insights; Bob D'Clancy for saving the lab while I worked on this book and forever reminding me that Excedrin works quite well just being in your pocket; and Joan Della Merrill, for always being "on call" for me and giving every success and failure the right perspective.

JPB

Contributors

The authors wish to express gratitude to the following people who provided insight, information, and peer review on the rapidly evolving subject of women and autoimmunity during the research and writing of this book.

William P. Arend, MD
Scoville Professor of Rheumatology
University of Colorado Health Sciences Center
Denver, CO

Henry C. Bodenheimer, Jr., MD
Chief, Division of Digestive Diseases
Beth Israel Medical Center
New York, NY

Laurence A. Bradley, PhD
Professor of Medicine
Division of Clinical Immunology and
    Rheumatology
University of Alabama at Birmingham

D. Ware Branch, MD
Professor and Chair, Department of Obstetrics
    and Gynecology
University of Utah School of Medicine
Salt Lake City, UT

Evelyn Bromet, PhD
Department of Psychiatry
State University of New York at Stony Brook

James B. Bussel, MD
Professor of Pediatrics,
Director, Platelet Disorders Center
Weill Medical College of Cornell University
New York, NY

George P. Chrousos, MD
Chief, Pediatric and Reproductive Endocrinology
National Institute of Child Health and Human
    Development
National Institutes of Health
Bethesda, MD

Daniel J. Clauw, MD
Professor of Medicine, Division of Rheumatology
Director, Center for the Advancement of Clinical
    Research
University of Michigan
Ann Arbor, MI

Terry F. Davies, MD
Chief, Division of Endocrinology
Mount Sinai School of Medicine
New York, NY

Madeline Duvic, MD
Professor of Medicine, Interim Chair,
    Department of Dermatology
Director, National Alopecia Areata Registry
M.D. Anderson Cancer Center
University of Texas
Houston, TX

Denise L. Faustman, MD, PhD
Associate Professor of Medicine,
Harvard Medical School
Director, Immunobiology
Massachusetts General Hospital
Boston, MA

Alan W. Friedman, MD
Associate Professor of Medicine
Division of Rheumatology
University of Texas Health Science Center
Houston, TX

Christine L. Frissora, MD
Assistant Professor of Medicine
Weill Medical College of Cornell University
New York, NY

Barbara S. Giesser, MD
Associate Clinical Professor of Neurology
University of California, Los Angeles

Peter H. R. Green, MD
Clinical Professor
Columbia University College of Physicians and
    Surgeons
Director, Celiac Disease Research Center
New York, NY

Bevra H. Hahn, MD
Professor of Medicine
University of California, Los Angeles

E. Nigel Harris, MD, DM
Dean, Morehouse School of Medicine
Atlanta, GA

Melanie J. Harrison, MD
Assistant Professor of Medicine
Weill Medical College of Cornell University
Director of Rheumatoid Arthritis Clinical
    Research, Hospital for Special Surgery

Sunanda V. Kane, MD, MSPH
Assistant Professor of Medicine
Section on Gastroenterology
University of Chicago

Robert Kimberly, MD
Chairman, Division of Clinical Immunology and
    Rheumatology
Professor of Medicine
University of Alabama at Birmingham

John H. Klippel, MD
Medical Director
Arthritis Foundation
Atlanta, GA

Mark Lebwohl, MD
Professor and Chairman of Dermatology
Mount Sinai School of Medicine
New York, NY

Arnold I. Levinson, MD
Chief of Allergy and Immunology
University of Pennsylvania School of Medicine
Philadelphia, PA

Carol J. Levy, MD
Assistant Professor of Medicine
Weill Medical College of Cornell University
Attending Physician, Cornell Diabetes Center
New York, NY

Michael Lockshin, MD
Director, Barbara Volcker Center for Women and
    Rheumatic Diseases
Hospital for Special Surgery
Weill Cornell Medical Center
New York, NY

Mary Loeken, PhD
Assistant Professor of Medicine
Harvard Medical School
Investigator, Research Division
Joslin Diabetes Center
Boston, MA

Judith Luborsky, PhD
Director of Reproductive Immunology
Rush-Presbyterian Medical Center
Chicago, IL

Noel Maclaren, MD, PhD
Director, Cornell Juvenile Diabetes Program
New York Weill Cornell Medical Center
Professor of Medicine
Weill Medical College of Cornell University
New York, NY

Susan Manzi, MD, MPH
Professor of Medicine
Department of Epidemiology
University of Pittsburgh Graduate School of
    Public Health
Pittsburgh, PA

Janice M. Massey, MD
Professor of Neurology
Director, Myasthenia Gravis Clinic
Duke University Medical Center
Durham, NC

Lloyd Mayer, MD
Professor and Chairman
Immunobiology Center
Dorothy and David Merksamer Professor of
    Medicine
Mount Sinai School of Medicine
New York, NY

Maureen D. Mayes, MD, MPH
Professor of Internal Medicine
Division of Rheumatology
University of Texas Health Science Center
Houston, TX

Joan T. Merrill, MD
Head, Clinical Pharmacology Program
Director, the Registry for the Anti-
    phospholipid Syndrome
Oklahoma Medical Research Foundation
Oklahoma City, OK

Hal J. Mitnick, MD
Clinical Professor of Medicine
New York University Medical Center
New York, NY

Lila E. Nachtigall, MD
Professor of Obstetrics and Gynecology
New York University School of Medicine
New York, NY

J. Lee Nelson, MD
Member, Immunogenetics Program
Fred Hutchinson Cancer Research Center
Professor, University of Washington at Seattle

David L. Olive, MD
Professor of Obstetrics and Gynecology
Director of Reproductive Endocrinology and
    Infertility
University of Wisconsin, Madison

Melissa Palmer, MD
Liver Specialist, Private Practice
Plainview, NY

Ann Parke, MD
Professor of Medicine
University of Connecticut Health Center
Farmington, CT

Michelle Petri, MD, MPH
Director, Lupus Clinic
Associate Professor of Medicine
Johns Hopkins Medical Institutions
Baltimore, MD

David Pisetsky, MD, PhD
Chief of Rheumatology, Duke University
    Medical Center
Codirector, Duke University Arthritis Center
Durham, NC

Anthony T. Reder, MD
Associate Professor, Department of Neurology
University of Chicago
Chicago, IL

Robert A. S. Roubey, MD
Director, National Antiphospholipid
    Syndrome Registry
Associate Professor of Medicine, Division of
    Rheumatology and Immunology
University of North Carolina, Chapel Hill

S. Gerald Sandler, MD
Professor of Medicine and Pathology
Georgetown University Medical Center
Washington, DC

Daniel W. Skupski, MD
Associate Professor of Obstetrics and Gynecology
Weill Medical College of Cornell University
New York, NY

Janine A. Smith, MD
Deputy Clinical Director, National Eye
    Institute (NEI)
National Institutes of Health
Bethesda, MD

Virginia D. Steen, MD
Professor of Medicine
Division of Rheumatology, Allergy, Immunology
Georgetown University
Washington, DC

David A. Sullivan, PhD
Senior Scientist, Schepens Eye Research Institute
Associate Professor, Department of
    Ophthalmology
Harvard Medical School
Boston, MA

Rhonda Voskuhl, MD
Associate Professor
Department of Neurology
University of California, Los Angeles

Sara E. Walker, MD
Professor of Internal Medicine
University of Missouri School of Medicine
Columbia, MO

Introduction

A New View of Autoimmunity

It is a pleasure for me to participate in the birth of this, the first book on the autoimmune diseases for women.

It is only recently that we have begun to think of autoimmune diseases as a single category, as we think of cancer or infectious diseases. Autoimmune diseases are seen and treated by different medical specialists, and it has not been the mind-set of either doctors or their patients to begin to think of these diseases together. Yet there are important reasons why they should be thought of as a single category of disease.

One of the common features of autoimmune diseases is a bias toward women. This observation emphasizes the important interrelationship between the hormonal system and immune responses. The fact that there are a few autoimmune diseases that are not more common in women may provide valuable clues that the disease actually began before the age of puberty. This book will outline some of the theories as to why there is a female preponderance in many of these diseases.

Clinically, these diseases also travel together. A single patient may have more than one autoimmune disorder. This is quite common and important for patients and their physicians to know. Autoimmune diseases cluster in families. And while that is an indication that genetics is involved, environment must also play a role.

In studies of the autoimmune diseases, we have found that in identical twins the chances of the second twin developing an autoimmune disease are about 30 percent, as opposed to 4 or 5 percent among nonidentical twins. This also tells us that even in identical twins, where genes are the same, the immune system does not react in identical ways.

Overall, genetics may account for about half the risks for autoimmune disease. However, what is inherited is not a specific gene that causes a defect that leads to disease, but several genes that collectively increase vulnerability or susceptibility.

While it is clear that there are environmental triggers for autoimmune disease, we don't know much about them or how they might cause disease. Probably the best documented triggers are drugs, such as those that cause lupus, and there is strong (but not conclusive) evidence that viruses and bacteria can also serve as triggers. Foods (such as gluten) can also serve as a trigger, as can hormones.

Even if one is genetically predisposed, the possibility exists that autoimmune disease can be avoided if the environmental trigger is eliminated. Indeed, the final victory over the autoimmune diseases may come from strategies to prevent rather than treat disease.

One of the common threads uniting all of the autoimmune diseases is the presence of *autoantibodies*. Finding autoantibodies in blood serum is a key first step in the diagnosis of autoimmune disease. At the same time, the presence of autoantibodies is not sufficient criterion for a diagnosis. It is a combination of clinical findings with laboratory data that helps a physician make a final diagnosis. In fact, many normal individuals have autoantibodies in their serum without any clinical evidence of disease.

Scientifically, we now know that many of the mechanisms involved in the development of one autoimmune disease pertain to others. Therefore, studying the common factors in these diseases may help us understand the underlying causes of autoimmune disorders as a whole—and begin to treat the causes of these diseases, not just the symptoms.

The common threads that connect the autoimmune diseases are woven throughout this important book, enabling readers to obtain a greater understanding of these illnesses individually and collectively. Together with new information contained in this volume about diagnostic and treatment advances, patients and their families will be better able to cope with these diseases and, as the title states, get on with their lives.

Noel R. Rose, MD, PhD
Chairman, AARDA National Scientific Advisory Board; Director, Johns Hopkins Autoimmune Disease Research Center; Professor of Pathology and Professor of Molecular Microbiology and Immunology; Director, PAHO/WHO Collaborating Center for Autoimmune Disorders

1

Autoimmune Disease— Facing Our Intimate Enemy

I had never heard the word autoimmune *before I was told that I had antiphospholipid syndrome. And that diagnosis was scary enough. Imagine having normal checkups all of your life, then having a stroke from an illness you never even heard of. You have to learn a whole lot in a very short time to understand what's happening to you and feel in control and not frightened.*

ELAINE, FIFTY-EIGHT

You probably bought this book because you've been diagnosed with an autoimmune disease, or you suspect you may have one. Perhaps someone in your family has an autoimmune disease, like rheumatoid arthritis, and you're worried about your own risk.

Maybe you're even wondering how it is that the body can declare war on itself. Simply put, somewhere along the line, your immune cells got the wrong message. Your body dispatched the battalions of cells that normally recognize and eliminate foreign invaders such as bacteria to instead destroy healthy tissue. The attack can target any area, including the joints (causing rheumatoid arthritis), the thyroid gland (causing it to become overactive or underactive), or nerve cells (leading to multiple sclerosis).

Often it's not a single assault; immune attacks may have several targets. If you have one autoimmune disease, you're at risk for a second or even a third disease. Immune attacks may also come in waves, with lulls in between; you can have symptoms for weeks, then feel perfectly fine. The specialist treating your particular problem may not be looking for these additional diseases, so it's important to be aware that they can occur.

This book is designed to give you the inside story of the battle within your body. We're focusing on what makes you special as a woman, and why simply being female may put you at risk of autoimmune disease. We'll examine those diseases more common in women and explore how they're interrelated. We'll look at treatments—some of them brand-new and generating excitement and optimism—and discuss the impact of autoimmune diseases during different stages of your life.

Most important, you'll learn some of the key signs and symptoms of autoimmune diseases, which may help you get a diagnosis more quickly. Lack of knowledge can lead to tragedy, such as the one endured by AARDA spokeswoman and actress Kellie Martin and her family. Martin recounts the story of her nineteen-year-old sister Heather, whose flulike symptoms initially led doctors to think she had a severe virus. But Heather had lupus, and by the time she was diagnosed, her kidneys had been irreparably damaged by the disease.

A few days after finishing her sophomore year at college, my sister Heather couldn't get out of bed. She experienced severe abdominal pain and leg cramping, had numerous sores in her mouth that prevented her from eating, and had a temperature of 102. The doctor said it was the flu, or just stress from her recent final exams. So we were told to wait it out; a flu or virus just needs to run its course. "There's nothing we can do, except give her some painkillers," they said. Three emergency room visits and three days later, the doctor finally admitted Heather to the hospital for observation and testing. In the hospital she was examined by an internist, an infectious disease doctor, and a hematologist. After running several tests and concluding that she did indeed have an unusual virus, the doctor discharged Heather.

They discharged Heather even though she still couldn't walk, eat, or sleep. After she was home for a few days, my mom and I took Heather to another doctor's office, where her condition was suspected two minutes after our arrival. The doctor looked disturbed at Heather's charts and medical history. After a brief physical exam, the doctor simply sat down and talked to Heather. He listened thoughtfully as she described exactly how she was feeling. The doctor suspected that she had an autoimmune disease called lupus.

The following day she was again admitted to the hospital because of dehydration and kidney failure, both caused by lupus.

We were given the list of treatments Heather would be receiving: steroids, vitamins, and fluids. During her first week at the hospital, the blood vessels in her lungs began to burst, and her breathing became increasingly labored. The doctors, who now included a pulmonary specialist, three rheumatologists, and an oncologist (and those are just the doctors I can remember at this point), found that the lupus had affected Heather's liver and bone marrow. Therefore, the list of treatments increased to antibiotics and chemotherapy. My family believed that once Heather's condition had a name, she would receive the treatment necessary to make her better. Unfortunately, that diagnosis came too late. She died not long afterward, at age nineteen.

Unfortunately, it's common to encounter difficulty in getting a diagnosis of an autoimmune disease. A survey conducted by the Lupus Foundation of America found that more than half of people with lupus had symptoms for at least four years and saw three or more doctors before they were correctly diagnosed. Misdiagnosis or late diagnosis, due to lack of awareness and understanding of symptoms, is a leading cause of death in autoimmunity. So it's imperative that you, the patient, be informed and alert.

To truly understand your disease and the others for which you may be at risk, you need to become familiar with the fundamentals of autoimmunity. So that's where we'll begin. Think of this chapter as Autoimmunity 101.

Our Immune System—and How It Goes Awry

Our immune system has several layers. The first line of defense from outside invaders is a physical barrier—the skin and mucous membranes. Harmful organisms, such as bacteria, can breach this perimeter when, for example, we get a cut.

Once inside, these bacteria must face a second line of defense called the *innate immune system,* cells produced by the bone marrow. If you remember the video game Pac-Man (or in this case, Ms. Pac-Man), you'll recall those little smiley circles that gobbled up everything in their path. The Ms. Pac-Men of the innate immune system are *neutrophils* and *macrophages* (in Latin, *macro* means big, *phage* means to eat . . . this cell is literally a "big eater"). Billions of macrophages and neutrophils patrol the bloodstream at any given time. When macrophages see an invader (like bacteria from that cut), they grab it, suck it in, and chew it up into little pieces that are destroyed by enzymes within the cell. They are messy eaters, though. They burp back fragments of their meal, and those "crumbs" signal other immune cells to join the fray. Not only that, but as they chomp away, macrophages produce chemicals that also cause inflammation that helps to heal but, if allowed to go on too long, can also hurt.

Now we come to the third (and most complicated) layer of the immune system, the one that's mainly involved in autoimmunity. It's called the *adaptive immune system*, which means cells in this system must be *told* how to do their job. *All* of these cells are intended to recognize what is *self* and what is *nonself*, or foreign.

When a nonself entity like a bacteria or virus enters the bloodstream, the macrophages sound the alarm and battalions of other white blood cells (*lymphocytes*) are mobilized to search out the invader, referred to as an *antigen*.

There are several types of lymphocytes in the adaptive immune system, and each has a specific job to do: *T-cells* help identify and eliminate antigens, and *B-cells* produce *antibodies* that attach to one special antigen and help destroy it.

B-cells, which develop in the bone marrow, must be activated in order to produce antibodies. First, B-cells encounter antigens in the circulation. Then, after a special signal from "helper" T-cells, B-cells multiply and intensify their antibody response, making it more lethal. In autoimmune diseases, susceptible women produce *autoantibodies*, antibodies that attack self. We can make dozens of these autoantibodies, which can interfere with the normal function of tissues and destroy them. Some antibodies specifically react with material inside the nucleus of a cell (think of the nucleus as the yolk of an egg). These are classified as *antinuclear antibodies*, or *ANAs*. These antibodies are associated with autoimmune diseases such as *systemic lupus erythematosus* (*SLE*). While ANAs can be an indication you may have an autoimmune disease, they're not diagnostic in and of themselves. Some antibodies attack the fluid of the cell surrounding the nucleus, called the *cytoplasm* (the white of the egg); these antibodies are also seen in SLE, and in *Sjögren's syndrome*.

Many other antibodies attack the surface or membrane of a cell—such as a red blood cell or platelet, or in a specific tissue such as the thyroid—causing the cell (or the target tissue) to malfunction. For example, an autoimmune assault on the thyroid gland can cause it to become overactive and produce too much thyroid hormone (*Graves' disease*), or to become underactive and secrete too little thyroid hormone (*Hashimoto's thyroiditis*). In *multiple sclerosis (MS)*, the target is the protective coating called *myelin* that's wrapped around nerve cells in the brain and spine, disrupting communication between nerves and causing disability. In *myasthenia gravis*, the immune system targets the nerves that control muscles, causing progressive damage and weakness.

There are three types of T-cells:

- Helper T-cells that signal B-cells to produce stronger antibodies
- Cell-killing (*cytotoxic*) T-cells that produce molecules that destroy cells carrying antigens
- Suppressor T-cells that down-regulate other immune responses

T-cells are activated when they encounter an antigen, "recognizing" it through a kind of antenna on its surface, called a *receptor*, that receives signals from molecules sitting on the surface of the antigen. Cells that signal the T-cells in this process are called *antigen-presenting cells (APCs)*.

A normal helper T-cell might signal a B-cell that it has found a *rhinovirus* (which causes the common cold); the B-cell would then produce the appropriate antibody to get rid of that virus. A self-reactive T-cell would tell the B-cell to produce an antibody against healthy tissue. A cytotoxic T-cell might mistake the body's own cells for a bacterium or a virus and target it for destruction. A suppressor T-cell might hamper protective immune responses. Many autoimmune diseases are *cell mediated*, meaning the T-cells are what cause the damage, not antibodies.

We encounter millions of antigens during our lifetime, and we have a vast array of T-cells capable of recognizing, responding to, and remembering these antigens. T-cells mature in the thymus gland, where their receptors are programmed to react against foreign antigens and tolerate *self-antigens*; T-cells with receptors that react to self-antigens are usually eliminated in the thymus. But sometimes self-reactive T-cells aren't eliminated, or, as some researchers speculate, the thymus may not properly eliminate enough self-reactive T-cells. Whatever the cause, rogue T-cells are able to roam the body, attacking healthy tissue or sending the wrong signals to B-cells.

T-cells send signals through messenger molecules called *cytokines* and *chemokines*, which can also be key players in autoimmune disease. Cytokines are proteins that can activate immune cells (including other T-cells) and affect nonimmune processes, directly causing inflammation and damage. A common inflammatory cytokine in autoimmune disease is *tumor necrosis factor* (*TNF*); new drugs that can slow or halt the progress of rheumatoid arthritis, Crohn's disease, and other autoimmune diseases block the destructive effects of TNF (see page 32). *Chemokines*, substances manufactured by cells and tissues, act like a magnet for other immune cells. Overproduction of chemokines attracts macrophages (who never refuse a meal) and other destructive innate immune cells called *neutrophils*.

As we mentioned, macrophages and neutrophils (also called *phagocytes*) normally patrol the bloodstream, killing foreign cells by engulfing them and destroying them with toxic molecules. After digesting antigens, macrophages spit out tiny bits of the antigen on their surface to alert T-cells to the presence of an enemy. Neutrophils fight off infectious agents by releasing granules of potent chemicals that destroy the invaders. In autoimmune diseases, these cells become overactive and release too many of these toxic molecules, which damage surrounding tissue and contribute to inflammation. This happens in rheumatoid arthritis, multiple sclerosis, and other autoimmune diseases.

Another cause of inflammation in autoimmune disease is the formation of *immune complexes*, latticelike structures created when antibodies bind to antigens. Immune complex accumulation, coupled with an invasion of immune cells and inflammatory cytokines, can block blood flow in small blood vessels, destroying instead of nourishing tissues and organs.

The *complement* system also aids antibodies. If you think of antibodies as the "guns" of the immune arsenal, then complement proteins function as the "bullets" that help destroy foreign antigens. The complement system also protects the body against damage from immune complexes by preventing their formation, helping to dissolve them, or reducing them in size so they don't create blockages.

But activation of the complement system can also cause problems; products of this process can themselves attract neutrophils, fueling inflammation.

As you can see, a lot is going on in autoimmunity, which is why treatment for autoimmune disease is not as simple as a single antibiotic pill that kills bacteria. These diseases may require multidrug therapies to affect the different processes causing the symptoms and damage.

What Causes Immune Mistakes?

Because the immune system is so complicated, it's hard to pinpoint a single cause for any autoimmune disease. You may need to be susceptible (usually a matter of genes), you may need to encounter some kind of trigger (maybe an infection), but for sure your immune cells have to misfire.

We normally have small numbers of autoreactive B-cells and T-cells floating around the immune system, but self-tolerance is usually maintained. However, in susceptible people, that tolerance can be disrupted. Some people may be genetically programmed to produce large numbers of overreactive immune cells or too many damaging cytokines. Faulty genes could also cause problems with T-cell education in the thymus. Some T-cells may turn traitor after exposure to viruses or other environmental factors. Infections, environmental toxins (such as mercury), medications, and even sun exposure may also activate B-cells. For example, excess iodine can be toxic to thyroid tissue, causing autoantibody production and thyroid disease. Studies have tied exposure to *Epstein-Barr virus* (*EBV*, which causes infectious mononucleosis) to lupus.

Some cells in the body actually resemble viruses or bacteria, so T-cells may mistake one for the other and attack both. Such *molecular mimicry* happens in rheumatic fever: proteins on the surface of strep bacteria have a similar structure to proteins in cardiac muscle. Recent studies suggest that a similar process may take place in kidney cells, contributing to their destruction in lupus.

Genes also play a role in autoimmune diseases, and more than one gene may be to blame for a single disease. Think of genes as minicomputers, packed with complex codes that deliver instructions to cells, telling them which proteins to produce to grow and which proteins to produce to perform different functions. The genetic code is made up of sequences of four letters: A, T, C, and G (which stand for the basic components that make up DNA). Sometimes there's a gene mutation, a "typo." Genes that predispose people to autoimmune diseases are often those controlling *human leukocyte antigens*

(*HLAs*), which contain the codes for proteins that label a cell self or nonself. In some autoimmune diseases, these HLA genes mistakenly identify cells as nonself, setting off an attack. Several autoimmune diseases may have in common genes in the same HLA group; for example, genes in the *DR4* group are linked to both rheumatoid arthritis and to type 1 diabetes, among other diseases. Other genes regulate cytokines, causing too many or too few to be produced.

Autoimmune diseases and their related genes can run in families, but the same faulty genes don't always produce the same problem. One family member may have immune cells that react against the thyroid, while another may suffer an autoimmune attack on the joints. Even if you're an identical twin, your chances of developing the same autoimmune disease can vary.

All told, autoimmune reactions either cause—or are involved in—more than eighty chronic illnesses. The most common are actually thyroid disorders, including Hashimoto's thyroiditis or Graves' disease, which affect at least 3 percent of all adult women.

> *I have Crohn's disease, an underactive thyroid, Sjögren's syndrome, and endometriosis. I've probably had some of these since I was a teenager. It's hard for me to believe all these things are not related. They all have to do with a screwed-up immune system. The problem is, your doctor never really sees it that way. He focuses on your gut or your joints and never sees the big picture. In my opinion, that's a really myopic view and one of the reasons so many of us don't have our diseases managed well.*
>
> LAURA, FORTY-SIX

Is Autoimmunity a Single Disorder?

Many of these illnesses share the same autoantibodies, feature tissue or organ destruction caused by the same hordes of immune cells and inflammatory molecules, or have common genes. So some scientists are beginning to believe that these are not so much different illnesses, but different manifestations of a single underlying problem—autoimmunity.

Some of the strongest evidence to support this idea has come from the increasing use of the same medication to treat different diseases. Long before the concept of autoimmune disease (or the common factor of inflammation) was recognized, the corticosteroid drug prednisone was used to treat a variety of these disorders.

More recently, medications developed to target a specific mechanism in one illness have been found to effectively combat that same factor in others. For example, patients with some autoimmune diseases have high levels of *tumor necrosis factor* (*TNF*), an inflammatory molecule that contributes to organ and tissue damage. One anti-TNF drug, *etanercept* (*Enbrel*), soaks TNF up like a sponge, inactivating it; another drug, *infliximab* (*Remicade*), uses a "smart bomb" molecule called a *monoclonal antibody* to disable TNF. Etanercept was initially approved as a treatment for rheumatoid arthritis, but is now being used to treat people with Crohn's disease, autoimmune inflammatory bowel disease, and vasculitis. Remicade was initially approved for patients with Crohn's disease, but is now being used to treat rheumatoid and psoriatic arthritis.

While autoimmune diseases may target different areas of the body, the genes that affect immune responses may be the same. For example, genes that govern cytokines may have a mutation that causes too many inflammatory molecules to be released. Defective genes common to autoimmune diseases may also affect the way T-cells are programmed to recognize antigens, the number of receptors they carry, the number of T-cells with a faulty memory, or how many defective T-cells are eliminated. Gene therapy to correct these mistakes may one day be possible.

Many autoimmune diseases have the same inflammatory molecules and immune cells that cause damage. For example, a small study from the Hospital for Sick Children in Toronto, Ontario, found the *same* autoreactive T-cells in people with type 1 diabetes and multiple sclerosis, targeting similar antigens in the pancreas and in the central nervous system (CNS). The researchers studied T-cell autoreactivity in 38 people with MS, in 54 children newly diagnosed with type 1 diabetes, and 105 of their close family members, comparing them to a group of healthy controls. To their surprise, they found T-cells from the MS patients also targeted self-antigens on insulin-producing islet cells in the pancreas, and T-cells from two-thirds of the children with diabetes and their parents or siblings also showed responses to at least one autoantigen seen in MS—including myelin basic protein, one of the building blocks of the "insulation" around nerve cell fibers. The research, pub-

Autoimmune Disease: Female-to-Male Ratios

Hashimoto's thyroiditis	10:1
Systemic lupus erythematosus	9:1
Sjögren's syndrome	9:1
Primary biliary cirrhosis	9:1
Graves' disease	9:1
Chronic active hepatitis	8:1
Mixed connective tissue disease	8:1
Antiphospholipid syndrome	3:1
Scleroderma	3:1
Rheumatoid arthritis	2.5:1
Myasthenia gravis	2:1
Multiple sclerosis	2:1
Immune thrombocytopenia purpura	2:1
Autoimmune hemolytic anemia	2:1

Sources: Institute of Medicine; American Autoimmune Related Diseases Association

lished in the February 2001 *Journal of Immunology*, not only suggests that type 1 diabetes and MS may be more closely linked than anyone thought, but that there may be a lengthy "clinically silent" phase in both diseases that could be a potential target for future preventive therapy. In fact, emerging knowledge about autoimmunity as a cause of disease may lead to treatments that could halt such reactions before they have a chance to cause serious damage.

Why Are Women More Vulnerable?

As you can see from the previous table, women are prime targets for many autoimmune diseases (although disease severity doesn't always differ between the sexes). One reason for the high incidence of some diseases may be that women are exposed more often to possible triggers, like viruses or medications. But explanations are likely found in sex-related (biological) differences in certain immune functions.

The most obvious difference is our ability to bear children. We're able to carry a baby in the womb without the immune system attacking a technically half-"foreign" body (a fetus has genes and immune components from both parents). Recent research suggests that fetal cells from past pregnancies can survive in some women's bloodstreams for more than twenty years and may trigger an immune response akin to the rejection of a transplanted organ— perhaps causing diseases like scleroderma or rheumatoid arthritis.

Key elements in this reaction are the human leukocyte antigens (HLAs), which, as you'll recall, are governed by genes. In a bone marrow transplant, both the donor and recipient must have compatible HLAs (also called *histocompatibility antigens*), otherwise the transplanted cells will see the recipient's body tissues as "foreign" and attack. This is called *graft-versus-host disease* (which can often resemble autoimmune disease). In fact, the HLA genes involved in graft-versus-host disease are also involved in autoimmune diseases.

While our *own* HLAs are *self*-antigens, the combination of self and non-self HLAs in fetal cells means they are part foreign. The fact that fetal cells remain in a woman's circulation results in a condition called *chimerism*, a word that derives from the mythical creature called a *chimera* that has the head of one animal and the tail of another. The existence of these fetal cells is called *microchimerism*, and it may contribute to an autoimmune reaction by confusing the immune system, speculates J. Lee Nelson, MD, of the Immunogenetics Program at the Fred Hutchinson Cancer Research Center and a professor at the University of Washington in Seattle. The greatest risk for autoimmune disease seems to occur when there's a close, but not identical, match between HLA molecules. This confusion between the two sets of HLA molecules may disrupt normal communication within the immune system and provoke a wrongful attack on self. "You can directly inherit genes from your mother or father that put you at risk for disease. But these are genes that come from *your prior pregnancy* that are in your bloodstream."

Those same HLA genes (some of which may be linked to susceptibility to autoimmune disease) may also determine whether fetal cells that survive in the mother's blood have a detrimental effect on the mother. For example, if a child has the same HLA gene as the mother, it seems to be a strong risk factor for some diseases in the woman (because the immune system allows fetal cells containing the gene to stick around). Dr. Nelson has found twenty times more persistent fetal cells in women with scleroderma, compared to women who'd also had children but didn't have the disease. Similar evidence of persistent fetal cells has been found in women with lupus, autoimmune liver disease, thyroid disease, and Sjögren's syndrome.

"The effect of persistent maternal cells is not yet known. However, the effects of persistent fetal cells are not all adverse. Interestingly, we know that for rheumatoid arthritis, which usually gets better during pregnancy, women carrying a child that is not HLA-compatible have a better chance of a remission," says Dr. Nelson. Also, having previously given birth provides a modest protective effect against RA. However, in other cases, it may be that in some women these cells gravitate to certain sites in the body, the thyroid for example, and contribute to an autoimmune reaction.

It may well be possible to "vaccinate" women against suspect HLA molecules to slow or halt the progress of disease, or even prevent it altogether in high-risk individuals, says Dr. Nelson.

The same foreign cell "transfer" might occur from maternal cells that get into fetal circulation while the immune system is developing, Dr. Nelson adds. Maternal cells may also transfer to male offspring, increasing their risk of some autoimmune diseases as well.

Microchimerism is probably only a small piece of the puzzle. Our immune systems are unique in other ways. Women produce more antibodies and autoantibodies than men (though they don't necessarily cause problems). Men and women also have differing responses to organ transplantation. Organs donated by women are more likely to be rejected, and women have a lower survival rate compared to men. This could be partly due to genes, partly due to hormonal influences, or perhaps caused by differences in cellular immune responses.

Estrogen can stimulate certain immune responses in animals. For example, it can stimulate the production of helper T-cell cytokines and enhance the production of others, remarks Michael Lockshin, MD, director of the Barbara Volcker Center for Women and Rheumatic Diseases at the Hospital for Special Surgery in New York City. Estrogen can also increase agents that protect cells against programmed cell death and foster a break in B-cell tolerance. Estrogen can induce autoimmunity in experimental animals in the lab. However, emphasizes Dr. Lockshin, estrogen *alone* cannot explain sex differences in autoimmune diseases.

Some autoimmune diseases may worsen in pregnancy, while rheumatoid arthritis and multiple sclerosis get better. There's actually strong evidence that pregnancy may decrease the risk of developing RA, or at least postpone the onset, and not having children may elevate risk. On the other hand, pregnancy can trigger autoimmune thyroid disease.

In some instances, the elevations in estrogen during the first part of your menstrual cycle (the *follicular phase*) may coincide with disease flares. In multiple sclerosis or myasthenia gravis, symptoms may worsen premenstrually (when progesterone is elevated). However, early data suggest that women do not have an increased risk of flares when undergoing ovulation induction (where potent hormones are given to stimulate the ovary to produce several eggs for assisted reproduction). Also, in pregnancy, very few lupus patients have a serious flare, even with estrogen levels one hundred times as high as during the peak menstrual cycle. Some diseases, like Sjögren's, occur more often after menopause, when estrogen levels are decreased.

"The effects, if any, of pregnancy on the different diseases, and of the menstrual cycle, menopause, or hormone therapy, are different in different diseases, and that isn't consistent with a single cause, like hormones," stresses Dr. Lockshin. "What's more likely is that hormones may act as an on-off switch in some autoimmune diseases."

That on-off switch may be estrogen or other hormones influenced by estrogen. For instance, studies at the National Institute of Child Health and Human Development (NICHD) suggest that inflammatory autoimmune diseases are influenced by *corticotropin releasing hormone* (*CRH*), produced by the hypothalamus in the brain and by the placenta and immune tissues. CRH triggers release of stress hormones like *cortisol* (a natural steroid) when we're under stress and during pregnancy. Cortisol modulates certain aspects of immune activity in the body, including inflammatory cytokines. (Synthetic versions of this *corticosteroid*, such as prednisone, are used to treat inflammation.) New research from NICHD and Greece suggests that CRH may also stimulate production of a protein that helps shield the fetus from an immune attack.

Studies led by George P. Chrousos, MD, at the NICHD suggest that estrogen-related fluctuations in CRH may help explain why some autoimmune diseases are more common in women than in men and why some women are more vulnerable to certain diseases. For example, says Dr. Chrousos, when cortisol is high, susceptible women may be more prone to develop antibody-mediated diseases like lupus, and when cortisol is low (and inflammatory cytokines are more active), they may be likely to develop T-cell related diseases, like rheumatoid arthritis and multiple sclerosis. The CRH-inflammation connection may also explain why rheumatoid arthritis and multiple sclerosis get better in pregnancy and why lupus can get worse (albeit rarely)—effects previously thought to be due to estrogen alone.

On the other hand, it may be that male hormones (*androgens*) like testosterone are protective in some way. Women with lupus and Sjögren's syndrome are known to have low levels of testosterone, and correcting the imbalance may help symptoms. For example, an androgen called *dehydroepiandrosterone* (*DHEA*) is being used to treat lupus (although it has not been approved), and the National Eye Institute is testing androgen eye drops in women with Sjögren's.

The questions raised by all this research are fascinating. We could get some answers over the next decade from a $20 million research project funded by the National Multiple Sclerosis Society and the National Institute of Allergy and Infectious Diseases to study sex differences in autoimmune diseases. Knowledge eventually gained from this project and other research going on around the world could eventually help find some of the underlying causes and, possibly, sex-specific treatments for autoimmune diseases.

> *You just know that you're bone tired, and you can't seem to get yourself out of bed. And everything seems worse because of it. You get your period, and the cramps seem much worse—every little muscle ache and pain seems intensified. Your joints hurt . . . but is it water retention or is the RA worse? You often don't know what's arthritis, what's PMS, what's fibromyalgia . . . and what's simply being tired. Any new symptom that crops up, you often just don't know what to make of it. Most of the time your doctor just says "Oh, it's your RA." And unless you make it your business to learn everything you can, you probably would think that, too.*
>
> CATE, THIRTY

Recognizing the Enemy Within

While immune attacks may produce similar symptoms early on, they don't always point to a particular disease. Early symptoms can be vague and transitory; illnesses often overlap and mimic each other. For instance, fatigue and joint pain can be symptoms of rheumatoid arthritis, lupus, and thyroid disease.

Sometimes there's a gap in time between your symptoms and the clinical signs of disease that doctors look for to help make a specific diagnosis. The day you see your doctor your joints may not look swollen and red if you have early rheumatoid arthritis. So there's often a time lag between the actual onset of a disease and a formal diagnosis. And that time lag can be considerable. The signs of autoimmune disease may be misdiagnosed and treated as another condition, such as depression and fatigue in MS or lupus. Or, in women like Cate, fatigue and pain may be mistaken for worsening symptoms of rheumatoid arthritis, when they're actually due to fibromyalgia, a non-autoimmune disorder that often occurs with autoimmune diseases.

Many women suffer infertility, miscarriages, and pregnancy complications because of autoimmune-related problems, even if they don't have a diagnosable disease. For example, autoantibodies that lead to blood clots in the placenta may cause second-trimester pregnancy loss. These same autoantibodies, called *antiphospholipid antibodies*, are found in women who have lupus or antiphospholipid syndrome, as well as many other autoimmune diseases.

Tests for autoantibodies and immune agents like complement can help your doctor in making a diagnosis. For instance, a low level of complement can indicate lupus, while a positive test for rheumatoid factor can be one indication of rheumatoid arthritis (and also of Sjögren's syndrome). It usually takes a combination of blood test results, an assessment of clinical signs and symptoms, and sometimes diagnostic imaging to make a definite diagnosis.

How This Book Can Help You

As you read each chapter of this book, you'll learn more about the kinds of tests you need to obtain a correct diagnosis and what the results mean. We'll also detail the diagnostic criteria doctors use.

If you're suffering from seemingly vague and unrelated symptoms, we'll help you sort them out and tell you where to go for help. One recent survey by the Sjögren's Syndrome Foundation (SSF) found that as many as three out of four women under age thirty-five may suffer at least two *potential* symptoms of Sjögren's, including dry eyes or dry mouth, yet never tell their doctor, or simply hope the problems will go away. The more quickly you act, the better your chances for a successful treatment.

This book is designed to give you the tools you need to manage your own diagnosis. But, again, be aware that having one autoimmune disease puts you at risk for others that cluster with it. So you need to be alert for other symptoms that can crop up.

We'll also tell you how autoimmune diseases—and their treatments—can affect you during different stages of your life. Some autoimmune diseases, like antiphospholipid syndrome, can make it hard to sustain a pregnancy. Other diseases, such as multiple sclerosis, improve so much during pregnancy that some doctors dub it a "therapy." A frequent treatment for autoimmune disease, corticosteroid drugs, may put you at risk for osteoporosis or high cholesterol, especially if you're older. Corticosteroid drugs can also produce psychological symptoms, such as depression and explosions of anger, that can be extremely upsetting if you're not aware that they can occur.

Throughout this book, you'll learn about the latest scientific and medical research, including research into genetics, environmental and viral triggers, possible ways of altering immune responses, and potential new therapies (such as stem cell transplants and gene therapy). We've called on the expertise of immunologists, rheumatologists, endocrinologists, neurologists, hematologists, and gastroenterologists from institutions leading the way in investigating these diseases. Autoimmunity is a rapidly evolving field, but we've tried to include the latest information available. Each chapter will feature sections on early signs and symptoms, provide answers to commonly asked questions about fertility and pregnancy management, and detail special considerations for midlife, menopause, and later life. You'll also find advice on getting the latest treatments, finding an appropriate specialist, and navigating the health care system, so you won't have to shuttle from specialist to specialist. In the back of this book you'll find an extensive list of resources, support groups, and information on the Internet.

This is an exciting time for autoimmune research. New treatments are emerging that may make these diseases easier to manage and maybe even stop them in their tracks. We're on the cutting edge, though most of us didn't choose to be here. But armed with information, we can take charge of our health care as this new era in understanding autoimmunity begins.

2

Those Aching Joints—
Rheumatoid Arthritis

Around ten years ago I was doing a film, Serial Mom, *and my feet started to swell terribly; all of the shoes that we had bought for the character suddenly seemed painfully small. I thought I must be retaining water or something, even though retaining water didn't explain the pain. And it hurt terribly. It hurt to put my feet in the shoes, it hurt to put anything on my feet. I would rip the bottoms of the covers off the bed because I couldn't stand to have the weight of the blanket on my feet. When I finished the film and came home, I found that I couldn't get into my own shoes. Even sneakers; I had to take the laces out. So I went to the head of podiatry at one of the major New York hospitals and he took x-rays, felt my feet, and told me I needed bigger shoes. He wasn't very helpful.*

Then it went to my neck; I couldn't turn my head. So I went and had an x-ray of my neck, and the doctors told me that I had lost the curvature of the first four vertebrae, and they had no idea why and there was nothing they could do. Then I couldn't open my left arm; it was locked in position. So I went to a hotshot doctor, a sports medicine specialist who treats some New York teams, supposed to be the best in the city. He took an MRI as well as an x-ray and couldn't see anything. He said perhaps we should do exploratory surgery. It was at this point that I got really freaked out. And by then I was feeling so ill, so tired, and so sick—like having the flu all the time. This was over the space of eight or nine months. Back then I wasn't that aggressive about my own health; I

*had never had anything seriously wrong with me. But I was frightened.
I didn't know what was happening to me.*

*I finally went to my GP, who I've been seeing for years and years, and
I said, "I think I'm dying and I'm terrified. You've got to help me." He
was the first doctor to take blood to be tested. And he called me up the
next day and said to get over to his office right away. My rheumatoid
factor was sky-high; he didn't know how I was walking at all. I had
access to the best doctors in New York, and he was the one who found
the RA. But I was lucky—it only took me a year to get diagnosed.
Many women I know take three to five times as long to find out what's
wrong with them.*

KATHLEEN TURNER, FORTY-SEVEN

Unlike the charismatic actress Kathleen Turner, rheumatoid arthritis (RA) may not have much stage presence in the beginning. It may come on so gradually that you can't even remember when the aching and stiffness in your joints began. Or it may announce itself loudly, with a sudden outburst of swelling and joint pain. But the character of RA is revealed in its symmetry— the immune system attack on the joint lining usually affects the same joints on both sides of the body.

The Arthritis Foundation (AF) estimates that rheumatoid arthritis affects some 2.1 million Americans, almost three times more women than men. RA usually strikes in the prime of life but can also affect children (as juvenile RA) and the elderly.

Arthritis is derived from the Greek word *arthron*, meaning "joint," and the suffix *itis*, meaning "inflammation." But inflammation itself doesn't start out to be destructive; it is actually the body's defense mechanism. When there's an injury or invasion, the immune system sends specialized white blood cells to the area to destroy anything foreign and repair damage. For example, when you get a cut, the immune system dispatches a repair crew of white blood cells to the scene to destroy harmful bacteria and heal the damaged tissue. The work done by the repair cells initially makes things red and swollen— inflamed. When the repairs are done, the area heals and the redness and inflammation go away. But if an attack becomes constant, the inflammation doesn't cease. And it eventually becomes chronic and destructive.

A joint (the place where two bones meet) is surrounded by a protective capsule. The ends of the bones are covered by a layer of rubbery material called *cartilage*, which acts as a shock absorber and enables the bones to move against each other smoothly (cartilage breaks down from wear and tear in another common form of arthritis, *osteoarthritis*). The joint capsule is lined with a thin layer of tissue called the *synovial membrane*, which produces a clear fluid that lubricates the joint. The synovium also acts as a filter to bring nutritional materials from the blood into the joint and the cartilage, which does not have a blood supply. So the synovium is very important for maintaining function of the joint.

In rheumatoid arthritis, immune cells for reasons unknown mistakenly attack the synovium, setting off a destructive cascade of events. As white blood cells pour into the synovium, extra fluid is produced and antibodies and inflammatory molecules (*cytokines*) inflame the joint lining. Eventually, this *synovitis* results in the warmth, redness, swelling, and pain that are the classic symptoms of rheumatoid arthritis.

As the inflammation continues to percolate, synovial cells start to grow and divide abnormally, thickening a membrane that was once just three or four

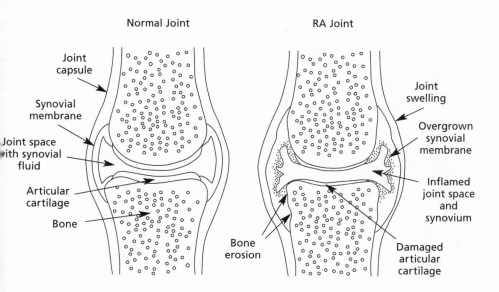

How RA Affects Joints

cells thick. As RA progresses, new blood vessels form to feed the growing mass of abnormal synovial cells and immune cells, which form a sheet (*pannus*) that spreads over the cartilage in the joint. This tissue begins to eat into the cartilage and also erodes and destroys the bone adjacent to the cartilage. This weakens the muscles, ligaments, and tendons that help support and stabilize the joint. When the support system is damaged, it can lead to pain, stiffness, and deformity.

This damage can begin during the first year or two of the disease, long before symptoms start to appear, and by the time RA is diagnosed the disease may have already become destructive. That's one reason early diagnosis and treatment are so critical.

In women, RA often starts in the fingers of both hands and progresses to the wrist joints and beyond, or it can begin in the feet (as in Kathleen Turner's case). The disease can affect any joint in the body, including those in the spine. Once it's set off, the inflammatory process takes on a life of its own and can reach beyond the joints. Inflammatory cytokines can cause reduced levels of *erythropoietin*, a hormone that stimulates the bone marrow to make red blood cells; if fewer red blood cells are produced, the result is anemia. Antibodies and inflammation in the eyes, mucous membranes, and salivary glands frequently cause dry eyes and mouth (*Sjögren's syndrome*). Inflammation may also affect the blood vessels (*vasculitis*) as well as the lining of the lungs (*pleuritis*), and the sac around the heart (*pericarditis*).

The inflammatory process of RA differs from woman to woman. In some, acute inflammation lasts only a few months or a year or two, then subsides without appreciable damage. Others have mild disease that periodically wors-

---

Warning Signs of Rheumatoid Arthritis

- Tender, warm, swollen joints
- The same joints hurt on both sides of the body
- Pain in the wrist and finger joints closest to the palm
- Pain in the neck, shoulders, elbows, hips, knees, or feet
- Fatigue, occasional fever, feeling unwell
- Morning pain and stiffness lasting more than an hour

---

ens (or flares) and then improves. For many women, RA improves during pregnancy and worsens in the postpartum period (initially leading many scientists to believe female hormones play a role in the disease). RA can become chronic and severe, causing serious joint damage and disability. But in recent years new drugs have been developed to block specific inflammatory molecules, slowing or even stopping the damage caused by rheumatoid arthritis.

What Causes Rheumatoid Arthritis?

RA appears to be caused by a combination of genetic vulnerability, environmental triggers (possibly infections), hormonal influences, and perhaps joint injury.

A number of genes are associated with RA, and they're found in healthy people and in women with other autoimmune diseases. These genes often control the *human leukocyte antigens* (*HLAs*), which contain instructions for the proteins that label a cell self or nonself. Women with rheumatoid arthritis may have the genes encoding the particular HLA group DR4, which may cause healthy tissues to be labeled as foreign. Different versions of the HLA-DR4 genes are associated with an increased risk of rheumatoid arthritis (and other autoimmune diseases that cluster with it, such as thyroid disease). "DR4 also predisposes to developing more severe disease. We don't quite understand why and how that occurs, but if you acquire rheumatoid arthritis, and you have this DR4 molecule, you may develop more severe disease," says William P. Arend, MD, professor of rheumatology and of immunology at the University of Colorado Health Sciences Center in Denver. Other genes linked to RA regulate the inflammatory cytokines like *tumor necrosis factor* (*TNF*) and *interleukin-1* (*IL-1*), leading to overproduction of these molecules, he adds.

But genes alone don't tell the story; some women with rheumatoid arthritis have *no* known RA-linked genes, while some who have these genes never develop RA. Even among identical twins (who share identical genes), if one twin has rheumatoid arthritis the other doesn't automatically develop it; the *concordance* (mutual occurrence) rate among identical twins is only about 12 to 15 percent.

But genetically vulnerable people need to encounter other factors, a combination of several "hits" required to set a disease in motion, says Dr. Arend. Those "hits" could include viral or bacterial infections, such as *Epstein-Barr virus* (*EBV*), which causes infectious mononucleosis. Suspect bacteria include *streptococci*, responsible for rheumatic fever; *salmonella*, a cause of food poisoning; *Escherichia coli*, responsible for urinary tract infections; *Helicobacter pylori*, which causes gastrointestinal ulcers; and *Borrelia burgdorferi*, the corkscrew-shaped bacterium carried by ticks that causes Lyme disease. Lyme disease triggers inflammation around the body and can cause an arthritis similar to RA (in fact, it's often misdiagnosed as rheumatoid arthritis). As many as 10 percent of people who've had a salmonella infection also develop a temporary, "reactive" form of arthritis, and a smaller number develop a more lingering and debilitating arthritis.

As we mentioned in Chapter 1, the structure of a virus or bacteria (or proteins they carry) and the structure of some cells and proteins in the body may appear similar, and immune cells react to both, a case of molecular mimicry. Studies have shown that T-cells taken from the joints of patients with RA react to proteins on the Epstein-Barr virus. A study by scientists from Johns Hopkins in the February 2000 *Nature Medicine* showed that the cell-killing (cytotoxic) T-cells that fight bacteria also attack normal cells carrying a molecule resembling a protein on salmonella. Even more intriguing, after a previous salmonella infection, the T-cells also targeted "bystander" cells that *hadn't* been infected. Normally cells will display bits of bacterial protein to show they've been infected, but these noninfected cells flashed a similar signal or molecular "flag." That flag was almost identical to a "housekeeping" protein found in normal cells, the researchers found. T-cells also attacked normal cells if they had been stressed in some way, perhaps by exposure to a toxin.

Population studies have also turned up links between environmental toxins and RA. Smoking cigarettes increases the risk of rheumatoid arthritis, and even coffee has been implicated. One Swedish study found that people who drank four or more cups of coffee a day were more likely to have rheumatoid factor (a marker for RA) in their blood and an increased risk of rheumatoid arthritis. An update from the Iowa Women's Health Study in 2001 found that women who drank four or more cups of *decaffeinated* coffee a day were more than twice as likely to develop RA as those who drank regular coffee. Conversely, those in the study group of 31,336 women aged fifty-five to sixty-nine who drank three or more cups of tea each day had a 60 percent reduction in their risk of RA. (While the study doesn't prove a cause and effect, the Arthritis Foundation says women might want to consider switching to tea.)

Then there's the question of hormones. The fact that rheumatoid arthritis improves in many women during pregnancy (when estrogen levels are very high) and worsens after delivery (when estrogen levels drop) has led some researchers to believe there's a hormonal factor in RA. It is known that estrogen can influence the activity of immune cells. The peak onset of rheumatoid arthritis is between ages forty and sixty, when estrogen levels may be wildly fluctuating or declining. But scientists believe estrogen may play only a small role.

Kathleen's story continues:

I was about two years into the RA and I kept on working despite the pain. I had no choice. If I didn't keep working my career would be over. I was offered a play, Indiscretions, *and I thought I'd be able to do it because the character was a diabetic, and the first and the third acts took place in her bedroom . . . I figured I'd be lying around a lot. It didn't turn out that way. In the second act of the play, there was a three-story spiral staircase that went up to a catwalk . . . we would sit up there until we heard the cues and start back down. By the time I got up to the catwalk I was sobbing every night—the pain was so terrible. So I kept tissues, powder, and a lipstick and a mirror up there so I could fix my face before I went back down. I only missed a few performances in the run. I didn't make my disease public at the time . . . because we didn't know at this point how much I was going to recover and if I was going to recover. And people don't understand rheumatoid arthritis. I was put on a whole cocktail of drugs and that was almost worse than the RA. I was on Plaquenil, I was on gold salts, I was on methotrexate, I was on prednisone, large doses of prednisone. It blew up my body, blew up my face. And the press had a field day—they decided that I had a drinking problem because I was so puffy. And I didn't even care if people thought I had an alcohol problem. I mean, they hire drunks, they hire repeated drug offenders every day in this business. But I knew they wouldn't hire me if they knew I had this disease.*

Symptoms of Rheumatoid Arthritis

The first symptoms of RA may be swelling and morning stiffness or just a general aching of the joints. In 90 percent of women, the first areas affected by rheumatoid arthritis are the feet and hands. The disease often affects the wrist and the finger joints closest to the palm, as well as joints in the jaw, neck, shoulders, elbows, hips, knees, ankles, and toes. Any joint in the body can be a target.

Inflammation can cause bodywide symptoms such as low-grade fever, flu-like body aches, and a general feeling of not being well (doctors call it *malaise*). You may also lose your appetite, lose weight, and feel like you have no energy. Fatigue is a very common symptom of RA and may first overtake you in the afternoon. Fatigue may also be a symptom of anemia, which often accompanies RA. Inflammation can affect the tear-producing glands in the eyes and saliva-producing glands in the mouth, so you may experience dry eyes and dry mouth. You can have muscle pain and stiffness after sitting or lying in one position for a long time. Depression is also common.

At first, these symptoms may not add up to much. "It takes a while for the symptoms to accumulate and for them to be obvious, in order for us to definitively state that this is rheumatoid arthritis," remarks Melanie J. Harrison, MD, a rheumatologist and the director of the Rheumatoid Arthritis Clinical Research Registry at the Hospital for Special Surgery in New York City. "In addition, there are other medical conditions, both rheumatic and non-rheumatic diseases, that can look a lot like rheumatoid arthritis, especially in the early stages, such as lupus and hypothyroidism. In fact, any infection that produces joint aches can look like rheumatoid arthritis."

Often a woman will complain of joint pain to her doctor, and all that can be seen is a puffiness of the hands, with no obvious redness or warmth. "You can see the swelling in the small joints of the hand, going across the knuckle. But some physicians might say 'What's the big deal? Take a little ibuprofen, and the swelling should go down.' But you can be developing erosions in the bone, and nothing may be apparent from examining the hand," says Dr. Harrison. "But the likelihood of developing erosions with chronic inflammation is very high, and it can occur very early on. It's a wearing away of the bone, almost as if bites were being taken out."

About one-quarter of women with RA develop raised, firm lumps called *rheumatoid nodules*. "Rheumatoid nodules are actually abnormal accumulations of cells, much like the synovial cells that we see accumulating within the joint, but they commonly occur just under the skin. Nodules often appear in an area where there's repeated pressure, such as on the elbows where you lean them on a table, or the finger joints," observes Dr. Harrison. "Because rheumatoid arthritis is a systemic disease, nodules can show up in other places, such as the eye, the heart, the lungs. They can be very destructive, very damaging, interrupting whatever is in their path of growth. And they can be disfiguring and disconcerting to patients."

Up to half of RA patients can develop inflammation in the linings of the chest and lungs (*pleurisy*), causing pain on taking a deep breath and breathlessness; rheumatoid nodules can also appear in the lung tissue itself, not just the lining. Inflammation can also affect the sac around the heart (*pericarditis*), producing fever, chest pain, a dry cough, and difficulty breathing. Blood vessels can also be inflamed (*vasculitis*); a common sign is tiny broken blood vessels in the cuticle area of the nail bed.

You may first notice the symptoms of RA during the winter, and symptoms often feel worse during the cold months and improve in warm weather.

While RA develops gradually in about 50 percent of women, with symptoms coming and going for months, a more continuous pattern eventually emerges. "It sort of locks in, and then there is a clear day-in, day-out pattern in which people are quite stiff for a long time when they wake up in the morning. The joints are swollen and red, and there's pain when the joint is moved. If this persists for a number of days or weeks, it should be a signal that a woman needs to see a doctor," stresses John H. Klippel, MD, medical director of the Arthritis Foundation. "This disease needs to be diagnosed very quickly and treatment needs to be started quickly. So that increases the importance of having women recognize the signs and symptoms."

Kathleen's story continues:
My disease took an incredible toll on my personal life. Making love was almost impossible. Just being touched hurt so bad. It's not like a muscle ache or something where you can lie down and relieve the pain on that part of your body . . . it feels like you've broken a wrist and never set it. And you're living with this and that's what it feels like . . . and you're depressed, you feel sick all the time, and you feel tired all the time. There's a huge fatigue factor in this disease. My daughter was about three and a half, four years old

and it was hard for me to even play with her. She'd stand on the stairs and say, "Mommy, catch me," and I'd have to scream, "Don't jump—I can't catch you!" One of the worst days, I remember, I had gotten out of the shower and I was sitting on the edge of the tub and I had this big plastic bottle of body lotion and I couldn't squeeze it to get any lotion out. And it was full. And I started to sob, I just started to cry . . . and Rachel walks in and says, "Mommy, what's wrong?" and I said, "I can't do this." And she said, "Oh, I can." And she took the bottle from me and squirted it all over my body like ketchup—which was wonderful and funny, but at the same time it was so terribly sad because I couldn't do what a four-year-old could do. My husband was wonderfully supportive . . . he and I had a code when we would go out for dinner or something, and if I had to get up to go to the bathroom or we would have to leave, he would come around to my chair and he would pull my chair back and in the guise of this great courtesy, would get his hands under my arms so that he could just lift me out of the chair because I couldn't get myself up.

Diagnosing Rheumatoid Arthritis

Rheumatoid arthritis can be difficult to diagnose in its early stages. For one thing, the full range of symptoms develops over a long period of time; in the early stages of RA only a few symptoms may be present, says Dr. Harrison. Symptoms can also vary widely from woman to woman; some have more severe symptoms, while others have only slight problems. Symptoms of RA can also mimic other types of arthritis and autoimmune diseases, such as lupus. So those conditions must first be ruled out.

The first thing your doctor will do is take a medical history, asking you to describe your symptoms, when they began, and how they may have changed or progressed over time. You'll be asked about the amount of joint pain you experience, how long you feel stiff in the morning, and how long episodes of fatigue last. The doctor will examine your joints for the classic signs of RA, including redness, swelling, and warmth; assess how flexible your joints are; and test your reflexes and muscle strength.

No single test can definitively diagnose RA, stresses Dr. Harrison. Diagnostic criteria set by the American College of Rheumatology (ACR) can help separate rheumatoid arthritis from other causes of chronic joint problems. They include:

- Morning stiffness lasting at least an hour
- Arthritis in three or more joint areas, with soft-tissue swelling
- Arthritis of the joints of the hand (including the wrist or knuckles)
- Symmetric involvement of joints
- Rheumatoid nodules
- A positive test for rheumatoid factor (RF) in the blood
- Erosions, bone loss, or other changes seen on an x-ray

You need to meet four of these seven criteria, and the first four must have been present for at least six weeks. Together with the results of a series of blood tests, these add up to a diagnosis of rheumatoid arthritis.

Tests You May Need and What They Mean

Rheumatoid factor (**RF**) is an antibody found in the blood of most rheumatoid arthritis patients. Not every woman with RA tests positive for rheumatoid factor—especially early in the disease, when it's detected in only 50 percent of patients. Eventually the test is positive in around 80 percent of people with RA. If you test negative, you're said to be *seronegative*. But RF can also be present in women with other conditions, like lupus and Sjögren's syndrome. So a positive test for RF can support a diagnosis of RA, but by itself isn't enough to diagnose the disease.

Erythrocyte sedimentation rate (**ESR or SED rate**) gauges how fast red blood cells settle out of the blood plasma. Any inflammation in the body (such as the flu or a severe infection) increases plasma proteins, such as the clotting factor *fibrinogen*, which makes red blood cells clump together. These clumps of cells settle faster than single cells. In healthy people, red blood cells fall at a rate of about 20 millimeters per hour; in women with inflammation, the SED rate speeds up to 100 millimeters an hour. An elevated SED rate is a nonspecific sign of inflammation, and is seen in rheumatoid arthritis and other autoimmune inflammatory conditions.

Antinuclear antibodies (**ANAs**), autoantibodies that react against the nuclear material of cells, are found in the blood of more than 95 percent of women with *systemic lupus erythematosus* (*SLE*) and a majority of women with Sjögren's syndrome, but less than half of women with RA. So a test for ANAs can help distinguish RA from lupus and help determine whether a woman suffering from dry eye has secondary Sjögren's.

A **complete blood cell count** (**CBC**) is a standard part of any medical workup. Using laser technology, a machine counts each type of blood cell one by one: red blood cells (RBCs), white blood cells (WBCs), and platelets (cells needed for blood clotting) are differentiated by their size. A CBC can detect anemia (low levels of red blood cells), which often occurs in RA. Your *hemoglobin* level reflects the oxygen-carrying capacity of red cells; the *hematocrit* tells how many red blood cells you have in a given volume of blood. Hemoglobin levels can vary from woman to woman, but the normal range is between 12 to 16 grams of hemoglobin per deciliter of blood (g/dL); a hematocrit ranges from 35 to 47. Either (or both) can diagnose anemia. (Reference ranges vary from lab to lab.)

A CBC also measures the number of key white blood cells, like neutrophils, that destroy invading bacteria and viruses by releasing granules of toxic chemicals. In RA, these cells are overactive and multiply. In some RA patients, neutrophils may be depleted (*neutropenia*), a disorder called Felty's syndrome which poses an increased risk of infection.

Other blood tests are done as part of an initial workup to assess organ dysfunction due to coexisting diseases. These tests include liver and kidney enzymes that indicate organ damage. This is important because some medications used to treat RA can be toxic to the liver or kidneys and can't be used if these organs are impaired.

X-rays (**radiographs**) are used to determine the degree of joint destruction. An x-ray can show damage to the bones, loss of cartilage, and distortion of the joints. Baseline radiographs are done to provide a reference to assess any future progression of the disease and to help judge the effectiveness of disease-modifying agents. In the early stages of the disease, bone damage will not be evident on an x-ray. In fact, the joints may appear normal except for signs of soft-tissue swelling and some thinning of the bone around the joints (*juxta articular osteopenia*). But there can be a rapid progression to the signs considered the hallmark of RA seen on x-ray—the start of bone erosion in areas close to the joint. "We've seen evidence of erosions developing on MRI within six weeks. So it can occur very early," remarks Dr. Harrison.

Kathleen's story continues:

I went to see a doctor in Boston who was horrified by the mixture of drugs I was taking, and the first thing he said was, "We have to get you off these drugs." And he told me to get into a pool, as much as I could as long as I could every day, and just try to swim. So I joined a club in midtown and I started to try to swim. My hands were OK enough that I could hold onto a kickboard, and my hips weren't affected very much, so I was able to kick straight-legged, and I went back and forth, back and forth, as long as I could stand it. The pain was unbelievable. One day I was able to let go of the kickboard and do a sort of half-breaststroke, and that was a great triumph. This was about four years in. One day I got my whole arm to do a stroke, and I stood there in this pool sobbing and yelling, and the poor lifeguard dove in and he grabs me, and I said, "No, no, you don't understand—I just moved my arm!" From then on I said to myself, "OK! I'm getting better."

When the new drugs came out I was in rehearsal for a one-woman show called Tallulah! *and my knees blew up . . . they were extremely painful, so my doctor gave me this new biological drug. I remember it was a Saturday and I injected the medication, and put my legs up and watched over the next four or five hours as my knee swelling went down, and I thought, "Oh God, I've got something really good here." I was on that drug for six months or so, and then I cut back, and now I just use it when I need it. I take a low-dose antibiotic and one of the new nonsteroidal anti-inflammatory drugs, and they keep me on an even keel. I'm in remission, and I know I'm incredibly lucky.*

Treating Rheumatoid Arthritis

The treatment of rheumatoid arthritis usually involves combinations of drugs to attack the disease process on several levels. "Number one is pain control. That's obviously what brings patients in, more than anything else, when they're first diagnosed; when they have flares, they're having pain," explains Dr. Harrison. "Second is to decrease the inflammation by using anti-inflammatory medications. We also try to modify the course of the disease, get at what's causing inflammation, stop that process and the destruction of

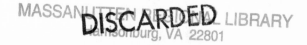

the joints. We're trying to avoid the development of deformity and disability that was previously seen in long-term rheumatoid arthritis, by getting in there earlier and more aggressively." Exercise and physical therapy are also important to prevent disability.

The choice of medication takes into consideration how active your disease is, how severe the symptoms are, and the risks and benefits of potential side effects. Treatments can contribute to premature cardiovascular disease and cause osteoporosis (see pages 47 to 50). The sections that follow reflect new guidelines for the management of RA, issued in 2002 by the American College of Rheumatology. (You can read the guidelines at www.rheumatology.org or in the February 2002 issue of *Arthritis & Rheumatism.*)

Analgesic (Pain) Medications

Nonsteroidal anti-inflammatory drugs (NSAIDs) are the drugs your rheumatologist will likely reach for first to treat joint pain and swelling. They include aspirin and aspirinlike drugs such as *ibuprofen (Motrin), naproxen (Naprosyn), indomethacin (Indocin), nabumetone (Relafen),* and *diclofenac sodium (Voltaren),* to name a few. NSAIDs have both painkilling and anti-inflammatory properties, but they can also cause gastrointestinal symptoms such as upset stomach or, in some cases, bleeding ulcers. That's because they work by blocking enzymes in the body called *cyclooxygenase-1 (COX-1)* and *cyclooxygenase-2 (COX-2).* While the COX-2 enzyme is related to inflammation, COX-1 protects the lining of the stomach and helps platelets to form clots. Because most NSAIDs block both COX enzymes, they can erode the stomach lining and lead to bleeding, especially among women using corticosteroids and women over age seventy-five who may have a thinned stomach lining. These complications can be minimized by taking NSAIDs with meals and using acid reducers like *omeprazole (Prilosec)* or *cimetidine (Tagamet),* or a prostaglandin such as *misoprostol (Cytotec).*

Newer NSAIDs, which only block the COX-2 enzyme, have a slightly reduced risk of serious gastrointestinal side effects (such as bleeding ulcers), but studies show around the same incidence of minor GI problems as the nonselective drugs. COX-2 inhibitors are also much more expensive, costing as much as $100 for a month's supply. Selective COX-2 inhibitors include *celecoxib (Celebrex), rofecoxib (Vioxx),* and *valdecoxib (Bextra). Meloxicam (Mobic)* is a less selective COX-2 inhibitor. Because COX-2 inhibitors don't have the blood-thinning properties of aspirin they do not lower the risk of blood clots and heart attack (and may potentially increase it). This is a special concern for women, since RA can lead to early heart disease (see page 47). If you already have heart disease and need antiplatelet therapy, the ACR recommends using low-dose aspirin (81 mg a day).

Disease-Modifying Antirheumatic Drugs (DMARDs)

Disease-modifying antirheumatic drugs (DMARDs) can alter the course of RA, preventing damage and destruction of the joints, bones, and cartilage. While many of these drugs work in nonspecific ways to modulate the immune system, newer DMARDs known as *biological agents* target specific cytokines. "We now believe that these DMARDs should be used early in the disease process, to stop the process, to arrest further bone and joint destruction from the beginning. And we believe that this early treatment leads to improved function and less disability," remarks Dr. Harrison. The choice of medication depends on a number of factors: the proven effectiveness of a drug in similar cases, how it's given, how much it costs (including the cost of monitoring its use, such as lab tests), how long it will take to work, and its side effects and risks. If you want to have children, that also restricts your choices, since some medications cause birth defects; you may have to modify your treatment regimen during pregnancy and breastfeeding (see pages 41 to 43).

The DMARD most commonly used is *methotrexate (Rheumatrex, Trexall)*, called MTX for short. MTX is a drug used to treat cancer that slows down abnormal cell growth (in this case the pannus, which invades cartilage and bone). A recent study found that MTX could help people with RA live longer. The study, in the April 4, 2002, *Lancet*, found that patients on methotrexate were 60 percent less likely to die prematurely than those not getting the drug. And, the researchers from the Arthritis Research Center Foundation at the University of Kansas School of Medicine found people taking MTX were 70 percent less likely to die from heart disease—a finding that supports the idea that inflammation and the immune system play a role in heart disease and that DMARDs may help prevent it.

"Methotrexate is the anchor, and everything else is added to it. This is the standard of care and what you will see most often," remarks Dr. Harrison.

Methotrexate is often chosen as the initial therapy, especially if RA is more active. The doses of MTX used to treat RA are much smaller than those used in cancer patients, so side effects associated with chemotherapy (like hair loss) seldom occur, but it cannot be used during pregnancy. MTX can produce toxic effects on the lungs and the liver (so you'll need to avoid alcohol while taking this drug), as well as bone marrow suppression. Taking supplements of the B vitamin folic acid may reduce those effects. MTX also has anti-inflammatory and immunosuppressant properties and usually begins working in one to two months. MTX may enhance the effects of other DMARDs. These include the antimalarial *hydroxychloroquine* (*Plaquenil*), *sulfasalazine* (*Azulfidine EN-tabs*), *leflunomide* (*Arava*), and newer "biological" agents like *etanercept* (*Enbrel*), *infliximab* (*Remicade*), and *anakinra* (*Kineret*).

Older DMARDs—such as *azathioprine* (*Imuran*), *D-penicillamine* (*Cuprimine, Depen*), *minocycline* (*Minocin*), *cyclosporine* (*Neoral*), and *gold salts* (*Myochrysine*, the first DMARD)—are effective but are used less frequently.

In women with early, milder disease, sulfasalazine (a sulfa drug that has anti-inflammatory properties) can quickly relieve symptoms—sometimes within a month—and has been shown to slow the progression of the erosions of RA seen on x-rays. It's an oral medication and requires some periodic monitoring with lab tests to detect low levels of white blood cells (*leukopenia*).

Leflunomide (*Arava*) is a newer, oral DMARD that suppresses immune responses and also affects rapidly growing cells. It may take four to twelve weeks to start relieving symptoms. Side effects include an increased risk of infections; it can be toxic to the liver and it also causes birth defects.

Biological Agents

Etanercept and *infliximab* are DMARDs, but they also specifically target *tumor necrosis factor alpha* (*TNFα*), the inflammatory cytokine causing damage in most cases of RA.

Infliximab is a *monoclonal antibody*, a molecular "smart bomb" that targets TNFα and inactivates it. Etanercept is a protein that blocks the receptor for TNFα on cells. Both drugs prevent TNFα from promoting inflammation, and both have been shown to dramatically slow the progression of RA and stop joint erosion.

Infliximab is given with methotrexate; infliximab is given intravenously every four to eight weeks, and MTX is taken orally once a week. This drug combination could start to produce benefits in a few days, or it may take up to four months. Etanercept is given by self-injection into the skin (subcutaneous) twice a week; it can also take a few days to four months to take effect.

Both infliximab and etanercept are quite costly; etanercept can run over $15,000 a year, and infliximab plus methotrexate can cost up to $30,000 a year, compared to just under $3,000 for leflunomide and between $500 and $750 for sulfasalazine (even less for the generic version).

These newer drugs carry a risk of serious side effects, including infection. Infliximab can also promote a lupuslike syndrome, promoting formation of antinuclear antibodies and other autoantibodies associated with lupus. There have been reports of new or reactivated cases of multiple sclerosis and tuberculosis. With etanercept, a few cases of the destruction of the protective coating around nerve fibers, which occurs in multiple sclerosis, have been reported. So close monitoring is needed.

Adalimumab is a newer TNF-blocking monoclonal antibody currently undergoing clinical trials. It's a fully human antibody (infliximab is an antibody that's partly human and partly mouse, a *chimeric* antibody) and it works by binding up excessive molecules of TNF and removing them from the body. Adalimumab is administered by subcutaneous injection once every two weeks. Clinical trials showed that the drug produced improvement in almost 70 percent of patients.

Anakinra (Kineret) is an entirely new type of biological agent. It's the first selective blocker of interleukin-1 (IL-1), another inflammatory cytokine elevated in RA. Anakinra, approved in November 2001, works by blocking the receptor for IL-1 on cells. Anakinra is a version of a molecule called the *IL-1 receptor antagonist*. In a normal joint it prevents IL-1 from binding to cells; in RA there's not enough of this antagonist molecule, so inflammation caused by IL-1 can lead to cartilage and bone erosion. By preventing IL-1 from locking onto cells, anakinra prevents joint damage. It's also given by subcutaneous injection.

Note: Some DMARDs and biological agents have been tested in people older than sixty-five and seventy-five. While older women excrete drugs more slowly and may need lower doses, the main consideration is the increased risk of infection. Again, different dosing, route of administration, and the risk of infection should be discussed with your physician.

Corticosteroid Drugs

Corticosteroids (glucocorticoids) are synthetic versions of steroid hormones normally produced in small amounts by your adrenal glands. Not to be confused with the *anabolic steroids* used by bodybuilders, these are drugs that reduce inflammation and suppress immune activity. Low-dose glucocorticoids (less than 10 milligrams of prednisone a day) can reduce the symptoms of RA very quickly, sometimes within a matter of days. They are also used to dampen disease flares. Recent studies show that low-dose corticosteroids may even slow the rate of bone damage, so they may have disease-modifying potential. They're often given with DMARDs. The most commonly prescribed corticosteroid for treating RA is *prednisone* (*Deltasone, Orasone*), but others may be used as well. These include *methylprednisolone* (*Medrol*), *prednisolone* (*Prelone*), and *dexamethasone* (*Decadron*). They are given as oral medication or as an injection into a joint. Corticosteroid injections can relieve pain, especially early in the disease, and can be used for disease flares in one or two joints. The benefits can be dramatic—but temporary. Because of the side effects of systemic corticosteroids, especially in doses equivalent to more than 10 milligrams a day of prednisone, their use must be closely monitored. Side effects can include weight gain (especially around the abdomen), a round face (so-called "moon face"), increased fat on the upper back ("buffalo hump"), increased appetite, acne, increased facial hair, easy bruising, bone thinning (*osteoporosis*, see page 49) and bone death. So if you're taking these drugs you also need to take calcium supplements, vitamin D, and possibly bone-building drugs (see page 50). Corticosteroids can also cause high blood pressure, cataracts, an increased risk of diabetes and infections, and sleep disturbances.

Prednisone and other glucocorticoids can also cause extreme psychological side effects, including depression, anxiety, hyperactivity, and outbursts of anger. So if you're on steroid medications, you'll need to be prepared. Anything you can do to help manage anger and stress—such as yoga, meditation, and regular exercise—will be important while you're taking steroids. Some women may be helped by psychological counseling to deal with the effects of the drugs and with their disease. While taking prednisone can cause physical and emotional stress, you should never stop it on your own. Prednisone and other glucocorticoids should be tapered slowly under a doctor's supervision.

What's Next?

Treatment approaches now being looked at in the lab include agents that target other cytokine pathways, drugs that block *costimulatory molecules* (molecules that send signals to activate different T-cells), and agents that inhibit subtypes of TNF (part of a "superfamily" of cytokines, so to speak), says Robert Kimberly, MD, chairman of clinical immunology and rheumatology at the University of Alabama at Birmingham and a leading researcher. "TNF is a general pro-inflammatory cytokine. Blocking it blocks inflammation, but also blocks other processes too, which is why there's an increased risk of infection with these agents," explains Dr. Kimberly. "So we are trying to develop strategies that are more selective, more specific. We are looking at aspects like signaling pathways between cells, molecules involved with cell death, and even eliminating specific types of T-cells. If you can eliminate specific cells involved in the immune response, then you can theoretically eliminate that aspect of the disease process."

One strategy currently being tested in patients involves using the cancer drug *rituximab* (*Rituxan*) to selectively target B-cells that produce antibodies that contribute to the disease process in RA. A clinical trial reported at the ACR annual meeting in 2002 showed that giving Rituxan, either alone or in combination with methotrexate or cyclophosphamide, resulted in significant improvements in symptoms among a small group of patients with active RA. More tests are needed, but Rituxan could be a potential therapy for RA as well as for other autoimmune diseases.

Since there are multiple processes in RA, there are multiple targets to aim at, and it's likely that some of the new agents in development would be used together. Affecting a single element in RA, while it can slow the disease and the destruction it causes, does not eliminate the disease itself, Dr. Kimberly points out. But what if a dysfunctional immune system could be *replaced* with a normal one? That's the idea behind stem cell transplantation. In this still highly experimental treatment, the immune system is destroyed with high doses of chemotherapy drugs and then reconstituted with stem cells, the cells that have the potential to grow into any kind of cell, including white blood cells. Before undergoing chemotherapy, patients have stem cells removed from their peripheral blood, purified, frozen, and then re-infused into the blood-stream to rebuild the immune system with "naïve" cells, immune cells that are not autoreactive.

So far, it's been tried in around 100 people with severe RA worldwide; most have responded, some with dramatic improvements. In clinical trials among patients with other autoimmune diseases, results have been mixed, and the death rate is around 8 percent in the year following the procedure. But since 20 percent of people with severe, progressive RA don't respond to any of the established therapies, at least one randomized clinical trial is being conducted to see whether it can help those kinds of patients.

A potential gene therapy, where genes in cells from an arthritic joint are coaxed into producing an antagonist to IL-1 and infused back into the joint, is also being tested.

Surgery

Joint replacement is the most frequently performed surgery for rheumatoid arthritis, and just about any joint can now be replaced with artificial parts made of metal and ceramic. New materials and cements to fix the new joint in place have increased the longevity of artificial joints. However, some artificial joints don't function as well as normal joints, and even the best materials can become worn and need to be replaced. "Most people want to get deformities corrected, more often for cosmetic reasons as opposed to functional reason, especially in the hands," remarks Dr. Klippel. "Surgeons are most interested in improving functional impairments, but they can certainly do things to make the hands cosmetically look better."

Because RA can damage or rupture tendons, the tissues that attach muscle to bone, **tendon reconstruction** is sometimes required. Done most often on the hands, the surgery attaches an intact tendon to a damaged one, helping to restore some hand function, particularly if done before a tendon is completely ruptured.

Synovectomy involves the removal of inflamed synovial tissue and is usually done as part of tendon reconstruction. Other procedures include carpal tunnel release, arthroplasty, and joint fusion. Studies are also under way to investigate the possible use of cartilage regeneration in RA.

Nondrug Therapies

Exercise is important for maintaining healthy and strong muscles to support the joints, preserve mobility, and maintain flexibility. It can also help you sleep and reduce pain. In addition, exercise has documented effects for boosting mood. Special exercise programs can be designed just for you by a physical therapist. But just as important as keeping active is balancing activity with *rest*. You may need more rest when your disease is active and fatigue starts to take a toll. Rest helps to reduce active joint inflammation and pain and fight fatigue. It's usually more helpful to take short rest breaks than to spend long periods of time in bed, since that can promote stiffness. (These strategies are also helpful for dealing with fatigue in other autoimmune diseases.)

Splints and assistive devices can help you function better and reduce stress on your joints. Splints are used mostly on wrists, hands, ankles, and feet to support the joint and reduce pain. They are often custom made by a doctor or a physical or occupational therapist. Self-help devices such as zipper pullers or long-handled shoehorns, special toothbrushes, and jar openers can help make everyday activities easier.

Rheumatoid Arthritis Clusters

Many other autoimmune diseases can cluster with rheumatoid arthritis, partic-ularly thyroid disease, which can compound the fatigue of RA.

- Sjögren's syndrome
- Raynaud's phenomenon
- Thyroid disease (underactive or overactive thyroid)
- Psoriatic arthritis
- Giant cell arthritis
- Pericarditis and endocarditis
- Autoimmune premature ovarian failure

Stress reduction is another important component in managing RA. While stress doesn't cause the disease, it can certainly make it harder to live with. So learning stress management, such as meditation or taking part in psychological support groups, can go a long way toward giving you more control over your life. Don't smoke to alleviate stress.

The Female Factor

Rheumatoid arthritis is almost three times more common in women than in men. Scientists have been exploring the role of estrogen and other steroid hormones in the body to see whether high or low levels of one or another hormone may make a woman more vulnerable to rheumatoid arthritis.

The observation dating back to 1938 that rheumatoid arthritis improves during pregnancy in 70 percent of women led to speculation that higher levels of estrogen (or certain estrogens) may somehow be protective. But studies using estrogen to improve symptoms have not worked. The improvement during pregnancy (and subsequent worsening during the postpartum period) may not be due to estrogen at all, says David Pisetsky, MD, PhD, chief of rheumatology at Duke University Medical Center and codirector of the Duke Arthritis Center. "The initial observation that a hormone produced during pregnancy might be protective actually led to the discovery of cortisol, corticosteroids. So we may be dealing with a steroid effect, but probably not from estrogen. And corticosteroids are anti-inflammatories," comments Dr. Pisetsky.

"There is research to find out which women will get this effect. One very interesting paper suggested that the more genetically different the mother and father, the more steroids, or immunosuppression, the body would produce. And the more similar the mother and the father were genetically, the fewer steroids, or immunosuppression, would be produced," remarks Dr. Pisetsky.

Cortisol is produced in response to a master hormone called *corticotropin releasing hormone* (*CRH*), which is produced by the hypothalamus in response to stress. It's also produced by the placenta and immune tissues. Cortisol also helps to suppress inflammatory cytokines like tumor necrosis factor and *interleukin-12* (*IL-12*), which are overactive in RA and multiple sclerosis. According to researchers at the National Institute of Child Health and Human

Development (NICHD), it appears that suppression of these two cytokines results indirectly from the CRH produced by the placenta. A small study headed by George P. Chrousos, MD, chief of pediatric and reproductive endocrinology at NICHD, found that after a woman gives birth, CRH drops off, stress hormones plummet, and levels of these two cytokines rise, resulting in a rebound of RA. Dr. Chrousos and colleagues speculate that the drop in CRH and cortisol and the sudden burst of TNF and IL-12 after giving birth may predispose some women to RA and other diseases related to cellular autoimmunity.

Immunomodulation during pregnancy helps ensure that a woman's body will not reject the fetus, which has genes from both parents and is technically not "self." Earlier research by Dr. Chrousos showed that CRH produced by the placenta and the uterine lining may play a role in preventing the mother's immune system from rejecting a developing embryo.

Other studies suggest that human leukocyte antigens (HLAs, the molecules that help define what's self and nonself) shared by a woman and her unborn child may be what alters the activity of the mother's immune system during pregnancy. Shared HLAs may also increase—or decrease—the risk of developing some autoimmune diseases. One study by J. Lee Nelson, MD, of the immunogenetics program at the Fred Hutchinson Cancer Research Center in Seattle, showed that greater differences in the genetic makeup between the mother and her fetus were associated with a greater chance of disease remission in RA. The exact mechanism for this is unclear, Dr. Nelson says, but is the subject of ongoing investigation.

At the same time, it has been suggested that the immune effects of pregnancy itself may somehow protect against rheumatoid arthritis (or at least delay its onset). Studies show a twofold increased risk of developing RA in women who have never had a child.

But research into estrogen's effects continues. Over the years, it has been suggested that oral contraceptives may be protective. A recent population study done by the Mayo Clinic in Rochester, Minnesota, found that taking oral contraceptives—even for as little as six months—cut the risk of RA in half. The study looked at forty years' worth of health data for all female residents of the city over eighteen years old, identifying 445 women with RA and comparing them to an equal number of healthy controls, and found that those women who used oral contraceptives reduced their risk by 54 percent, with the strongest protective effect among women who used oral contraceptives earlier in their reproductive years. Estrogen replacement therapy (ERT) did not have the same protective effects (but other studies show it may influence the severity of RA). "We think it might be either the estrogen dose or the progestogen dose. The doses used in oral contraceptives are much higher than the doses used in ERT, and some women taking ERT do not receive progestogen at all," comments the study's lead author, Michele F. Doran, MD, of the Beaumont Hospital in Dublin, Ireland. "So it might be that it's either the higher dose of the estrogen that's protective or the progestogen component of the oral contraceptive pill. But that's speculation at this point."

"Based on the data we have so far, unless a woman is at high risk for rheumatoid arthritis, it doesn't really pay to take birth control pills for prevention. For most women, the chance of RA is only around 1 in 100," comments Dr. Pisetsky.

All of the research into sex-related factors in rheumatoid arthritis is speculative, he adds. But it could one day lead to specific treatment strategies for women with RA.

Kathleen's story continues:
We had always wanted another child. But they told me that I'd have to go off the medications if I were to get pregnant. They told me my symptoms would probably improve while I was pregnant, but that afterward most women with RA not only go back to a fully active state but also usually get worse. So we're talking about my choice of having another child of my body or being able to walk, and move, and work. And to me the choice was very clear. That was the choice I was presented with—to put off childbearing until I had this disease under control. And by then, I was in my middle forties. We did try again and were not successful. And then I was forty-five and I was trying in-vitro, and the drugs almost put me back in an active state. It was a real risk taking them, but we really wanted another child. So that's part of the cost of this disease.

How RA Can Affect You Over Your Lifetime

As Kathleen Turner found, rheumatoid arthritis (and the drugs used to treat it) can profoundly affect a woman's life during her childbearing years.

Menstruation and Fertility

Women with rheumatoid arthritis may have reduced fertility that often predates the diagnosis of the disease. This may be the beginning of autoimmune *premature ovarian failure* (*POF*; see pages 191 to 194).

However, the medications you take can have effects on the menstrual cycle and your ability to become pregnant. Some drugs (like cyclophosphamide) may cause infertility, while others may interfere with ovulation. Methotrexate may cause irregular or stopped periods. Contraception is advised for women taking DMARDs. Because of the potential for birth defects, some drugs may need a "wash-out" period. For example, with infliximab, the usual advice is to stop the drug and wait six months before trying to conceive.

With Arava, contraception is required while taking the drug (for men who are taking the drug, as well). If you want to become pregnant and have taken the drug within the past two years, you (and/or your partner) must undergo a specific drug elimination procedure. You'll be given 8 grams of *cholestyramine* three times a day for eleven consecutive days, and then blood levels of Arava will be measured with two blood tests fourteen days apart until they are below a specific level (0.02 milligrams per liter of blood).

"We stop drugs that are likely to cause trouble like methotrexate. How long the wash-out period should be can become a guess. For methotrexate, most people would say three to six months for a wash-out period," remarks Dr. Pisetsky. "If a patient's disease becomes active, I'll give more prednisone on the grounds that it's probably safer. Most of the time that works out pretty well."

The effects of fertility drugs in women with RA have not been well studied, but the high doses of hormones needed to stimulate the production of multiple eggs by the ovary may make RA symptoms worse, adds Dr. Harrison.

Pregnancy and Breastfeeding

As we mentioned before, your symptoms will likely improve during pregnancy, but could recur within the first eight weeks after delivery. After six to eight months, you'll return to whatever level of disease severity you had before you became pregnant.

The major issue when you contemplate pregnancy is the effect of medications. The U.S. Food and Drug Administration (FDA) currently categorizes drugs A, B, C, D, and X, according to whether studies or case reports show risks to the fetus, such as birth defects, and whether those risks outweigh the benefits to the mother. Category A drugs demonstrate no risks, while category X drugs cannot be used during pregnancy because they've been shown to cause harm. Many newer drugs, such as biological agents, fall into category B. A listing in category B can mean that animal studies of the drug have not shown harm to a fetus, but there are no data or well-controlled studies of pregnant women—or that animal studies have shown adverse effects, but well-done human studies have *not*. Drugs listed in category C may have demonstrated adverse effects in animal studies, but there are no well-controlled studies in humans—or there have been neither animal nor human studies of the drug. Category D drugs may have shown risks to the fetus in studies of pregnant women, but sometimes the benefits of a drug may outweigh the risks for a particular woman. As you can see, prescribing drugs in these categories during pregnancy must be individualized.

Drugs that you take during pregnancy, including those considered "safe," may cross the placenta, and many pass into breast milk, stresses Dr. Harrison. "The most sensitive time during pregnancy for any drug effects is the first trimester, when the embryo is growing into a fetus. This is the period where birth defects are likely to occur." The third trimester, since it is closest to delivery, carries different risks.

In general, experts say NSAIDs appear safe during most of pregnancy, but physicians try to avoid their use too close to delivery since they inhibit hormones called *prostaglandins*, which affect uterine contractions and can prolong labor. Drugs like Vioxx can close off the placental artery supplying the baby, and may affect the function of a baby's heart; it could also cause pulmonary hypertension in the fetus. Corticosteroids are generally considered safe at any time during pregnancy but carry a slight risk of infections, says Dr. Harrison.

Azathioprine is a category D drug, meaning it can cause fetal harm and should not be given during pregnancy unless the benefits strongly outweigh the risks. Although this drug is designated category D, it should be emphasized that women taking azathioprine after transplants who have become pregnant have had successful pregnancies. However, its use is not recommended in nursing mothers. Methotrexate should never be used during pregnancy.

Remicade is classified as a category C drug, but since risk can't be completely ruled out, the *Physicians' Desk Reference* (*PDR*) advises that it should be given to pregnant women only if clearly needed.

Azulfidine is a category B drug, as are penicillamine and Enbrel. No harmful effects have been shown for Azulfidine on fertility or on a developing fetus. However, sulfa drugs like Azulfidine are excreted in breast milk and can cause liver toxicity in infants. Even though no harm was seen in developing fetuses in animal studies, the *PDR* advises that Enbrel should be used only if clearly needed.

As with other drugs used to treat autoimmune diseases, some women do inadvertently become pregnant while taking them. For example, one study of 102 women with RA, Crohn's disease, and other rheumatic diseases who either became pregnant while taking Remicade or were taking it during the first trimester found that almost half delivered successfully. One of the women gave birth to a child with a correctable birth defect; another delivered prematurely. There was one case of eclampsia, in which the baby died after being delivered at twenty-eight weeks. There were ten miscarriages among the group. However, the researchers pointed out that the rates of live births and miscarriages were similar to those among healthy women. But more research is needed before the labeling might be changed for Remicade.

Since there's little experience with new treatments like Kineret, you need to discuss their use with your physician. Carefully read *every* package insert that comes with any medication, and ask questions.

Menopause and Beyond

The peak years for a diagnosis of RA are those just before and after menopause, and recent research suggests that when RA is diagnosed after menopause the disease may progress at a faster rate.

A study from Holland reported in the August 2001 *Journal of Rheumatology* used a disease activity score to track disease progress over six years in 209 women and 123 men aged seventeen to fifty-three. Compared with the men, joint destruction seen on x-ray was more progressed in female patients at the start of the study, and postmenopausal women had significantly worse disability than premenopausal women, both at the outset of the study and three years later. While older men also had more joint destruction and disability than their younger counterparts, the researchers concluded that "the menopausal state was responsible for the major part of the differences in outcome between men and women. Postmenopausal state in early RA influences future disability and damage, especially in older patients."

Menopause *itself* is still uncharted territory where autoimmune diseases are concerned. Many rheumatologists focus on treating the disease and leave the management of menopausal symptoms up to a woman and her gynecologist. "A woman with RA who is going through menopause should be treated like any other woman as far as estrogen and hormone replacement decisions would go," states Dr. Klippel.

Hormone replacement therapy (HRT) should be considered for post-menopausal women with severe hot flashes and other symptoms in whom there are no contraindications, say the 2002 ACR guidelines on managing rheumatoid arthritis. Estrogen replacement therapy (ERT) is considered safe for women with RA, and there have been some hints over the years that estrogen can even make RA a little better.

"Women with rheumatoid arthritis do much better with estrogen; sometimes they even go into remission," observes Lila E. Nachtigall, MD, a reproductive endocrinologist and professor of obstetrics and gynecology at the NYU School of Medicine who has studied estrogen for almost thirty-five years. "However, you need to do a complete evaluation, including blood tests to see if women have any autoantibodies that make them prone to clotting. If the tests come back positive, those women should not be given any form of estrogen, since it does have a risk of clotting such as deep vein thrombosis."

Women with RA who are candidates for and wish to take estrogen replacement should be taking lower-dose preparations, such as conjugated equine estrogens (*Premarin*) or esterified estrogens (*Estratab, Menest*) in a 0.3 milligram dose, compared to the standard dose of 0.625 milligram. Estrogens are now available in even lower doses.

"We have to individualize therapy, depending on the drugs a woman is taking. For example, we know that corticosteroids interact with estrogen. They lessen the effectiveness of estrogen and often cause bleeding. This is because drugs like prednisone may interfere with estrogen receptors and can cause fluctuations in estrogen. So instead of the steady effects of your regular daily dose you get ups and downs that may cause you to bleed or spot," says Dr. Nachtigall.

Short-term estrogen replacement therapy (less than five years) has not been shown to increase the risk of breast cancer.

Women with an intact uterus need to take progestin along with the estrogen to prevent precancerous overgrowth of the uterine lining (*endometrium*).

These include micronized *progesterone* (*Prometrium*) and *medroxyprogesterone acetate* (*Provera*).

However, progestins carry risks as well. In 2002 the Women's Health Initiative (WHI), a major prevention trial of a combined estrogen/progestin drug (Prempro) among 16,608 healthy women aged 50 to 79, was stopped after five years because of an increased rate of heart attacks, strokes, deep vein clots, and invasive breast cancer among women taking the drug. There were fewer cases of colorectal cancer and bone fractures among women on HRT, but the WHI Data Safety and Monitoring Board (DSMB) concluded that the health risks of HRT outweighed the benefits and stopped the study. However, the actual risks were small. According to the WHI data, over one year, 10,000 women taking Prempro might experience seven more coronary heart disease events, eight more breast cancers, eight more strokes, and eight more pulmonary emboli (but six fewer colorectal cancers and five fewer hip fractures), compared to women not taking hormones.

The estrogen-only arm of the WHI was continued, with no increased risk of breast cancer seen among that group (all of whom had had hysterectomies). It's now recommended that women who take progestins take low doses (and not on a continuous basis).

On the strength of the WHI and other recent studies, the U.S. Preventive Services Task Force recommends that estrogen or estrogen/progestin therapy not be used to prevent heart disease and other chronic conditions, and that women should explore other therapies to prevent bone loss. Experts say the main indication for hormone therapy is to ease menopausal symptoms, and therapy has to be tailored to the individual.

Will you do well if you choose to take HRT? It's hard to say. Sometimes you have to try several different hormonal preparations to find the one that's best for you. Menopausal symptoms like hot flashes may get better, but there may be absolutely *no* difference in your disease. "There are no scientific studies. Physicians do say that in their experience estrogen replacement is helpful. But you can never be sure that it's really doing something for the disease, or whether it's improving a woman's sense of well-being, helping her mood, or lessening her pain perception, and so on," comments Duke University's Dr. Pisetsky.

If you can't (or don't want to) take systemic oral estrogens, estrogen is also available in patches (including *FemPatch*, *Alora*, and *Climara*) that are changed once or twice a week. For local estrogen therapy in the vagina there are creams (*Premarin, Estrace, Ogen*), rings (*Estring*), and tablets (*Vagifem*) that gradually release estrogen into vaginal tissues to prevent drying and thinning (*atrophic vaginitis*). Local estrogen therapy may also help with vaginal dryness in women who have Sjögren's syndrome secondary to their RA (see page 155).

Nonhormonal therapies for menopausal symptoms include the herbs *black cohosh* (*Cimicifuga racemosa*, sold in health food stores and under the brand name *Remifemin*) and *red clover* (sold as *Promensil*); both have been tested in clinical trials, but not specifically in women with autoimmune disease. These herbs are believed to contain plant estrogens, or *phytoestrogens*, and some studies suggest that they can relieve hot flashes, night sweats, irritability, insomnia, vaginal dryness, and mood disturbances, without any estrogenic effects on the breasts or uterine lining. Do not use black cohosh if you're also taking blood pressure medication. Red clover can interfere with blood thinners like aspirin, so do not use it if you have antiphospholipid antibodies or a bleeding disorder.

Soy protein contains phytoestrogens called *isoflavones*; some short-term studies suggest that they can relieve hot flashes. A study reported in the journal *Obstetrics and Gynecology* in March 2002 found that 100 milligrams of soy isoflavones a day significantly reduced menopausal symptoms and lowered harmful cholesterol, without affecting the uterine lining. However, other studies find little or no effect. Soy advocates recommend 20 to 50 grams a day from soy milk, soybeans, meat substitutes, or tofu.

As for vitamins, Dr. Nachtigall notes that anecdotal reports over the years have indicated that 400 to 600 International Units (IU) of vitamin E can help douse hot flashes. (Vitamin E, along with fish oil capsules, may have anti-inflammatory effects in RA.)

B vitamins, especially vitamin B_6 (200 milligrams a day), seem to help alleviate the emotional symptoms of menopause, including mood swings and anxiety. Another B vitamin, folic acid (recommended daily intake 400 micrograms a day), has the added advantage of lowering levels of *homocysteine*, a substance in the blood that can damage blood vessels and lead to atherosclerosis, a major risk for women with RA (see page 47).

Wild yams grow on vines all over North America and contain *diosgenin*, a precursor to natural progesterone (used to make some prescription progestins).

Creams containing progesterone made from diosgenin are said to help relieve hot flashes and other menopausal symptoms. According to the North American Menopause Society (NAMS) no adequate clinical trial data confirm these claims. If you want to try wild yam progesterone creams, do so only with your doctor's supervision.

Evening primrose oil (EPO) is made from the seeds of a North American wildflower that, true to its name, opens in the evening. EPO is rich in essential fatty acids, including *linoleic acid.* Some studies suggest that EPO may help lessen hot flashes and lower blood pressure and cholesterol. Side effects include inflammation, blood clots, nausea, and some immunosuppression, according to NAMS. EPO is best taken as capsules; the accepted dose is 2 to 3 grams a day (make sure it's "standardized to 8 percent gamma-linoleic acid"). Keep EPO refrigerated to prevent it from becoming rancid. It cannot be used with anticoagulants.

Cardiovascular Disease

The risk of premature *atherosclerosis* (thickening of artery walls with cholesterol-laden plaques) and coronary artery disease is greater among women with rheumatoid arthritis. The risk may be even greater for younger women with RA, notes Susan Manzi, MD, MPH, associate professor of medicine and epidemiology at the University of Pittsburgh School of Medicine. Dr. Manzi notes that mortality ratios for women with RA aged fifteen to forty-nine show an increased risk of death from heart attack and congestive heart failure as high as three times that of healthy women.

According to Dr. Manzi, potential risk factors for women with rheumatoid arthritis may include inflammation (as measured by *C-reactive protein*) related to RA that not only speeds up the development of plaque, "but it makes the plaque more vulnerable to rupture, leading to clot formation and blockage of the blood vessel." Other potential risk factors include elevated homocysteine (a common side effect of methotrexate), the effects of immune complexes that may stick to the blood vessel lining, and the action of those "big eater" macrophages (which can pull cholesterol into the blood vessel wall).

"Medications used to treat RA, like prednisone, may also speed the development of diabetes and atherosclerosis. There's also the issue of physical inactivity due to disability that increases risk. There are many factors that could be contributing," adds Dr. Harrison. Among those risk factors could be higher levels of harmful blood fats like *low-density lipoprotein (LDL) cholesterol* (which is more prone to stick to artery walls). One recent study from Sweden showed that thickening of the inside of the arteries with cholesterol-laden "plaques" was worse in people with rheumatoid arthritis and that their cholesterol levels were higher, compared to people the same age without the disease. The researchers, writing in the January 2002 issue of the *Journal of Rheumatology*, recommended that people with RA be screened and treated for cardiovascular risk factors like high cholesterol.

Federal guidelines set in 2001 recommend keeping LDL at an "optimal" level of 100 milligrams per deciliter of blood (mg/dl) or below, and recommend lifestyle changes and drug therapy when LDL tops 130 mg/dl in people at higher risk for coronary heart disease. Low levels of *high-density lipoprotein (HDL)* cholesterol are also a risk factor, since HDL helps remove LDL from the bloodstream. Under the guidelines, low HDL for women is under 40 mg/dl.

As for blood pressure, experts recommend staying at or near the "optimal" level of 120 millimeters of mercury (mm Hg) for *systolic* pressure (the higher number, measured while the heart is beating) and 80 mm Hg *diastolic* (blood pressure between beats). High blood pressure is considered to be above 140/90 mm Hg.

So make sure your doctor—whether it's your internist or rheumatologist—assesses your blood pressure at every visit. Each year your doctor should order blood tests to measure levels of

- LDL and HDL cholesterol,
- triglycerides (another harmful blood fat), and
- blood glucose (if it's elevated, that's a sign your body isn't using insulin properly—a red flag for type 2 diabetes, an independent risk factor for coronary disease).

Tests to measure homocysteine are becoming more widely available; ask your doctor about adding it to your annual bloodwork. A physical exam should include an *electrocardiogram (ECG)*.

Making lifestyle changes can also help. These include

- avoiding obesity,
- getting thirty to sixty minutes of moderate exercise most (if not all) days of the week,
- eating a diet rich in fruits, vegetables, whole grains, and lowfat dairy products, and
- getting no more than 10 percent of calories from saturated fat.

You may need advice from a nutritionist to help you work out a heart-healthy diet that you can follow.

Dr. Manzi says TNFα blockers are also being studied in the treatment of heart failure, and more widespread use of these drugs in rheumatoid arthritis may be a more effective way of controlling inflammation—and a potential means of preventing coronary disease in women.

Osteoporosis

Bone loss is a threat for any woman with RA, indeed *any* woman with an autoimmune disease who takes corticosteroids or other drugs that thin the bones. Postmenopausal women are already at increased risk for osteoporosis, and steroid treatment increases the risk even further; bone loss can begin as early as six months after starting steroids, says Dr. Harrison. Osteoporosis risk is doubled among women with RA, and it may not all be related to corticosteroids.

Most recently, a study from Norway measured bone mineral density (BMD) in the hip and spine of 394 women with RA aged fifty to seventy and compared them with healthy women in the same age groups from the U.S. and Europe. The researchers found that over 31 percent of the RA patients had BMD reductions in the hip, and 19 percent had bone loss in the upper spine. Current use of steroids was one factor predicting lower BMD, but rheumatoid factor predicted lower bone mass in the top of the thigh bone in the hip (which may reflect bone erosion in that joint).

Corticosteroids cause bone loss because they interfere with calcium absorption. Even "low"-dose prednisone (10 milligrams a day) taken long term can cause significant bone thinning, so rheumatologists look for ways to minimize these effects (such as giving other drugs with corticosteroids that allow lower doses to be used, or *steroid-sparing* drugs). But often the only way to stave off osteoporosis is bone-building drugs.

According to the ACR's guidelines for preventing steroid-induced osteoporosis, *bisphosphonates* should be given to women when they begin short-term corticosteroid treatment. Bisphosphonates slow the resorption of bone and have been shown to reduce both hip and spinal fractures. For women on long-term therapy, bisphosphonates should be prescribed, along with bone density scans every one to two years and hormone replacement, if needed.

The bisphosphonates approved for treating osteoporosis are *alendronate* (*Fosamax*) and *risedronate* (*Actonel*), which are available in daily and weekly oral preparations. In addition, the ACR guidelines recommend that women take 1,500 milligrams a day of elemental calcium (in diet and supplements), plus 400 to 800 IU of vitamin D (which aids calcium absorption). The ACR guidelines say women who can't take bisphosphonates should be given *calcitonin*, another antiresorptive agent in nasal spray form.

I've always had this sense from doctors and other people that because this is not life threatening, because you're not going to necessarily die from this disease, it's not important. It's just some kind of inconvenience, just creaky joints. But it's lifestyle threatening . . . your sex life, your parenting, your work. Everything is affected by this disease. The most important thing is to know you can fight it—that you can fight it and you can pretty much beat it. There's so much that can be done to alleviate this disease and to fight it and to feel that you're not this victim, that you're not helpless in the face of this disease.

KATHLEEN TURNER

3

The Shadow of the Wolf—
Systemic Lupus Erythematosus

I probably started developing lupus when I was in high school. I remember I had all these weird symptoms my sophomore year. I had red splotches on the bottoms of my hands and the soles of my feet; I thought they were blisters and would actually poke them with a pin. Then I started getting swollen joints, and I was terribly stiff. I remember one time I was at the beach with my friends, and I couldn't even lift myself off the blanket. My parents got worried and took me to a big hospital, and I was told I had juvenile rheumatoid arthritis. I was put on prednisone for a year. It made my face look all puffy and really wrecked my self-esteem, but the symptoms went away. I basically forgot about it until I went away to college and started feeling ill. I had fevers, I was fatigued, I had difficulty concentrating. At first I thought it was stress. But then my joints started to feel swollen and painful. And no one seemed to know what was wrong with me. I'm trying to cope with college life, I wanted to keep my grades up, and here I was constantly seeing doctors, getting tests. It still took them a while to finally tell me I had lupus. Eventually, it affected my kidneys, my intestines, and my brain. Now when I think back, I think this disease was sort of shadowing me for years.

DEANNA, THIRTY-THREE

*L*upus means "wolf" in Latin, and, as it did with Deanna, it can stalk you silently over a period of years or strike suddenly without warning, snarling and scratching the skin of the face and vital organs. *Systemic lupus erythematosus*, or *SLE*, is a leading cause of kidney disease in younger women, and it can lead to premature heart disease. In recent years, there has been a troubling rise in deaths from lupus, especially among middle-aged black women. However, in most cases lupus is a chronic disease that can be managed with medication. Many women—like Deanna, who's now married and teaching full time—live active lives. However, it can be a complicated disease, sometimes requiring multiple medications, some of which can put you at risk for other health problems, like osteoporosis.

Lupus emerges most often between ages fifteen and forty, affecting nine times as many women as men. More African-American, Latina, Asian, and Native-American women are affected than Caucasians, with a rate as high as 1 in 300. Figures vary, but according to the National Institutes of Health, between 350,000 and 500,000 people may be affected.

Unlike other autoimmune diseases that target a single organ, like thyroid disease, lupus can affect just about any organ or tissue in the body—including the joints, the kidneys, the heart, the blood, the lungs, and even the nervous system. Some forms of lupus are limited to the skin, like *discoid lupus* (which can occur by itself or as part of the systemic disease). Ten percent of women initially diagnosed with discoid lupus may eventually develop systemic disease.

As with other autoimmune diseases, lupus can be challenging to diagnose because the signs (what the doctor can see) and symptoms (what you may experience) can occur separately over time. So it may be months or even years before enough symptoms are present to unequivocally meet the diagnostic criteria for lupus (see page 58). A survey conducted by the Lupus Foundation of America found that half of lupus patients had symptoms for five years before obtaining a diagnosis, consulting three or more doctors before being correctly diagnosed.

Lupus can often mimic other diseases. It may be initially diagnosed as rheumatoid arthritis because the first problems seen were joint pain and stiffness of the hands, wrists, and knees. Fatigue and depression may be mistaken for chronic fatigue syndrome or major depression. Pain and color changes of the fingers in the cold weather, called *Raynaud's phenomenon*, which can occur in lupus but are common in scleroderma. In fact, as many as a third of women

---

Warning Signs of Lupus

- Achy but not swollen joints (arthralgia)
- Painful and swollen joints, which can be warm and red (arthritis)
- Fever
- Extreme or prolonged fatigue
- Unexplained rashes on the face, neck, or scalp
- A butterfly-shaped rash across the cheeks and nose
- Anemia
- Pain on deep breathing or when lying down (possible inflammation in the lining of the lungs or heart)
- Skin rashes after sun exposure
- Hair loss
- Raynaud's phenomenon
- Depression
- Painless mouth or nose ulcers

---

with lupus may have other autoimmune diseases. Symptoms of a second disease may often be attributed to lupus, resulting in a delay in diagnosis.

What Causes Lupus?

The precise cause of lupus is not known. And it's a complex disease. Antibodies attack healthy cells—even specific parts of those cells. These include antibodies to DNA and to the cell nucleus, the yolklike structure in the center of each cell that contains your DNA. That's one reason lupus can strike just about anywhere in the body. Various forms of antinuclear antibodies can produce skin rashes or damage the kidneys. Other antibodies attack proteins involved in blood clotting, causing abnormal blood clotting.

The B-cells that produce autoantibodies first need to be activated by helper T-cells. In lupus these B- and T-cells may be hyperactive, and the regulatory mechanisms that normally rid the body of abnormal cells may not be working properly.

One theory involves the "suicide program" built into every cell. Programmed cell death, or *apoptosis*, is necessary to eliminate defective cells, cancer cells, cells produced because of too-rapid growth in certain tissues, and lymphocytes that are no longer needed once a particular immune response has ended. This suicide program can be activated by genes within a cell, damage to DNA (such as sun damage from ultraviolet light that can lead to skin cancer), signals sent to cells by cytokines, or even by an infection.

During apoptosis, the contents of the dying cells are spilled out into the bloodstream to be gobbled up by macrophages and eliminated by the body. In lupus, that clearance system may not be working properly. So the debris from these dying cells—which contain fragments of the cell nuclei—may cause the body to produce those antinuclear autoantibodies, which then attack healthy tissues, explains Bevra H. Hahn, MD, professor of medicine at the University of California, Los Angeles, a noted lupus researcher.

Conversely, a problem with the suicide programming of the B-cells that produce ANAs (or the T-cells that send instructions to pump out ANAs), may lead to the survival of too many abnormal lymphocytes, which react against healthy tissue. Such problems could be genetic; a person could be born with a defect in a gene that controls apoptosis. In some women genetically destined to get lupus, self-reactive cells may escape destruction during fetal development and produce autoantibodies later in life.

Immune complexes also play a major role in lupus. These latticelike structures are formed when antibodies bind to their targets and build up in tiny blood vessels. Accumulation of immune complexes causes blood vessel inflammation and even blockage, and blood clots (caused by lupus anticoagulant antibodies) can also block off vessels supplying vital organs.

Proteins called *complement* normally dissolve immune complexes, or prevent them from growing too large. Women with lupus may have genetic defects in the complement system, producing too little complement to keep up with rapidly forming immune complexes, or it gets used up too quickly. "Lupus seems to be a problem of regulation that allows increased rates of cell death in circulating lymphocytes, decreased clearance of cellular debris, sustained production of autoantibodies, and the increased formation of immune complexes, which cause organ damage," concludes Dr. Hahn. Simply put:

lupus both clogs and corrodes aspects of the body's plumbing system—be it in blood vessels or other tissues.

The genes that control these processes may be among many that contribute to lupus. So far, around a dozen genes have been linked to lupus. One gene, called *C1q*, encodes a protein that coats apoptotic cells and helps them to be cleared before antigens on their surface are recognized by the immune system, so antibodies are not made against them. When this gene is absent, people can develop a lupuslike illness. Another genetic problem may be with a receptor called Fcγ which clears immune complexes.

The genetic defects that contribute to lupus appear to run in families. The chance of two sisters having lupus is around 10 percent, but if they are identical twins (who share the same genes), the chances of both having lupus increase to 25 percent. Currently, several centers around the country are investigating genes involved in lupus, and more information should be available in the next few years.

But genes alone are not enough. An environmental trigger like a drug or a virus could also play a role in triggering lupus in genetically vulnerable women. A virus that inhibits normal cell death could allow infected cells to multiply. A number of studies have implicated *Epstein-Barr virus (EBV)*, which infects B-cells and is periodically reactivated. This reactivation could be a source of chronic immune system stimulation and, in theory, could cause increased production of lupus autoantibodies (and possibly disease flares), says Dr. Hahn.

A recent study in the journal *Arthritis & Rheumatism* by researchers at the Oklahoma Medical Research Foundation and Case Western Reserve University in Cleveland, Ohio, looked at 196 lupus patients and compared them to 392 healthy people matched for age and sex; all but one of the lupus patients had been exposed to EBV at some point, compared to 94 percent of the control group.

In rare cases, lupus can be triggered by drugs, including antibiotics like *minocycline*, often used to treat chronic acne; *procainamide*, prescribed for irregular heartbeats; and *isoniazide*, used to treat tuberculosis. In these cases, the disease usually disappears when the drug is stopped.

Then there are hormones. Some studies have suggested that women with SLE have abnormalities processing estrogen and testosterone. Although estrogen is the main female sex hormone, women also produce male hormones, or *androgens*, including testosterone. Androgens play a variety of roles in the body, affecting bone density, muscle strength, energy, well-being, sex drive (*libido*), and possibly immune system function. Women with lupus appear to have low levels of testosterone. (For more, see pages 68 to 69.)

Deanna's story continues:
I chiefly remember how difficult it was for me my first two years of college. I was under enormous pressure. Keeping my grades up was very important to me, but it was a struggle just to get out of bed some days. I had a lot of joint pain; I had headaches. At this point I was running back and forth to hospitals, getting all kinds of tests done. It was so hard for me to concentrate on anything. I usually grasp things pretty quickly, but even the simplest things would take me hours to absorb. I know now that I was experiencing a lupus flare. But my doctors still hadn't figured out what was wrong. I also developed skin lesions on my buttocks—raised red marks, like scabs. I had every test you could think of. It was very stressful. First they said I had vasculitis and that I needed to take steroids. So I found myself back on prednisone and I had the side effects again, the moon face, the hair loss, the weight loss . . . at one point, I was down to ninety pounds. I took steroids my entire sophomore year, but they didn't help. I was getting progressively worse. And I started experiencing blurry vision in my right eye. It was very frightening. I just figured I was stressed out with all the tests and the medication. Then they did more tests and said I had optic neuritis, my blood pressure was up, and they found blood and protein in my urine. The lupus had moved into my kidneys. Only then was I finally diagnosed with lupus.

Symptoms of Lupus

Any one of the warning signs we've listed may herald lupus, but the disease shows itself differently in each woman. It often begins with vague joint pains and fever. You may almost feel like you have the flu—achy and feverish, with swollen glands and fatigue. For some women, like Deanna, there are memory and concentration problems, a lupus "fog."

Approximately half of women with lupus will have skin rashes, including a classic "butterfly" rash. This is a raised, red rash that spreads across the bridge of the nose (the body of the butterfly) and across the cheeks (the wings). Lupus actually got its name from this rash; some people thought it made the face look like it was mauled by a wolf. (*erythema* means "red skin.") This rash is quite different from acne, but may be confused with rosacea. In acne, you see redness and pimples anywhere on the face; the lupus rash does not extend into the folds alongside the nose and mouth. Discoid lupus usually has plugged follicles, patchy hair loss, and scaly lesions. In *subacute cutaneous lupus erythematosus*, you develop a very sun-sensitive, red rash.

In fact, a rash or other skin problem is often the first clue that a woman may have lupus. Sensitivity to the ultraviolet rays of the sun (*photosensitivity*) can also produce or worsen skin rashes (sunscreen is a *must* when you have lupus).

Fatigue is a common symptom of many autoimmune diseases. In lupus it may be due to anemia (a lowered red blood cell count), difficulty breathing, or muscle weakness. You may also have lower white blood cell counts (*leukopenia*), which make you more susceptible to infections, or a low platelet count (*thrombocytopenia*) that causes unexplained black-and-blue marks and increases the risk of bleeding after something as routine as a dental visit. More than three-quarters of women with lupus may have some signs of depression. This may be due to fatigue or feeling unwell. Migraine headaches may also be a problem.

You may have arthritis, with tender, swollen, and painful joints. Hair loss (*alopecia*) may accompany a lupus flare. If your kidneys are affected, you may see some fluid retention, most commonly as swollen ankles. The kidneys are responsible for filtering waste products from the body and excreting them; when the kidneys aren't functioning well, it affects the balance of fluid and salt in the body. When the kidneys' filtering system is damaged, it can cause too much protein to leak into the urine (*proteinuria*). Blood pressure may also be elevated.

Ethnicity may affect your symptoms and play a role in how quickly your disease progresses. A study in the December 2001 *Arthritis & Rheumatism* suggests that Latina women are more likely than African-American or Caucasian women to have disease worsening and organ impairment. The study, which included 258 patients (82 Caucasians, 104 African-Americans, and 75 Latinas) in Houston and Birmingham, Alabama, who had SLE for less than five years, found that although African-American women had slightly more organ damage than the other two groups, after a followup period of sixty-one months, more than 60 percent of the Latinas had additional organ damage, as well as more eye damage and mental impairment. However, the study authors stress some good news: half of the women studied did *not* have any organ damage by the end of the followup period, suggesting that some women have mild disease and more severe cases are being treated before organ damage can occur.

Diagnosing Lupus

To be classified as having SLE, a woman needs to have four of the eleven criteria defined by the American College of Rheumatology (ACR). Those four criteria need to be present at some point in time, but need not occur together. (Note: These criteria are typically used for patients who wish to enter into clinical trials.)

- Malar rash (the classic raised, red rash that looks like a butterfly over the nose and cheeks)
- Discoid rash (red, raised patches with scaling and plugged follicles)
- Photosensitivity (an unusual reaction in the skin after being in the sun)
- Oral or nasal ulcers (usually painless ulcers, in the mouth or nose, most often the upper palate)
- Arthritis (tenderness, pain, and swelling in two or more joints)
- Serositis (fluid around the lining of the lungs or heart; this can be called *pleurisy* if it affects the lungs, *pericarditis* if it affects the heart)
- Kidney disorder (proteinuria)
- Brain disorder (psychosis or seizures)
- Blood cell disorder (hemolytic anemia, lymphopenia, leukopenia, or thrombocytopenia)
- A positive test for antinuclear antibodies (ANAs)
- Evidence of other autoantibodies (like anti-dsDNA antibodies, anti-SM antibodies, or antiphospholipid antibodies) including a false-positive venereal disease research laboratory test (VDRL)

Some doctors may diagnose SLE even if only three of these criteria are positive. These classifications were originally intended for clinical trials.

ANAs can be positive in healthy women. A positive ANA is not specific for lupus, although it's the reason most patients are referred to a rheumatologist.

In contrast, the autoantibodies to double-stranded DNA (*anti-dsDNA antibody*) are very specific and with rare exceptions signify lupus. If two of the symptoms listed are present, a diagnosis of lupus is uncertain until more symptoms develop, or other more specific blood tests produce positive results.

Tests You May Need and What They Mean

Blood tests are an integral part of the workup for lupus. They help to pin down a diagnosis because your symptoms can overlap with other diseases.

A complete blood count (CBC) is a standard blood test in any diagnostic workup, measuring white blood cells, red blood cells, and platelets. In a lupus workup, it can flag problems such as leukopenia (a total white blood cell count below 4,000 cells per cubic millimeter) or lymphopenia (fewer than 1,500 lymphocytes per cubic millimeter) or thrombocytopenia (fewer than 100,000 platelets per cubic millimeter). Because white blood cell counts can fluctuate in healthy women, it's important that leukopenia and lymphopenia be detected on two or more occasions to satisfy the ACR classification. A CBC can also detect hemolytic anemia (a condition in which autoantibodies react against targets on red blood cells and destroy them, resulting in low red cell counts).

Antinuclear antibodies (ANAs) will be positive in more than 95 percent of women with SLE. However, since the test can be positive in other autoimmune conditions, the results have to be considered along with a woman's medical history and any clinical signs and symptoms of lupus that may be present. Since discoid lupus does not usually involve internal organs, the ANA test may be negative (or show very low levels of antibodies).

ANA test results include a *titer* (or quantity) of the antibody; this is a number based on how many times an individual's blood must be diluted to get a sample free of antinuclear antibodies. So a titer of 1:640 shows a greater concentration of antinuclear antibodies than a titer of 1:320 or 1:160. As it turns out, the ANA titer doesn't really indicate whether the disease is active. Once the ANA is found to be positive, it's not that useful to repeat. Patients in extended remission can actually have no detectable ANAs, but others may always retain these antibodies, even in remission.

Antibodies to double-stranded DNA (anti-dsDNA) target DNA, which contains the genetic instructions in every cell. A positive anti-dsDNA test is considered highly specific for lupus. If this test is positive, you have a very strong chance of having SLE. Anti-dsDNA antibodies are found in 30 to 70 percent of women with lupus.

Antibodies that target DNA may sound pretty dangerous. Yet these antibodies rarely cross into the cell itself, but rather bind to DNA when it's released from the cell and an immune complex is formed. Anti-dsDNA antibodies are usually associated with kidney disease, and that is why women with these antibodies need to have urine samples tested several times a year to check for protein (it's done with a simple urine dipstick). These antibodies also appear to track lupus activity, they can come and go with disease flares. So patients are tested frequently for anti-dsDNA antibodies in an attempt to predict disease flares.

Anti-SSA/Ro and **anti-SSB/La antibodies** are antibodies directed against normal cellular components called *Ro*, or *Sjögren's syndrome A* (*SSA*), and *La*, or *Sjögren's syndrome B* (*SSB*). SSA and SSB are detected in approximately 40 percent and 15 percent, respectively, in individuals with SLE. Common clinical features associated with these antibodies are skin rashes worsened by sun exposure, and dry eyes and mouth (these antibodies are detected in 75 percent of women with Sjögren's syndrome). It's important to know about antibodies to Ro and La when planning a pregnancy, since some women with anti-Ro and anti-La antibodies can have children with heart problems and transient skin rashes (page 75).

Anti-Smith antibodies (anti-Sm) are present in around 25 percent of women with SLE. They are also directed against nuclear material in the cell (they're related to and coexist with *anti-ribonucleoprotein antibodies, anti-RNP*). Anti-Smith antibodies are specific to lupus and constitute one of the criteria for a diagnosis. Anti-Sm antibodies occur more frequently in African-American and Asian women than in Caucasians.

Anti-Ro, anti-La, and anti-Sm antibodies are usually detected by an *enzyme-linked immunoabsorbent assay* (*ELISA*), in which serum (the clear part of blood not containing any cells) is analyzed. ELISA is capable of detecting very small quantities of these antibodies.

Antiphospholipid antibodies (APLs) are increased in a third of women with SLE, as well as in women with antiphospholipid syndrome. Antiphospholipid antibodies can cause damage to blood vessels and act against proteins in blood to promote clotting problems. There are several types of antiphospholipid antibodies, each of which can be related to an increased risk of clotting anywhere in the body and/or low platelet counts. These antibodies are also associated with miscarriages, since they can cause blood clots in the placenta.

There are four basic types of antiphospholipid antibodies, and each is detected by a different test. The most common are *anticardiolipin antibodies* (*aCLs*) and the *lupus anticoagulant* (*LA*); both proteins on platelets are involved with clotting abnormalities. As many as half of patients who test positive for LA have lupus; up to 47 percent of lupus patients have elevated aCLs. A third type of antiphospholipid antibody is actually detected by a test for syphilis.

The **venereal disease research laboratory test** (**VDRL**) is the test for syphilis, but a positive VDRL does *not* mean you have syphilis. The anticardiolipin antibody in a lupus patient recognizes a similar structure on the syphilis bacteria (another case of molecular mimicry). A positive VDRL is actually a positive test for the presence of that antibody. In the overwhelming majority of patients, when tested against more specific components of syphilis bacteria, the test is negative (so lupus patients have a false positive VDRL).

Complement levels are used to gauge lupus activity, usually by measuring two specific components, C3 and C4. Again, it's helpful to think of complement as the bullets of a gun. When levels are low, it may mean the complement "bullets" have been fired and caused tissue damage. In some cases, women may be born with a low C4, and it may be hard to tell whether that stems from an inherited deficiency or actual disease activity. It's like a bank account: it can be low because you didn't deposit enough money or because you withdrew too much (as in the case of active lupus). Your doctor may measure these levels at all visits to see if they predict disease flares.

Skin biopsy is done if you have a rash (often a sign of discoid lupus). A small biopsy of skin will be taken from the rash area to look for markers of inflammation.

A **urine dipstick test** is simple, but extremely important. Excessive protein in the urine means the kidney is losing protein. To more accurately measure the quantity of protein lost, it may be necessary to collect urine over a period of twenty-four hours. A microscopic examination of the urine may reveal abnormalities, such as red blood cell or white blood cell casts (abnormal elements derived from red and/or white cells, and kidney *glomerular* cells). A kidney biopsy may be done if urine or blood tests indicate evidence of kidney disease.

I was diagnosed with lupus when I was twenty-three—that was more than thirty years ago. Back then, very little was really known about lupus. I was passed around from one doctor to another. I was told I had multiple sclerosis, I had a malignant brain tumor, I had rheumatoid arthritis, it was a psychosomatic illness . . . just about any illness you can think of, depending on what symptom I was having at the time. I was having seizures. And I went through a lot of torturous tests because they thought I had a brain tumor. I was sent to a rheumatologist, a neurologist, and a neurosurgeon, and I was even sent to a psychiatrist, who said a lot of it was all in my head. Unfortunately, I went home and I tried to convince myself that my symptoms were imaginary. But of course that was the wrong thing to do; nothing was imaginary.

My symptoms just kept getting worse . . . I went from specialist to specialist, and no one tried to put together a whole picture. I was finally diagnosed through a kidney biopsy in 1967. I remember when they told me I had lupus, they said I wouldn't live a year. Well, I'm still here. I've had heart trouble, and the lupus has affected my lungs and my kidneys . . . I also have back problems and I have some trouble getting around these days. But I don't let anything drag me down. And I was fortunate to finally find a doctor who knew something about lupus, and who was aggressive in treating it. I credit my longevity to aggressive doctors, to good treatments, and to God.

JANE, SIXTY-THREE

What's a Lupus Flare?

The most important thing to keep in mind is that lupus is a fluctuating disease; you can experience periods of remission in which the disease is quiet, and flares in which the disease is active, like the swing of a pendulum. The pattern varies from one person to the next. However, a lupus flare does *not* necessarily mean that your disease is progressing or that permanent damage to the internal organs is occurring.

Flares can have a number of triggers, including emotional stress, exposure to sunlight, infections, and certain medications. The stress connection is very real. A preliminary study from Germany, reported in September 2001, looked at blood levels of cytokines after acute psychological stress in women with lupus, rheumatoid arthritis, and healthy women, and found stress-induced increases in interferon gamma and interleukin 4 (IL-4) in the women with SLE and RA, suggesting that changes in cytokine patterns may be responsible for flares. Lupus flares also occur in a minority of women during pregnancy or the postpartum period (see pages 70 to 72), suggesting some hormonal influence.

During a lupus flare, disease *activity* can be measured. In most cases, flares involve physical changes that may be accompanied by abnormalities in the blood analysis. So your doctor will assess lupus activity by taking a history, performing a physical exam, and drawing blood for testing. The degree of activity can actually be quantified, and there are several scoring systems developed for this purpose. One such "score sheet" is the *SLEDAI* (*SLE Disease Activity Index*). This is a list of various physical findings and blood tests. The SLEDAI score literally adds up the number of problems; the more points, the more disease activity. This scoring system is generally used for clinical trials, but some physicians do use the system for keeping track of disease. While keeping score is not the point, it may be helpful to understand just how sick you are by reviewing how the SLEDAI score sheet is used (and you may find it useful for tracking your own symptoms). Many of the symptoms are the same as those in the ACR diagnostic classification (page 58).

A mild flare (less than three points) is likely to consist of any one of the following: new or recurrent facial rash, hair loss, photosensitivity, mouth or nose ulcers, and unexplained fevers. Increased fatigue can be part of a lupus flare, but the SLEDAI doesn't factor it in, although other lupus activity score sheets do. A moderate flare might include joint swelling and pain in more than two joints, pleuritis, or pericarditis. A severe flare (SLEDAI scores greater than twelve) generally indicates more internal organ involvement, such as the kidneys or brain, and almost always requires treatment with glucocorticoids. But the degree of a problem also varies. Depending on the degree of activity, flares are treated differently.

On the other hand, disease *progression* (and any potential damage) is assessed using the SLE damage index, which records damage or permanent injury to a particular organ that has occurred after the diagnosis of lupus. The damage may be due to lupus itself or may have been caused by treatments. For example, cataracts are a side effect of glucocorticoids, not lupus per se. The purpose of a damage index is to have an assessment of the total health status of a patient over time. Like the SLEDAI, the damage index is generally used only in clinical studies and academic centers where lupus is being researched.

While the SLEDAI and damage index are useful, a careful physical examination and the appropriate lab tests will usually provide all the information your rheumatologist needs. Even without scales and scoring, physicians must assess lupus from at least two perspectives—how sick a patient is or how active her disease is at the time of a visit, and how the lupus has affected the patient's health over time until the visit. It's hoped that early treatment, where necessary, can prevent permanent damage to organs or tissues.

You can take preventive measures to reduce the risk of flares. Learning stress-reduction techniques can help you minimize stress-induced flares. Getting regular exercise should help combat fatigue and muscle weakness. If you're photosensitive, avoiding excessive sun exposure and using sunscreen when you're out in the sun will usually prevent rashes. If you smoke, stop smoking. Not only can it trigger flares, but it's the number-one risk factor for heart and blood vessel disease . . . and cardiovascular disease can follow lupus like a shadow.

Living with the unpredictability of lupus flares can be difficult. Which symptoms are the hardest, and who does best? A study of four hundred patients with SLE, run by the University of Texas-Houston Health Science Center and the University of Alabama at Birmingham (now in its eighth year), found that fatigue and pain were the two most difficult symptoms from the patient's point of view. But the women who were able to cope with their disease from the time they were first diagnosed did much better. "It's not so much disease activity, or disease damage, or individual organ system dysfunction (lupus nephritis or CNS lupus) that predicts how women say they're doing. It's more things like pain and fatigue, which are difficult to fix, and feeling helpless that make for poorer outcomes," comments Alan W. Friedman, MD, an associate professor of rheumatology, one of the study's investigators. Because stress can also play a major role in lupus flares, learning stress reduction exercises can be very beneficial, as can joining a support group where women can learn more effective coping strategies to help manage both the physical and emotional effects of their disease.

Treating Lupus

Treatments are aimed at reducing symptoms, decreasing the number and severity of flares, stopping progression of the disease, and minimizing permanent organ damage.

Pain medications, most frequently *nonsteroidal anti-inflammatory drugs* (*NSAIDs*), are given to reduce muscle and joint pain and inflammation. NSAIDs include *aspirin, ibuprofen (Motrin), naproxen (Naprosyn), indomethacin (Indocin), nabumetone (Relafen).* However, these drugs can cause gastrointestinal problems, including bleeding. They can also affect kidney function and cause liver abnormalities.

Newer NSAIDs, called *COX-2 inhibitors* (see page 30), are less likely to cause serious GI bleeding. They include *celecoxib (Celebrex), rofecoxib (Vioxx),* and *valdecoxib (Bextra). Meloxicam (Mobic)* is a partially selective COX-2 inhibitor. There's a special precaution, however. Selective COX-2 inhibitors do not have the anticlotting properties of aspirin (and therefore don't reduce the risk of a heart attack), so it's important that women who take these drugs first be checked for antiphospholipid antibodies, which may add to the risk of clotting. Celecoxib also contains sulfa, and this may be a problem because lupus patients have a tendency to be allergic to sulfa.

Glucocorticoids (corticosteroids) are used to reduce inflammation and suppress immune activity (see page 34). Among the most commonly prescribed are *prednisone (Deltasone, Orasone)* and *methylprednisolone (Medrol).*

Corticosteroids have a number of major side effects (see pages 34 to 35). The biggest risk for side effects occurs when higher doses of steroids are taken for long periods of time. However, corticosteroids are extremely effective in treating lupus, and may be needed for long periods in cases of life-threatening complications.

Prolonged use of corticosteroids also leads to a shutdown of the adrenal glands. To get the adrenal glands working again, steroids must be slowly tapered.

Antimalarials are drugs originally used to treat malaria that suppress the inflammation leading to skin rashes, joint pain, hair loss, and fatigue in lupus. They include *chloroquine* (*Aralen*), *hydroxychloroquine* (*Plaquenil*), and *quinacrine* (*Atabrine*). Hydroxychloroquine is the most commonly prescribed. The side effects include nausea, diarrhea, bad taste in the mouth, and rashes (in rare cases), most of which can be avoided by taking the drug just before bedtime. One potential side effect of these drugs, eye damage, is extremely rare; problems can be avoided by seeing an eye doctor once a year. Keep in mind that it may take months to see a benefit from antimalarials, so patience is important. Recent studies suggest that hydroxychloroquine may also have protective effects on bone mass, preventing bone loss at the hip and spine, areas vulnerable to fracture. They may even protect against blood clotting and high lipids.

Immunomodulating drugs belong to a class of drugs called cytotoxic (cell-killing) drugs that can help suppress the immune system by reducing populations of immune cells. These drugs include *azathioprine* (*Imuran*), *cyclophosphamide* (*Cytoxan*), and *mycophenolate mofetil* (*CellCept*), and are generally used when there's more serious kidney or other organ involvement.

Side effects include anemia, a low white blood cell count, and an increased risk of infection. There are suggestions these drugs may increase the risk of cancer (but this has not been proven). Cyclophosphamide can also cause sterility (premature menopause).

Anticoagulants are prescribed for women with clotting abnormalities to prevent clots in leg veins (*deep vein thrombosis*) or in the lungs, as well as in coronary arteries. Low-dose aspirin prevents platelets from sticking together to form clots. *Warfarin* (*Coumadin*) interferes with some of the proteins that regulate clotting that depend on vitamin K. Heparin affects another clotting mechanism. It's important to remember that blood thinners must be monitored carefully to avoid bleeding episodes.

Intravenous immunoglobulin (**IVIG**) may be used to raise platelet counts in women with thrombocytopenia (see pages 307 to 308).

Dehydroepiandrosterone (**DHEA**) is an androgen, or male hormone, normally produced by the adrenal glands and converted by the body into estrogen and testosterone. Some scientists believe that women with lupus have low levels of androgens (which have anti-inflammatory properties). DHEA may be helpful if you have mild lupus, especially skin rashes, hair loss, and joint pain. It does not appear to be effective for more serious manifestations of lupus, such as kidney disease. DHEA is usually well tolerated with only minor side effects, including mild acne.

While DHEA is available in health food stores as a dietary supplement, a pharmaceutical preparation of DHEA (*prasterone*, *Aslera*) is still being tested in lupus patients and has not yet been approved. The first U.S. multicenter trial of prasterone found that taking 200 milligrams a day stabilized the course of the disease over a one-year period. A trial conducted in Taiwan found that it reduced the incidence of flares by almost half, compared to a placebo. Another study found that it improved bone density in a small group of women taking prednisone. DHEA may allow you to reduce the amount of prednisone you're taking. As this book went to press, prasterone had yet to be approved by the FDA for women with lupus. Don't buy DHEA supplements in a health food store or take it without a physician's supervision.

What's Next?

Future treatments, including newer drugs called *biologicals*, are currently in clinical research trials and are hoped to have a more specific effect on the immune abnormalities of lupus, not just global immunosuppression. Among these are agents that block production of specific antibodies, such as anti-DNA antibodies, or drugs that suppress the "cross-talk" between B-cells and T-cells in hopes of reducing production of autoantibodies. One drug currently being tested in many clinical centers across the country is *LJP394*, designed

---

Lupus Clusters

A recent survey by the Lupus Foundation of America found that a third of patients had another autoimmune disease in addition to their lupus. Among the most common are:

- Thyroid disease
- Sjögren's syndrome
- Raynaud's phenomenon
- Antiphospholipid syndrome

---

to modulate the production of anti-DNA antibodies by B-cells. Preliminary evidence indicates that LJP394 may help prevent or reduce the recurrence of kidney flares.

Preliminary studies also suggest that low doses of *thalidomide* (*Thalidomid*) may help improve rashes in women with cutaneous lupus who have failed other therapies. Thalidomide has some anti-inflammatory effects, but doesn't put lupus in remission. Side effects include a cessation of menstrual periods, weight gain, drowsiness, and blood clots in women who have risk factors for clots. The drug can also cause irreversible nerve damage, so nerve conduction tests must be done at baseline and periodically during treatment. Because of its devastating effects on a developing fetus, thalidomide cannot be used by women who wish to become pregnant (so planning is essential).

Deanna's story continues:
The high doses of steroids I was on made my muscles very weak, and I was in physical therapy to try to get my strength back. There was a period when I couldn't even lift myself off the toilet. I was emotionally a mess from the steroids. I would have temper tantrums. I had an inflamed esophagus, so I had difficulty swallowing food. But the joint pain got better. When my doctor told me I had lupus nephritis, he said I probably would not be able to go back to school . . . that made me furious . . . I was determined to get better. Eventually, they reduced the steroids. My face was going back to normal, my hair was growing in again, and my self-esteem was coming back. I had to go back to college that fall on crutches at first . . . but I worked even harder in school. I felt I had a lot to make up for. I graduated summa cum laude. Highest honors. I couldn't control the lupus, but I could try to control everything else. I graduated from college, taught for a while, and eventually got my master's degree.

The Female Factor

Ninety percent of patients with lupus are women, and numerous studies suggest a role for estrogen in the disease. Unlike rheumatoid arthritis, which gets better during pregnancy when estrogen levels are high, lupus can sometimes flare during or after pregnancy. Some studies suggest that women with lupus may have an abnormality in the way their bodies process naturally occurring estrogens, while others find that women with SLE may metabolize testosterone at a faster rate than men, so high levels of estrogen may go unopposed by androgens. Male hormones may play a protective role in lupus; women with low levels of androgens may be more vulnerable to SLE.

Prolactin (produced during lactation) is another hormone that may play a role. It not only stimulates the flow of mother's milk, but it's also produced by immune cells and can act as a cytokine. In this role, prolactin triggers the release of other cytokines and stimulates immune reactions. About 20 percent of lupus patients have higher prolactin levels than the body would normally produce, says Sara E. Walker, MD, professor of internal medicine at the University of Missouri. "My theory is that if a woman has lupus, if she has high prolactin, this might fuel the disease process," says Dr. Walker. "Prolactin levels also increase during pregnancy and postpartum, times when some women are vulnerable to lupus or have lupus flares."

Dr. Walker has been testing treatment with the drug *bromocriptine* to lower prolactin levels and reduce symptoms in women with lupus, with some success. "Bromocriptine is an extremely safe drug. But we don't yet have the studies to prove it will work as a treatment for lupus," she adds.

There are also studies that suggest a role for *microchimerism* in lupus, where cells from the fetus get into the mother's bloodstream and may trigger a reaction by the immune system (see page 11). However, it may be the *maternal* cells that get into the fetal circulation and persist into adult life that increase the risk of lupus and neonatal lupus, suggests Anne Stevens, MD, PhD, a pediatric rheumatologist working with Dr. J. Lee Nelson at the Fred Hutchinson Cancer Research Center and the University of Washington. These cells could travel to certain sites in the body and provoke immune reactions. Dr. Stevens notes that biopsies of heart muscle have found maternal cells in babies with neonatal lupus, and that studies also show that you can create lupus in mice by injecting parental cells. However, this area of research is still very much in its preliminary stages.

How Lupus Can Affect You Over Your Lifetime

Lupus can affect women in many ways during their reproductive years, especially during and after pregnancy, and their children also face an increased risk of neonatal lupus.

Lupus and Your Menstrual Cycle

You may find that lupus symptoms flare during different times of the menstrual cycle. For some women, flares occur just prior to menses (when estrogens are lowest), while in others, flares occur at the time of ovulation (when estrogens are highest). It may be the change in hormone levels that triggers a flare, not the absolute level itself. Birth control pills create steady levels of hormones and may help prevent these cyclic flares (although not proven).

Menstrual periods can stop during times of severe disease activity. A study from Brazil reported at the 2001 Scientific Meeting of the American College of Rheumatology (ACR), found that disease activity was a major factor associated with menstrual disturbances. The study, which included thirty-six SLE patients ages eighteen to thirty-nine years, determined half of the women had menstrual dysfunction, with increased menstrual flow being the most frequent. About 11 percent had elevations in *follicle-stimulating hormone* (*FSH*), with or without menstrual disturbances, suggesting there may have been subclinical ovarian damage. The study found no significant association of low-dose prednisone with menstrual changes. But other studies have shown that women being treated with high-dose steroids do have menstrual cycle irregularities, with a temporary loss of periods being most frequent. Unfortunately, treatment with cyclophosphamide (especially in women older than thirty-five) can result in permanent sterility.

Lupus and Pregnancy

Fertility and sterility rates for women with SLE are comparable to those for women who don't have SLE when the disease is in remission. However, your fertility may be depressed during times of severe disease activity.

One recent study that followed 173 women with SLE for a period of six years (1991 to 1997) found that those with inactive disease at the onset of pregnancy had the least amount of subsequent disease activity. The study found that pregnant SLE patients with inactive disease had less activity during pregnancy and the postpartum period than women with more active disease.

Although pregnancy is always considered high risk in a woman with SLE, you should know that outcomes for you and your baby are quite encouraging, provided you get proper treatment. Complications can arise, however. A recent study from the University of New Mexico Health Sciences Center that examined data from 358 women with SLE (during 726 pregnancies) found that one-third of the women experienced fetal loss. Losses during the first trimester were associated with blood clotting (deep vein thrombosis and strokes). Losses that occurred in the second and third trimester were associated with kidney disease.

There is a higher risk of preeclampsia (abnormally high blood pressure during pregnancy). The risk is greater when there's preexisting hypertension and kidney disease. Women with SLE-related kidney disease are also more likely to have protein in the urine, or *proteinuria*, which may signal a lupus flare or preeclampsia. Regular monitoring for these conditions is a must. As soon as you know you're pregnant, a baseline measurement of protein in the urine over twenty-four hours should be done; after that, dipsticks should be done at each obstetrical visit, and twenty-four-hour urine collections should be done each trimester.

If you've been in remission for six months, this is the best time to consider having a baby. This usually means being clinically well without major organ involvement such as active kidney, heart, lung, or brain disease, and taking less than 20 milligrams per day of prednisone. Taking greater than 20 milligrams of prednisone, despite feeling well, is not likely to represent a true state of remission. In fact, the definition of remission is quite individual. For example, blood tests may indicate a minor degree of disease activity (slightly low complement levels and slightly elevated anti-DNA antibodies), but a woman may have no other signs of a problem. So you needn't always wait for a complete absence of evidence of lupus activity in your blood work before getting pregnant. If you're planning a pregnancy, you also need to make sure that you're not anemic or have a very low platelet count. Minor joint or skin involvement is usually not a reason to avoid pregnancy.

Ideally, you should be cared for by a team consisting of a rheumatologist and a high-risk obstetrician with prior experience in managing patients with SLE. The obstetrician should be affiliated with a neonatal intensive care unit, in case your baby needs special attention.

In general, lupus patients can do well during pregnancy. While some investigators have found flare rates as high as 60 percent, these scary statistics usually include even minor problems such as fatigue and joint aches. So the situation is not as discouraging as it seems. What's important to realize is that severe flares probably occur in less than 20 percent of cases, and most often among women with prior kidney disease and low platelet counts. These two problems can recur during pregnancy and women must be carefully monitored for them. While minor flares—such as joint pains, increased skin rashes, and fatigue—may be uncomfortable, they usually don't pose a significant threat to mother or baby. Overall, very few patients have permanent deterioration in any aspect of their disease during or after pregnancy. However, it's critical that you be seen frequently by your rheumatologist, as well as your obstetrician.

A woman with problems becoming pregnant may need hormonal stimulation to produce multiple eggs for implantation with in-vitro fertilization (IVF). A small study at three lupus centers in New York City found that ovulation induction, ovarian hyperstimulation, and in-vitro fertilization resulted in increased disease activity in 25 percent of women with SLE. The small study, analyzing data from 19 women with SLE and primary antiphospholipid syndrome who had undergone 68 cycles of ovulation induction and IVF, also found some associated complications during pregnancy and postpartum. Pregnancy complications included toxemia, lupus flares, and diabetes; postpartum problems included a flare in kidney disease, cartilage inflammation (*costochondritis*), and depression. "I believe that ovulation induction and so-called 'superovulation' are potentially dangerous, especially superovulation, where you try to produce as many eggs as possible. You are pushing a woman's estrogen levels very high. Women with lupus who desperately want to have children should fully understand the risks, or explore other alternatives," cautions Dr. Walker.

Tests you'll need if you're pregnant. Once you're pregnant, you will need routine blood tests, such as a complete blood count and urinalysis. The standard tests to assess lupus activity should also be done, such as measuring complement levels and anti-DNA antibodies.

During your first trimester you'll need several other blood tests. The first set of tests assesses the risk of a spontaneous miscarriage and measures antibodies to phospholipids, which may cause blood clotting in the placenta. One of the tests you'll need is the VDRL (a standard test for syphilis that can also detect anticardiolipin antibodies). A traditional ELISA for direct measurement of anticardiolipin antibodies will also be done, along with special clot-ting tests. One type of clotting test is called a *Dilute Russell Viper Venom Time* (*DRVVT*), which checks for the presence of the so-called lupus anticoagu-lant (that actually promotes clotting, not bleeding).

A second set of antibody tests is done to assess the rare risk of permanent cardiac damage in the developing fetus and/or skin rash and liver disease in early infancy. These are antibodies to SSA/Ro and SSB/La proteins. Of course, a positive test for any of these antibodies does not mean you'll have problems with the pregnancy, but your doctors need to know so they can be prepared. Also, as a precaution, during each trimester you should be tested for anti-DNA antibodies and complement levels, and have twenty-four-hour urine collection to test for protein and creatinine. Protein in the urine means the kidneys are leaky—think of a colander in which the holes might be too big and spaghetti can leak out. The creatinine level tells you how well the kid-neys are filtering waste products.

Before the third trimester, a fetal sonogram is done to assess growth and general health. If there are signs of fetal distress, it may be wise to hospital-ize the mother and consider early delivery, because there is a higher rate of prematurity in babies born to women with lupus. Patients with lupus have a high risk of preeclampsia (toxemia of pregnancy), high blood pressure, and protein in the urine.

Medications during pregnancy and breastfeeding. Keep in mind that *all* drugs taken during pregnancy could have potential harm to the growing baby since they may cross the placenta. However, certain drugs are necessary even if there are risks, since they're intended to either keep your lupus at bay or prevent a problem in the baby.

In general, low-dose aspirin (81 milligrams per day) is not likely to cause harm but may be helpful in preventing a clot in the placenta. High-dose NSAIDs are not recommended during pregnancy because they may be asso-ciated with high pulmonary pressures in the fetus. NSAIDs can prolong labor and are generally avoided close to the time of delivery; because of the risk of bleeding, aspirin is also generally stopped when you're close to term.

Prednisone at doses less than 20 milligrams daily is generally not a problem for the fetus, since the placenta inactivates the drug. At higher doses, slightly more active drug is available in fetal circulation, but still may not be dangerous. Possible side effects of steroids to the fetus include decreased amniotic fluid, decreased growth, and suppression of the adrenal glands. The mother needs to be closely monitored for hypertension and gestational diabetes.

Hydroxychloroquine (*Plaquenil*) does cross the placenta, although the available literature shows very few problems. Concerns about Plaquenil have declined to such an extent that most rheumatologists with experience in treating pregnant lupus patients suggest staying on the drug. The reason is that there is a risk of a flare if it's discontinued, and this may override any potential harm to the fetus. Keep in mind that Plaquenil is an extremely long-acting medication, so if you do want to stop it, it must be done months before getting pregnant.

Azathioprine (*Imuran*) is a category D drug, and while it's actually been used during pregnancy to treat women who've had kidney transplants and there have been few adverse effects, its use should be avoided unless considered absolutely necessary. Some lupus specialists have prescribed it for severe flares during pregnancy. Cytoxan is a category X drug and cannot be taken during pregnancy. Unfractionated heparin and low-molecular weight heparin for treatment of clotting problems is commonly used in the special situation of recurrent fetal loss.

Drugs can be passed to your baby if you breastfeed. NSAIDs are generally safe, since they do not pass easily into breast milk. However, high doses of NSAIDs can pose a problem, since babies eliminate them more slowly than adults do and they can accumulate in an infant's system. Hydroxychloroquine is excreted in small amounts in breast milk but seems to pose no risk. Lower doses of prednisone appear to be safe.

Using immunosuppressive agents is controversial. Small amounts of azathioprine have been found in breast milk, but it seems to be safe. Cyclophosphamide and cyclosporine cannot be used if you nurse because they are toxic to an infant.

Maternal autoantibodies can pass to the baby via breast milk but only during the first few days of life, so this is not likely to pose problems. Breastfeeding may increase fatigue, but don't let that stop you.

Neonatal lupus. During pregnancy, antibodies in the mother's circulation travel across the placenta into the bloodstream of the developing fetus, starting at about twelve to fourteen weeks of gestation. The fetus is unable to make antibodies on its own and is dependent on maternal antibodies to fight infection. Mothers with antibodies SSA/Ro and SSB/La can have children with neonatal lupus. Two concerns in neonatal lupus are heart problems and skin rash.

The most concerning heart problem is in congenital heart block, in which there is literally a block in the electrical signal coming from the *sinus node* located at the top of the heart to the *atrioventricular* (*AV node*) in the middle of the heart. This electrical signal is responsible for normal cardiac rate and rhythm. Blockage of the signal causes the ventricles to contract more slowly, and the overall result is an abnormally slow heartbeat. In congenital heart block, the AV node is damaged by the maternal autoantibodies or other as yet unidentified associated factors. This cardiac dysfunction (slow heartbeat) is most often detected between eighteen to twenty-six weeks of gestation, with the twenty-third and twenty-fourth weeks being the most vulnerable.

A slow fetal heart rate can be identified by routine examination using an amplified stethoscope, an obstetrical sonogram, or a special fetal echocardiogram. In almost all cases, heart block occurs as an isolated problem (there are no structural deformities of the heart itself). Curiously, the presence of these autoantibodies is *not* associated with heart problems in the mother, only in her offspring. The risk of having a child with heart block is 2 percent if you have antibodies to SSA/Ro and SSB/La. If you have had one baby with heart block, there is a 17 percent risk of having a second affected child.

The skin rash of neonatal lupus is most commonly noted at about six weeks after delivery, but can be detected at birth. The rash often involves the eyelids, face, and scalp. It is generally very red and can have a circular appearance. The skin rash can be triggered by sun exposure, so babies born to women with lupus should not be exposed to the sun without the use of sunscreen during the first months of life.

Liver abnormalities and low white blood cell and platelet counts are extremely rare problems, but need to be checked. Most affected children have either heart block or skin rashes, but some do have both. Studies to date suggest that girls may be more prone to the rash than boys, but both sexes are equally susceptible to congenital heart block.

Actually, the term *neonatal lupus* is misleading. The name came about because the skin rash seen in infants resembled that seen in adults with SLE. While many mothers do have lupus, some mothers of affected children are totally asymptomatic themselves and have only the anti-Ro and/or anti-La antibodies in their blood. It's important to note that just because you may have anti-Ro or anti-La antibodies and your baby has neonatal lupus does not mean *you* have lupus or Sjögren's syndrome. Even more important to know: a child with heart block or skin rash does *not* have SLE, but rather a temporary disease acquired from the passage of maternal autoantibodies. Neonatal lupus is not a true systemic disease.

Helping mothers at risk. If you're found to be at risk for having a child with neonatal lupus, it's best to take precautionary steps, whether it's a first pregnancy or you have previously had a baby with heart block or other signs of neonatal lupus.

It's recommended that you have a fetal echocardiogram (a sonogram of the heart that gives a far better picture of the heart structure and function than routine obstetrical ultrasound) between the sixteenth and eighteenth weeks of pregnancy. This should be done every week, if possible, until about the twenty-sixth week. After that, it should be done every other week until about thirty weeks. After that, just listening with a stethoscope may be sufficient.

Should a problem in the fetal heart be detected, therapies may be needed to lower antibody levels or to treat the inflammation in the heart. However, once established, complete heart block (sometimes the block is not complete, which is better) is not likely to be reversed. Most children will eventually need a pacemaker.

In the situation of a mother with known antibodies who has already had a child with heart block, the risk of having a second affected child may be as high as one in six. In studies from the National Research Registry for Neonatal Lupus, there have only been thirteen cases of a recurrence of heart block in eighty-four subsequent pregnancies. However, it's possible to have one child with heart block and a second child with a rash and vice versa. At this time, no data suggest a benefit to prophylactic therapies, such as *plasmapheresis* (to filter antibodies from the blood) and/or steroids, *prior* to the detection of a problem.

If the fetus *is* diagnosed with heart block, and the block has been present for more than three weeks, the baby is watched and weekly echocardiograms are performed to determine if there are signs that heart function is deteriorating (for example, if fluid builds up around the heart or lungs).

If the heartbeat is second-degree block (incomplete), it is theoretically possible (but not yet proven) that treating the mother with a steroid such as dexamethasone, which can cross the placenta and be available in the fetal circulation, will reverse the block before it progresses to third-degree heart block. Unfortunately, the block is usually complete when it is first detected. If the fetus shows signs of inflammation, such as fluid around the heart or lungs or abdomen, this may be a more serious sign and dexamethasone may be initiated.

What's the outlook for your baby? The prognosis for the child with heart block is generally good. However, heart block is permanent, and in 20 percent of cases the condition is fatal (most often before three months of age). Most children will require pacemakers, probably for life. Pacemakers are commonly implanted within the first three months after birth. In a child whose only manifestation of neonatal lupus is a skin rash, the situation is generally excellent since the rash usually disappears by about eight months to one year. In most cases no medications are needed and no scars or marks are left.

Although any child born to a mother with SLE does have a higher risk of developing SLE later in life (approximately one in ten if it's a girl), no data persuasively indicate that the risk is increased if the child also had neonatal lupus.

Lupus and Estrogen

For both healthy women and women with SLE, there are times when estrogen may be needed. A woman may want birth control, and the best method may be oral contraceptives (OCs). After menopause, women may need the symptom relief estrogen replacement therapy can bring.

It's been suggested that OCs may even be useful in controlling cyclical disease activity in some patients. The estrogen in oral contraceptives may be useful in preventing steroid-induced osteoporosis and may preserve fertility in women taking cyclophosphamide.

For years, the conventional wisdom was that estrogens might provoke lupus flares. Clinical trials are being conducted to see whether postmenopausal hormone replacement and oral contraceptives do affect disease activity. Preliminary data from a clinical trial among 100 women in Mexico City found that ERT did not definitively increase disease activity. However, the study was not large enough to determine the safety of ERT.

The Safety of Estrogens in Lupus Erythematosus, National Assessment (*SELENA*) trials, randomized double-blind placebo-controlled trials, one for hormone replacement and one for oral contraceptives, should definitively answer the questions about the safety of hormones for women with SLE and whether estrogens change the rate of flares.

Lupus and Menopause

You need to discuss with your doctor the risks and benefits of taking estrogen for menopausal symptoms. The Women's Health Initiative (WHI), a major clinical trial of one form of hormone replacement therapy (*Prempro*) among healthy women, was halted in 2002 because of slight increases in heart attacks, strokes, blood clots, and invasive breast cancers among women taking the drug (although there was a reduced risk of colon cancer and benefit to the bones). Given the consideration that HRT may further increase the already elevated risk of cardiovascular disease in women with lupus, the HRT arm of the SELENA trial was also stopped. However, 285 women had already completed the study and the results should be quite informative. In the meantime, you should not take HRT if you have antiphospholipid antibodies.

There are a number of nonhormonal remedies for menopausal symptoms, among them vitamins E and B, soy, and herbs like black cohosh (see pages 46 to 47). However, you should avoid some menopausal remedies: Evening primrose oil promotes clotting and cannot be used by women who have antiphospholipid antibodies; red clover can interfere with blood thinners used to treat antiphospholipid syndrome and promotes bleeding.

Dr. Sara Walker says women with lupus should be extremely cautious about plant estrogens like soy or black cohosh. "We simply do not know the effects of phytoestrogens in women with lupus. We know that these substances act like estrogens in the body, binding to the same receptors. But could they stay around long enough to potentially cause harm?" she says. "Herbal products are not well regulated, and contents can vary quite widely. I would urge women not to try anything without talking it over with their rheumatologist."

Lupus and Your Heart

If you have lupus, you should be aware that you're at increased risk for cardiovascular disease, and the risk may be greater before age forty-five. One study found that women aged thirty-five to forty-four were actually fifty times more likely to have a heart attack than women of similar age in the general population, but women with SLE aged forty-five to sixty-four had only two to four times the risk.

The natural estrogen present in your body that usually protects women before menopause may actually promote blood clotting in younger women with SLE who have antiphospholipid antibodies, high blood pressure, or kidney disease. Immune complexes in the blood may irritate the lining of blood vessels and cause inflammation, promoting atherosclerotic lesions. These fatty plaques narrow the carotid arteries—the major blood vessels supplying the brain—more often in premenopausal women with SLE, says Susan Manzi, MD, MPH, an associate professor of medicine and epidemiology at the University of Pittsburgh School of Medicine. A recent study by Dr. Manzi and colleagues also found that stiffness in the aorta might be an early marker of atherosclerotic disease. As women become perimenopausal and develop more heart disease risk factors (such as high cholesterol, high blood pressure, and obesity), this process may speed up, adds Dr. Manzi. Having antiphospholipid antibodies increases the risk of stroke.

A study from Britain in the February 2002 issue of the *Annals of the Rheumatic Diseases* also found that antinuclear antibodies are much more common in people who have severe atherosclerosis, suggesting that systemic autoimmunity may play a role in the development of fatty plaques in coronary arteries.

Taking corticosteroids causes abnormalities in blood fats, including cholesterol, and may promote insulin resistance. Homocysteine, a naturally occurring by-product of normal metabolism of food, can damage blood vessels if it's present in high levels. Some women with SLE have been shown to have elevated homocysteine levels, possibly because of the effects of treatment with methotrexate. Cholesterol-lowering drugs may be one way to lower the risk of heart attacks.

Other steps you need to take to protect your heart include keeping your weight under control, getting regular exercise, and following a heart-healthy diet (see pages 48 to 49). Blood pressure should be monitored carefully, and levels of LDL and HDL cholesterol, triglycerides, and homocysteine should be measured once a year. Your annual physical exam should include an electrocardiogram (ECG).

The Threat of Osteoporosis

Any woman taking corticosteroid therapy for autoimmune disease is at risk for bone loss. Studies among women with lupus indicate that taking bone-building drugs like *alendronate* (*Fosamax*) can help prevent osteoporosis in those on long-term glucocorticord therapy.

Hormone replacement is also an effective therapy for preventing bone loss in women taking corticosteroids. A small study among younger women with early menopause, who were taking more that 30 milligrams a day of prednisone for more than 130 months and suffered mild bone loss (*osteopenia*), found that those taking HRT had increased bone-mineral density in the lumbar spine after two years. But those women taking *Calcitriol* (*calcitonin*) showed little effect and even lost bone in their wrists. In this study, HRT consisted of 0.625 milligram of conjugated equine estrogen (Premarin) and 5 milligrams of medroxyprogesterone (Provera).

The antimalarial drug *hydroxychloroquine* may help protect against bone loss due to corticosteroids. Researchers at the University of Connecticut Health Center in Farmington studied ninety-two women with SLE to identify factors associated with low bone-mineral density and, surprisingly, found that 68 percent of those taking hydroxychloroquine appeared to be at least partially protected against bone loss in fracture-prone areas in the hip and spine. The drug also appeared to protect against further bone loss in women with osteopenia.

The one important thing is not to let it get you. Make sure you get the proper care, take care of yourself, eat right and exercise, and you can beat it. I firmly believe that. I've met women in the support groups who let lupus consume them, and their disease just gets worse and worse. I've had kidney problems, intestinal problems; I had bone death because of the steroids I was on, and I have had both hips replaced. But I focused on my work, on living my life no matter what, and that kept me going. I got married last June, and I look at the wedding pictures and outwardly, you'd never know anything was wrong. I look healthy. Sometimes when I don't feel well, my husband will still say, "But you don't look sick." Despite all the problems I've had, I try not to think of myself as being sick. Maybe you can't control the disease, but you can control your attitude. I really believe the power of the mind can be stronger than the disease.

DEANNA

4

The Elusive Butterfly Gland— Thyroid Disease

I really had no idea anything was wrong with my thyroid until I literally passed out in the street and had to be taken to the emergency room. The doctors said it was a "thyroid storm." The way they explained it, it was like driving a car with the gas pedal pushed all the way down to the floor. My body was speeding along and just crashed. I had always been a "hyper" person, always active, always fidgety. I had a high pulse rate, I was skinny. But up until I collapsed, I didn't think anything of it. That's just the way I was.

ANNE MARIE, THIRTY-SIX

The thyroid is a butterfly-shaped gland located in the neck, just below your voice box. Although it's small—a little more than two inches wide—the thyroid gland plays a big role in the body. Thyroid hormones influence almost every organ and regulate *metabolism*, the rate at which the body converts food into energy. Having thyroid disease is akin to living in a house where the thermostat doesn't work properly—it's either set too high, turning up the heat and making you feel jumpy, or set too low, making you feel cold and tired.

The thyroid is part of the *endocrine system*, a network of glands that secretes hormones right into the blood, rather than piping them through a network of ducts. The other endocrine glands are the pancreas, the pituitary, the adrenals, the parathyroids, and the ovaries—all of which can be the targets of autoimmune attacks.

83

The *pituitary gland* (located in the brain just behind the eyes) is known as the "master gland" because it regulates the other endocrine glands, including the thyroid. The master gland has a master switch, and that's the *hypothalamus*, a tiny area in the base of the brain connected to the pituitary. Secretion of just the right amount of thyroid hormones is governed by a feedback system between these three structures.

The hypothalamus sends out a hormone called *thyrotropin releasing hormone (TRH)*, which prompts the pituitary to release *thyroid stimulating hormone (TSH)*, triggering the secretion of thyroid hormones by the thyroid gland. There are two thyroid hormones: *thyroxine (T4)* and *triiodothyronine (T3)*. Thyroxine is produced by the *follicular* cells of the thyroid and converted to T3 by enzymes in various organs (some T3 is produced by the thyroid, too). If thyroid hormones in the bloodstream rise above normal levels, they cause a decrease in TRH and TSH that prompts the thyroid to cut back on the amount of hormones it secretes. If thyroid hormone levels drop below normal, the hypothalamus increases secretion of TRH, which prompts the pituitary to pump out TSH to stimulate the thyroid.

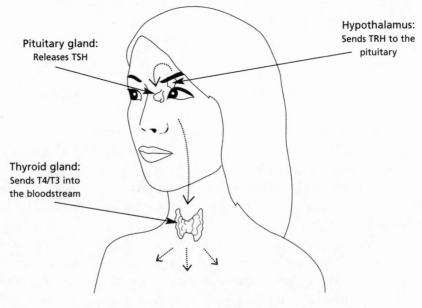

Pituitary gland:
Releases TSH

Hypothalamus:
Sends TRH to the
pituitary

Thyroid gland:
Sends T4/T3 into
the bloodstream

The Thyroid Feedback Loop

This feedback loop is like a thermostat, constantly keeping thyroid hormones at just the right level. When the immune system attacks the thyroid, it leads to overproduction or underproduction of thyroid hormones. Either the heat's too high, as excess thyroid hormone speeds up energy use and causes weight loss, hyperactivity, sweating, and nervousness; or the heat's too low, as too little thyroid hormone slows energy use, causing weight gain, fatigue, coldness, and depression.

Thyroid diseases are the most common of all autoimmune diseases, affecting more than ten million people. *Hashimoto's thyroiditis*, an underactive thyroid gland, affects ten times more women than men. *Graves' disease*, in which

---

Warning Signs of Thyroid Disease

Hashimoto's Thyroiditis (Underactive Thyroid)

- Fatigue
- Intolerance to cold
- Dry skin, dry hair
- Depression
- Unexplained weight gain
- Constipation
- Weakness
- Muscle cramps
- Impaired memory

Graves' Disease (Overactive Thyroid)

- Anxiety, nervousness
- Rapid heartbeat, palpitations
- Trembling hands
- Unexplained weight loss
- Feeling warm, heat intolerance
- Difficulty concentrating
- Muscle weakness
- Brittle or thin hair, hair loss
- Protruding eyes

---

the thyroid becomes overactive, is five times more common in women. Both can lead to infertility and miscarriage, emerge during or after pregnancy and present a threat to an unborn child, and, in older age, be mistaken for signs of aging. Untreated hyperthyroidism can also lead to bone loss since excess thyroid hormone activates bone-eating cells called *osteoclasts*.

What Causes Thyroid Disease?

In Hashimoto's thyroiditis, T-cells attack the follicular cells, causing inflammation that hampers production of thyroid hormones. Healthy thyroid cells are replaced by lymphocytes and macrophages and, eventually, by scar tissue so little or no hormones are secreted. Autoantibodies (sometimes called *thyroid autoantibodies*) are directed against the contents of the thyroid cells, either *thyroglobulin* (*TG*) or *thyroperoxidase* (*TPO*), two proteins needed for the production of thyroid hormones. "Whether these antibodies cause the disease, worsen it, or are simply results of thyroid disease has not been fully established," remarks Noel Rose, MD, PhD, director of the Autoimmune Disease Research Center at Johns Hopkins. "Many people have these antibodies with no evidence of clinical disease. So there must be additional factors triggering thyroiditis."

In Graves' disease, antibodies attack receptors for thyroid stimulating hormone on the surface of thyroid follicular cells, triggering overproduction of thyroid hormones. These autoantibodies, *thyrotropin receptor antibodies* (*TPO*) (also called *thyroid stimulating immunoglobulins* or *thyroid stimulating antibodies*), affect every cell in the thyroid, causing the gland to enlarge as it becomes hyperactive. So Graves' is also called *diffuse toxic goiter*. Antibodies to thyroglobulin and thyroperoxidase are also found in Graves' disease.

Both Graves' and Hashimoto's are closely related; women with thyroiditis may eventually develop Graves' and vice versa. "There's a phenomenon we call *Hashitoxicosis*, where patients with Hashimoto's disease become hyperthyroid because they have the thyroid stimulating antibody as well as the typical thyroid inflammation. And you also have a phenomenon where patients start out hyperthyroid and become hypothyroid," says Dr. Rose. "There may be separate autoimmune processes taking place in the thyroid, but one may be clinically dominant over the other, and this may shift over time."

Autoimmune thyroid diseases tend to run in families. It's not uncommon for one family member to have Hashimoto's and another to have Graves' disease. A woman with autoimmune thyroid disease in close relatives may have a five- to tenfold risk of developing thyroid disease. Thyroid diseases frequently occur with other autoimmune diseases (see page 99).

It's not known just what sets off the process that destroys or overstimulates the thyroid. One possibility is that excess iodine in the diet triggers the autoimmune response. Another theory proposed by researchers at Mount Sinai Medical Center is that fetal cells that enter a woman's circulation during pregnancy may play a role in thyroid disease (see page 98). Other factors, such as severe stress, could be involved.

In some cases, a woman may develop Graves' disease or Hashimoto's after giving birth (see page 101). It's thought that the immune system rebound after pregnancy causes production of autoantibodies (or increases levels of previously undetected antibodies), leading to dysfunction of the thyroid.

Symptoms of Hashimoto's Thyroiditis

When the thyroid produces too little thyroid hormone, it not only slows metabolism but also decreases production of body heat. The body tries to conserve heat by diverting blood flow from the skin, which keeps the skin cool and reduces sweating, preventing the loss of body heat. So women with an underactive thyroid often feel cold (even though their body temperature is normal) and look somewhat pale. Skin may become dry, nails and hair may become brittle, and there may even be hair loss on the scalp and elsewhere on the body (including the eyebrows, eyelashes, and pubic hair). Hair loss may be so gradual that you don't even notice it at first.

As the body slows down conversion of food to energy, you may gain weight and feel tired and drowsy. Some of the weight gain comes from fluid accumulation. Muscle contractions in the intestines, which move digested food along for absorption and waste excretion, also slow down, so you may experience hard stools and constipation. An underactive thyroid also leads to elevated cholesterol.

A key symptom of Hashimoto's is depression, and if you have a persistent low mood you should be tested for low thyroid hormones. Depression is also common in women with multiple sclerosis and lupus, as is difficulty concentrating. Clinical depression is a separate illness and does *not* accompany thyroid disease. However, women being treated with the mood stabilizer lithium for a form of depression called *bipolar disorder* (*manic depression*) may develop hypothyroidism.

Nerve problems can also occur in Hashimoto's. You may feel tingling or a pins-and-needles sensation in your hands and feet (which may also occur in MS). *Carpal tunnel syndrome* can also occur, because of tissue swelling and pressure on the median nerve, which passes through a tunnel-like space in the wrist. Carpal tunnel syndrome causes tingling in the hands and fingers, especially at night. The problem is often blamed on repetitive stress, especially if you work at a computer, but it may in fact be caused by an underactive thyroid. You may also have shortness of breath because of a lowered heart rate, muscle aches or cramps caused by decreased blood flow to the muscles, and slow reflexes. These symptoms may be attributed to a coexisting autoimmune disease.

As Hashimoto's becomes progressively worse, the thyroid can become enlarged, causing a feeling of pressure around the throat when swallowing, and the voice can become hoarse. Menstrual flow can increase and periods may become longer. There may be bleeding between periods and a failure to ovulate, leading to infertility. Women with undiagnosed hypothyroidism are also at risk for miscarriage, premature delivery, stillbirths, and certain birth defects (see pages 100 to 101).

All of these symptoms can come on very gradually. "The reserve of the thyroid is huge. So before you may actually present with symptoms of hypothyroidism, a large proportion of the gland would need to be destroyed," remarks Dr. Rose.

Anne Marie's story continues:
After I collapsed, they tested me for everything under the sun. And it was then that I noticed how much weight I was losing and how much I was eating. I was eating everything and dropping weight so quickly. A pound or so every few days. I weigh 120 now, but eight years ago I maybe weighed 99, 100 pounds. I would feel like I was jumping out of my skin. When I had a "thyroid storm" I felt a kind of madness, and my pulse was pounding. And I had this stare. My eyes were protruding and I was very self-conscious about

it. Now I realize I must have had thyroid symptoms for a long time; they must have started very gradually. After I was told my thyroid was overactive, it all made sense to me. But truthfully, I didn't pay much attention until I had a problem.

Symptoms of Graves' Disease

While Hashimoto's causes a slowing down of body functions, Graves' disease speeds things up. Metabolism increases, causing weight loss. Because the body needs more blood to compensate for increased energy use, the heart must pump faster. So you can have a rapid pulse, palpitations (heightened awareness of a pounding heartbeat in the neck or chest, or a brief episode of rapid heartbeat, even at rest, or a sensation of a skipped heartbeat), sometimes accompanied by shortness of breath. Excess thyroid hormone can lead to the development of an irregular heartbeat (*arrhythmia*), including *atrial fibrillation*, a rapid fluttering of the upper chambers of the heart. Atrial fibrillation, which occurs in 10 to 15 percent of women with an overactive thyroid, can increase the risk of stroke. Because the atria are not pumping properly, blood may stagnate, forming clots that can break off and block blood flow to the brain.

As the body produces more heat, sweating increases. If you have an overactive thyroid you may feel warm and flushed and feel uncomfortable in hot weather or warm environments. The gastrointestinal system speeds up passage of food through the intestines, so bowel movements become more frequent. As metabolism increases, you feel more energetic, even hyperactive, jumpy, or "wired." It can become hard to sit still and concentrate, and you jump from task to task (some women describe this as feeling like their "motor is always running"). You may even talk rapidly. The motor doesn't slow down properly at night, so it may be hard to fall asleep and stay asleep; your mind may still feel like it's racing. Since you don't sleep properly, you can become fatigued.

Muscle weakness is also common, especially in the muscles of the hips, thighs, and shoulders. It can be so bad you may have difficulty raising your arms to brush your hair, climbing stairs, or even getting out of a chair. Changes in the skin and nails also occur. Your nails may grow faster, causing them to get soft and tear easily. Skin feels thin and almost silky, and there may be areas of increased (or decreased) pigmentation. In rare cases, women may develop reddish, lumpy, and thickened skin in front of the shins (*pretibial myxedema*). Hair becomes softer and finer and may begin to fall out. Hair loss may be related to another autoimmune disease, *alopecia areata*, which causes roundish bald spots on the scalp (pages 133 to 139). But more often, it's thinning hair, which can be extensive. Treatment with thyroid hormone usually stops hair loss.

The emotional symptoms of Graves' include irritability and wide mood swings. Small annoyances may set off a major reaction. Or you may act manic, with bursts of energy and intense activity. Since this can also be a sign of bipolar disorder, if no other symptoms of hyperthyroidism are present, an evaluation by a mental health professional may be needed.

The thyroid gland often becomes enlarged in Graves' disease, but may not cause discomfort. In severe cases, where the thyroid grows three to four times its normal size, you may have a feeling of pressure in the neck when swallowing or turning your head.

Menstrual flow may become lighter if you have Graves' disease, and periods may become shorter; some women may stop having periods altogether (page 100).

The hallmark symptom of Graves' disease is eye inflammation and the development of protruding eyes (*Graves' orbitopathy*). This occurs in about 50 percent of women with Graves' as the eyes are pushed forward because of swelling and inflammation of muscles around the eye and tissues behind the eyeballs. It can cause major vision loss if it damages the optic nerve. Increased pressure behind the eye hampers normal blood and fluid drainage, causing swelling of the tissues around the eye and aching or pressure. The eyes may also be red and inflamed. Weakened eye muscles can hamper movement of the eyes, leading to double vision or impaired vision. Eyelids may not close completely at night over protruding eyeballs, causing the cornea to become dry and prone to ulcerations. The severity of these problems usually has nothing to do with the degree of hyperthyroidism and may even occur without significant elevation of thyroid hormones.

In some cases, symptoms gradually get better over six to twelve months, but there's no way to predict whether eye problems will improve. Inflammation is usually not permanent, and less than 1 percent of women have serious or permanent problems. Most often, problems are mild, requiring artificial tears to prevent dryness; more severe cases may necessitate steroid medications, radiation therapy, or surgery (see page 97).

Diagnosing Thyroid Disease

A diagnosis is made by assessing physical symptoms, examining the thyroid gland, and doing key blood tests. The thyroid becomes enlarged in both Hashimoto's thyroiditis and Graves' disease, but feels different in each. In Hashimoto's, the gland feels hard and rubbery (sometimes pebbly in texture); in Graves' it feels smooth and soft to firm in texture. During your physical examination, your doctor will palpate the thyroid, often while having you slowly swallow a cup of water, and listen with a stethoscope for a sound called a *bruit*, caused by increased blood flow in the thyroid (characteristic of Graves' disease). Signs like cold, dry skin or hand tremor and a fast pulse rate, along with clinical symptoms (such as depression or anxiety), will usually point to a specific diagnosis, but blood tests are needed to assess thyroid function.

Tests You May Need and What They Mean

A **complete blood count** (CBC) and metabolic profile are needed to rule out anemia, abnormal liver function, and excess calcium in the blood (*hypercalcemia*), and other possible causes of symptoms.

Thyroid stimulating hormone (TSH) levels are the best indicator of thyroid function. TSH is increased in women with hypothyroidism and is low or undetectable in women with hyperthyroidism, says Dr. Rose. The most sensitive test, capable of detecting very low levels of TSH, is called a *third generation assay*. The normal range for TSH is 0.4 to 5.5 micro international units per milliliter of blood (micro IU/ml), but ideally a young, healthy person should have a TSH below 3.0. A woman with hyperthyroidism usually has a TSH below 0.1 micro IU/ml; in hypothyroidism, TSH is elevated above 5 micro IU/ml.

Total and free thyroxine (T4) are measured separately. A test for total T4 measures all of the circulating thyroxine; a test for free T4 measures only the biologically active thyroxine (the amount that is not bound up by *serum-*

binding proteins and can attach to hormone receptors in cells). This test can be done either by direct analysis or by a dialysis technique. The normal reference range for free T4 in nonpregnant women is 0.8 to 2.7 nanograms per deciliter of blood (ng/dl). The normal range for total serum T4 is 4.5 to 12.5 micrograms per deciliter of blood (mcg/dl). A woman with Graves' disease would have a total T4 above 12 mcg/dl; a hypothyroid woman would have a T4 below 5 mcg/dl.

Total triiodothyronine (T3) measures the amount of circulating T3, which can be influenced by factors that change levels of *thyroxine binding globulin* (including estrogen). Normal levels of T3 range from 0.4 to 4.2 micro IU/ml. This blood test may only be done if additional information is needed about thyroid function.

Thyroid antibody blood tests look for autoantibodies to components of the thyroid cells (*thyroid antibodies*), such as antibodies to *thyroglobulin* (*TG*) and *thyroperoxidase* (*TPO*). "As many as 80 percent of women with Hashimoto's thyroiditis also have elevated antibodies to TG," says Dr. Rose. "As many as 80 percent of women with Hashimoto's thyroiditis also have elevated antithyroid antibodies." High levels of thyroid stimulating autoantibodies, thyrotropin receptor antibodies (TPO), can confirm the diagnosis of Graves' disease.

Radioactive iodine uptake may normally be ordered if a woman has thyroid nodules or a goiter (and may be done in conjunction with a thyroid scan). The iodine that we take in from food is absorbed by the thyroid gland and is a key building block of thyroid hormones. The test involves giving a small amount of oral radioactive iodine and measuring the amount absorbed by the thyroid gland; the normal range of absorption is 8 to 30 percent after twenty-four hours. Radioactive iodine will be elevated above 30 percent in women with Graves' disease. It will also be elevated in postpartum thyroiditis, and in women taking replacement thyroid hormone.

A **thyroid scan** uses a special detector that's able to see how much radioactive iodine has been taken up by the thyroid and how evenly it's dispersed in thyroid cells. If the radioactive iodine is taken up by the entire thyroid, it rules out the possibility that overactive nodules are causing hyperthyroidism. A benign nodule producing too much thyroid hormone will be "hot" on the scan, in contrast to a "cold," hypofunctioning nodule, which can be benign or malignant.

Ultrasound examination of the thyroid may be done if your doctor feels nodules when examining your thyroid. Ultrasound uses sound waves to create pictures of thyroid nodules felt on examination, to determine whether they are solid or fluid-filled (it can also show nodules that can't be felt).

Needle aspiration biopsy may be performed if a nodule looks suspicious. In this procedure, a small needle is inserted into the nodule to withdraw a small amount of fluid or cells for analysis. This test is 90 percent accurate in detecting cancer.

Anne Marie's story continues:

After I was diagnosed with Graves' disease, they gave me drugs to slow down my thyroid. I would go through periods of feeling very tired and periods of feeling very awake, hyperawake. Then they ablated my thyroid with radioactive iodine. You go into a hospital, down to nuclear medicine, and they give you this tablet. It looks like an ordinary pill, but it's radioactive. And it made me feel very strange. It makes you feel like you're sweating out of your pores, you feel lethargic, kind of out of it. At least that's how I felt. I had some thyroid tissue left over after the ablation, and it was very hard to regulate my thyroid. I needed blood tests every few weeks. But I take my thyroid pill religiously every day. Sometimes my numbers are out of whack and they have to give me less, and sometimes they have to up the dose. It's been a long process.

Treating Autoimmune Thyroid Disease

Treating an underactive thyroid is very straightforward: giving replacement thyroid hormones. Graves' disease is easily treated, but several steps may be needed.

Treating Hashimoto's Thyroiditis

Hypothyroidism is treated with synthetic *levothyroxine sodium* (synthetic T4) to normalize levels of thyroid hormone. It may take some time to find the right dose. If the dose isn't high enough, symptoms of hypothyroidism may persist; if the dose is too high, you may have symptoms of an overactive thyroid. So doses are gradually increased until blood levels of TSH are in the normal range (when this happens, you're said to be *euthyroid*). Hashimoto's goiters may shrink by almost a third over a two-year period with T4 supplementation. Annual physical exams and blood tests are needed to make sure thyroid hormone levels stay in the normal range.

Around 10 percent of women may have a spontaneous remission four to eight years after starting treatment. But in some cases thyroid failure is progressive, and levothyroxine doses may need to be increased as the thyroid continues to slow down.

Levothyroxine is sold by prescription under a number of brand names, including *Synthroid, Levothroid, Levoxyl,* and *Unithroid.* It can interact with several other drugs, including male hormones (androgens); antacids containing *aluminum hydroxide* (such as *Rolaids*); antidepressants like *fluoxetine (Prozac), amitriptyline (Elavil),* and *phenelzine sulfate (Nardil)*; blood thinners such as *warfarin (Coumadin)*; insulin; digitalis-type drugs such as *digoxin (Lanoxin)*; iron supplements; and *cholestyramine (Colestid, Questran)*. Postmenopausal women taking hormone replacement therapy (HRT) may need higher doses of thyroid hormone (see page 103).

You will need periodic bone scans after menopause to check for bone loss, and because mild thyroid hormone excess over many years may increase the risk for heart rhythm problems, you may also need periodic electrocardiograms.

Treating Graves' Disease

In Graves' disease, the overactive thyroid gland must be calmed down or destroyed and then replacement thyroid hormone is given.

Antithyroid drugs, including *propylthiouracil (PTU)* and *methimazole (Tapazole)*, make it harder for the thyroid to use iodine to make thyroid hormone, which lowers secretion of thyroxine. PTU and methimazole are typically used in mild Graves' disease (or when Graves' occurs in children or young adults) and are often prescribed for elderly women who also have heart disease. Women over age sixty-five who have chest pain or irregular heart rhythms may suffer heart damage if they become more hyperthyroid. Treatment with radioiodine (page 95) may temporarily boost levels of thyroid hormone; giving antithyroid drugs prevents this increase. Between 20 and 30 percent of women with early, mild Graves' disease will experience a prolonged remission after twelve to eighteen months of treatment with antithyroid drugs. As many as 40 percent of patients may achieve a permanent remission.

However, PTU and similar drugs sometimes provoke allergic reactions. About 5 percent of women may develop skin rashes, hives, or, less commonly, fever and joint pain. In some cases, these drugs may cause a decrease in certain white blood cells (*neutrophils*), which may increase the risk of infections. In rare instances, white cells may actually disappear entirely, causing *agranulocytosis*, which can be fatal if you get a serious infection. If you're taking an antithyroid drug and develop an infection (such as strep throat) call your doctor immediately and ask if you need to get a white blood cell count. If white blood cells have been decreased, stopping the drug can return the neutrophil count to normal. During therapy you should also avoid immunizations, as methimazole can lower the body's resistance and may lead to the very infections vaccines are designed to prevent.

If you go into remission, antithyroid drugs will be continued for another year or two. Signs of a remission include a decrease in the size of the thyroid and a near-normal or higher TSH. But neither is a reliable predictor, and more than half of patients will develop a recurrence within five years. You'll need to be monitored by your doctor every three months for the first year of treatment and annually after that.

Radioiodine/radioactive iodine (or iodide) accumulates in the thyroid and damages thyroid cells, reducing the amount of hormone-producing tissue. Radioactive iodine emits two types of radiation: gamma rays, which travel through tissue and can be seen with a special detector (as in thyroid scans); and beta rays, which travel only a few millimeters and are absorbed by thyroid cells. The beta rays don't kill the thyroid cells but cause enough inflammation and DNA damage to prevent them from producing too much thyroxine and from reproducing. The dose is determined by how much radioactive iodine is absorbed by the thyroid during an uptake test.

Radioactive iodine is given in capsule form (taken with lots of water). Within twenty-four to forty-eight hours, most of the radioactive iodine will be taken up by the thyroid, and the remainder is excreted in urine (or decays into a nonradioactive state). The level of radioactivity of the iodide left in the thyroid declines by 50 percent every five to seven days. It's not going to be harmful to family members, but it might be wise to limit contact with infants and pregnant women for the first week after taking the radioisotopes, just to be safe.

Because of increased inflammation (and possibly increased autoantibodies) in the thyroid caused by radioactive iodine, secretion of thyroxine will be greater for a few weeks, and may heighten symptoms, especially in older women and those with heart disease (for that reason, antithyroid drugs are given beforehand—see page 104). You'll likely begin to improve in three to six months, but there's a chance you may remain hyperthyroid and need a second or third dose. A majority of women become hypothyroid after treatment, and need replacement thyroid hormone.

The word *radioactive* may sound scary, but no serious complications from treatment have been seen in fifty years of using the drug. In fact, more than 70 percent of American adults with hyperthyroidism are treated with radioactive iodine, with no increased risk of cancer.

If you plan to become pregnant, you must wait three to six months after treatment before trying to conceive. This is to ensure your baby will not be exposed to radioactive iodine, which can cause developmental problems and destroy the baby's thyroid.

Thyroidectomy, surgical removal of the thyroid, may be advised if you're allergic to antithyroid drugs, don't wish to take radioactive iodine, have a large goiter, or are pregnant. First, hyperthyroid symptoms need to be brought under control with an antithyroid drug or a beta-blocker (which controls the effects of too much thyroid hormone), so that there is not an abrupt increase in hormones. The drugs are usually given a week or two prior to surgery. Surgery cures hyperthyroidism, but you still can become hypothyroid afterward and will need yearly blood tests to measure thyroid function and levothyroxine.

Beta-blockers may be needed if you're undergoing any of these treatments to reduce symptoms until the therapy takes full effect. These drugs—including *propranolol* (*Inderal*), *atenolol* (*Tenormin*), or *metoprolol* (*Lopressor*)—block the effects of circulating thyroid hormone in the body, helping to slow heart rate and lessen anxiety and nervousness. Patients who can't take beta-blockers include women with asthma and heart failure (which may be worsened by beta-blockers) and people with diabetes who take insulin (because symptoms of low blood sugar may not appear while on these drugs).

Treating Graves' Orbitopathy

Most of the time, Graves' orbitopathy is a mild problem that does not damage the cornea or impair vision. However, if your lids do not completely close, your eyes can dry out at night. Special adhesive tapes normally used for first aid can be used to tape the lids closed while you sleep, or you can wear an eye patch. Artificial tears can also be used during the day for added lubrication (see page 91), side panels for glasses lessen air flow around the eyes to prevent dry eye, and tinted glasses can ease light sensitivity.

Surgery to remove swollen tissue and decrease the opening of the eyes can lessen the appearance of a prominent stare. You'll need to consult an ophthalmologist to determine the type of surgery and its timing.

Corticosteroids are used to reduce inflammation and lessen swelling of tissue around the eye in cases of severe congestive orbitopathy. Oral steroids such as *prednisone* (*Deltasone*) and *methylprednisolone* (*Medrol*) can be used for short periods, or in low doses for longer periods, to relieve redness, swelling, and eye pain. Side effects include weight gain, muscle weakness, and, with long-term treatment, an increased risk of osteoporosis, bone fractures, diabetes, high blood pressure, and infection (discussed on page 34).

Radiation therapy, which directs low doses of radiation to the area around the eyeball, has been widely used for decades. A 2001 study by the Mayo Clinic concluded that radiation therapy is not effective for mild or moderately severe orbitopathy. According to the study, corticosteroids and corrective surgery should be used instead. The researchers did not look at women with severe orbitopathy causing damage to the optic nerve.

Corrective eye surgery removes or repairs swollen muscles around the eye that can cause pressure on the optic nerve and double vision. The surgery should be performed by an ophthalmic surgeon only after orbitopathy has been stable for three to six months.

Orbital decompression surgery, which enlarges the bony opening around the eyes to provide more space for the eye and eye muscles, is done only when other treatments fail.

The Female Factor

While the ratio of males to females is about equal in juvenile thyroiditis, after puberty it's more common in females, suggesting that female hormones play a role in thyroid disease.

Estrogen and progesterone both exacerbate thyroid inflammation, and thyroiditis can be reversed with testosterone, as shown in experiments with mice bred to have an animal model called *experimental autoimmune thyroiditis* (*EAT*). "When the testes were removed in the mice and we gave them estrogen, they became more susceptible to thyroiditis. When we removed the ovaries of the female mice and gave them testosterone, they became less susceptible to thyroiditis," says Dr. Rose.

During pregnancy autoimmune thyroiditis gets better, but in the year after giving birth it worsens. Some studies show that in women with mild thyroid inflammation, the increased immune response after pregnancy tips the balance and causes thyroid dysfunction (*postpartum thyroiditis*). And up to 25 percent of women may develop a permanent autoimmune hypothyroidism within ten years after delivery. There's also an increased risk of developing Graves' disease in the postpartum period. However, estrogen is not the whole story. There are other hormonal influences, such as stress hormones, that may come into play.

Fetal cells that enter the maternal circulation during pregnancy may contribute to autoimmune thyroid disease, says Terry F. Davies, MD, chief of the division of endocrinology, diabetes, and bone diseases at the Mount Sinai School of Medicine in New York City. In one study of mice, Dr. Davies's research team found fetal cells in the thyroid glands of mice with EAT during pregnancy and the postpartum period but none in mice without EAT. Dr. Davies and other researchers have also isolated cells containing the male chromosome in thyroid tissue from women undergoing thyroid surgery who had previously given birth to boys.

"The theory is that during pregnancy the fetal cells actually suppress thyroid disease, in the same way that the immune system is suppressed and doesn't attack the fetus. And that may be why the thyroid disease improves during pregnancy," explains Dr. Davies. "Once the placenta and the baby are gone, then the number of fetal cells starts to fall rapidly and their ability to suppress the thyroid disease decreases, and you get a recurrence."

The fetal cells may be attracted to the thyroid by inflammation. "The inflammation would be organ specific. If you start off with thyroid inflammation, thyroiditis, fetal cells may accumulate in the thyroid. If you start out with beta cell destruction in diabetes, then fetal cells may be attracted to the pancreas," he adds.

However, the exact relationship between fetal cells and autoimmune thyroid disease is still unknown, as is the relationship between environmental factors such as stress or infections and female hormones.

It wasn't until years after I was diagnosed with Hashimoto's that I found out I had a strong family history of thyroid disease. My father had a goiter, one of his first cousins had Graves' disease, and another has Hashimoto's. Their children also had thyroid disease; one of them also has lupus. But until I asked questions, no one had ever mentioned it. It wasn't regarded as important, not like if someone had cancer. I got my period late, around age fourteen, and maybe that was the beginning of it. Back then, and we're talking thirty years ago, no one even thought to look.

LYNNE, FIFTY-FOUR

Thyroid Disease Clusters

Hypothyroidism is very common in other autoimmune diseases; up to 30 percent of women with type 1 diabetes may develop thyroid disease after many years. Among the diseases that cluster with thyroid problems are the following:

- Rheumatoid arthritis
- Myasthenia gravis
- Lupus
- Type 1 (insulin-dependent) diabetes
- Vitiligo
- Alopecia areata
- Pernicious anemia (an inability to absorb B_{12} in the stomach)
- Addison's disease (adrenal insufficiency)
- Premature ovarian failure
- Celiac disease
- Primary biliary cirrhosis

How Thyroid Disease Can Affect You Over Your Lifetime

Thyroid disease can impact a woman's health throughout the various stages of her life.

Menstruation and Fertility

Women with Hashimoto's thyroiditis often have heavier periods that last for longer than a week. They may also have bleeding between periods, because of a failure to ovulate (*anovulation*). Normally, the ovaries are stimulated to produce an egg in the first part of the menstrual cycle, the *follicular phase*. After ovulation, in the *luteal phase*, the uterine lining builds up an extra layer of blood vessels in preparation for a fertilized egg. If pregnancy doesn't occur, the lining is shed as menstrual flow. In Hashimoto's, the normal hormonal feedback between the ovaries, the pituitary, and the hypothalamus is disrupted. So a woman may fail to ovulate, but the uterine lining will continue to be stimulated, so bleeding can occur outside the normal cycle. Anovulation is common in hypothyroidism. Hashimoto's is also associated with premature ovarian failure (see page 191). In women with Graves' disease, an increase in metabolism causes a decrease in menstrual flow and a shorter cycle. A woman whose period normally lasted four or five days may see it decrease to two or three days. In severe hyperthyroidism, some women stop having periods altogether.

Taking oral contraceptives containing estrogen can also increase the amount of serum thyroxine binding globulin, which makes T4 less available to cells. Women with normal thyroid function will secrete more thyroxine to compensate, but women with Hashimoto's can't produce the extra T4, remarks Dr. Rose. This also occurs during pregnancy, mainly because of increased estrogen levels, and in women taking estrogen replacement therapy (ERT) after menopause (see page 103).

Pregnancy

Until the fetal thyroid gland is developed, at approximately twelve weeks' gestation, the mother's thyroid is the only source of thyroid hormone for the baby (transferred through the placenta and amniotic fluid). If you were diagnosed with thyroid disease before you conceived you'll need to be monitored closely during pregnancy. If you're hypothyroid you'll probably need to have your thyroid hormone dose increased by an average of 45 percent to normalize TSH. "I recommend that pregnant women with thyroiditis have their TSH checked once every six weeks," says Mount Sinai's Dr. Terry F. Davies.

Untreated thyroid disease during pregnancy may negatively affect a child's psychological development. In Graves' disease, thyroid stimulating hormone receptor antibodies can cross the placenta and cause neonatal hyperthyroidism. Women with untreated thyroid deficiency during pregnancy may be up to four times more likely to have children with lower IQ scores, as well as deficits in motor skills, attention, language, and reading abilities, according to a 1999 study from Harvard. In the study, 19 percent of the children born to mothers with undetected hypothyroidism scored 85 or lower on the IQ testing, compared to only 5 percent of children born to women without thyroid disease. (Scores below 85 typically signal that a child will have difficulty in school.)

Infants can develop a temporary form of neonatal thyroid disease, which is related to the transfer across the placenta of antibodies from the mother. Research from Japan has found that a subset of women with autoimmune thyroiditis make what are called *TSH inhibiting antibodies*, and these antibodies can cross the placenta, resulting in transient hypothyroidism in the baby. In Graves' disease, stimulating antibodies also cross the placenta, temporarily causing an overactive thyroid in the baby. However, all infants are routinely screened for thyroid problems.

There are no increased instances of birth defects in children born to mothers who took radioactive iodine and waited the recommended six months before becoming pregnant. Women who have trouble conceiving because of hyperthyroidism often have fertility restored after treatment.

Postpartum Thyroid Disease

Some women have antithyroid antibodies in their blood for years, but never develop a problem until after giving birth. Immune function is modulated during pregnancy, and the normal rebound after delivery may elevate levels of antithyroid antibodies during the third to eighth months postpartum.

In some women, this may not produce noticeable symptoms. Others may blame their symptoms on normal fatigue, the "baby blues," or postpartum depression. "I think thyroiditis is much more common than is reported, because a lot of postpartum depression may actually be postpartum thyroiditis," remarks Dr. Noel Rose. And postpartum depression can be worsened by thyroiditis.

If the thyroid gland is severely inflamed, it may become overactive, causing a sudden onset of hyperthyroid symptoms. Once the thyroid hormone stored in the gland is depleted, hypothyroidism sets in. In some women, the thyroid may eventually normalize. Symptoms typically last six months or less.

As many as 8 to 10 percent of women may develop thyroid problems after giving birth. Radioactive iodine uptake will be low in women with postpartum thyroid inflammation; in women with Graves' disease there will be an increased uptake of radioactive iodine due to overproduction of thyroid hormone. Before the test, breastfeeding should be discontinued for three to five days, as radioactive iodine can pass into breast milk. Having a prior episode of postpartum thyroiditis increases the risk of recurrence with each pregnancy. Women with recurrent postpartum thyroiditis have a 20 to 30 percent chance of developing permanent hypothyroidism five to ten years afterward. Antithyroid antibodies may help identify those women at increased risk.

The hyperthyroid phase of postpartum thyroiditis doesn't usually require treatment. But hypothyroidism will require replacement thyroid hormone for six to twelve months. If you have a goiter, it will usually shrink in response to treatment. Only tiny amounts of thyroid hormone pass into breast milk, so you can continue breastfeeding.

Hypothyroidism may become permanent after pregnancy in as many as 30 percent of women who have a preexisting problem, says Dr. Rose. So treatment is usually stopped for four to six weeks to do blood tests for T4 and TSH, to see whether the hypothyroidism has resolved. Women may need annual thyroid testing to see whether a thyroid problem recurs.

Menopause

As many as 14 percent of women will develop chemical or subclinical hypothyroidism in the years just before and after menopause, most of it due to Hashimoto's. During perimenopause, production of estrogen and progesterone becomes erratic and may disrupt pituitary-thyroid function and even interfere with the action of thyroid hormones. Autoantibody production might also increase. "It's really not clear what is going on. The age, sex, and postpartum distribution suggest that there's some connection between the immune system and the endocrine system," remarks Dr. Rose.

Hypothyroid symptoms, especially depression, may be mistakenly attributed to perimenopause or menopause, he adds. Therefore many experts say routine screening for underactive thyroid may be needed at menopause and afterward.

A recent study found that menopausal women taking hormone replacement might need an increased dose of levothyroxine. The study, which appeared in the *New England Journal of Medicine* in June 2001, looked at the effects of estrogen on pituitary-thyroid function in eleven postmenopausal women with normal thyroids and twenty-five women being treated for chronic hypothyroidism. In the normal women, ERT produced an increase in thyroxine binding globulin, prompting an increase in thyroxine production. But in those with hypothyroidism, there was a significant drop in the amount of free thyroxine, requiring an increased dose of medication. An accompanying editorial suggested that in women taking thyroid hormones, thyroid function should be checked after starting ERT and the dose of levothyroxine adjusted accordingly. Conversely, if a woman discontinues ERT, her dose of thyroid medication may need to be reduced.

Thyroid Disease in Later Life

Some studies estimate that as many as 15 to 20 percent of women over the age of sixty have elevated TSH (often with antithyroid antibodies), even if they don't have symptoms of hypothyroidism. One study suggested that 20 percent of these women will develop Hashimoto's. The risk is greatest if TSH is high and antithyroid antibodies are present. Symptoms may be difficult to recognize in older women. Depression, dry skin, hearing loss, muscle cramps, numbness and weakness of the hands, unsteadiness of gait, anemia, and constipation may simply be blamed on aging. Hyperthyroidism can also be easily overlooked. Few of the classic symptoms, such as an enlarged thyroid, may be present in older women. Additional symptoms may include shortness of breath, palpitations, depression, nervousness, and muscle weakness.

Treatment has to be adjusted in later life, as well. Levothyroxine is metabolized and excreted more slowly in older women, so smaller doses are needed. Antithyroid drugs are often used before radioactive iodine treatment in older women, especially if they have other medical problems, such as chest pain (angina) or an irregular heart rhythm. Radioactive iodine can trigger a temporary rise in thyroid hormone that can cause complications or heart damage. Beta-blockers may also be needed to dampen the effects of excess thyroid hormone before treatment with radioactive iodine.

All patients over age sixty-five need long-term followup with annual blood tests for TSH and T4 because thyroid function may continue to decline over the years.

5

The Body Snatchers—Scleroderma and Autoimmune Skin Disorders

I developed an overwhelming fatigue, and when I got up in the morning my fingers would swell and feel tight when I tried to bend them. Within a few weeks, my feet were so swollen I couldn't put my shoes on, one leg was bigger than the other, and I developed such shortness of breath I couldn't stand. I saw two rheumatologists when I first started having the fatigue and joint stiffness, but the tests were all negative and both doctors said maybe I wasn't handling stress very well. One doctor even said I might be imagining some of my symptoms and suggested that I talk to a therapist. At the time, I was twenty-seven and I was in a difficult master's degree program, putting in sixty- to eighty-hour weeks. So at first I thought maybe they were right—maybe it was stress. But when my symptoms got much worse, I knew something was wrong. My skin started to harden all over my body. When I would reach up into the cupboard, the inside of my arm was like webbing. When I tried to smile, the skin on my face would pull. I felt like I had been put into this nightmare body with no way out.

KAREN, FORTY

Some autoimmune disorders profoundly affect the skin, connective tissue, and hair, causing pain, damage, and disability. These "body snatchers" include *scleroderma*, which causes skin to harden and scar, and *alopecia areata*, which can lead to total hair loss. All told, they affect hundreds of thousands of women, altering their appearances and their lives.

105

Warning Signs of Scleroderma

- Patches of thick, hard skin
- Extreme sensitivity of the fingers to cold, with pain and color changes (white, blue, then red)
- Small ulcerations on the fingertips
- Swollen hands or feet
- Joint pain
- Fatigue
- Trouble swallowing
- Chronic heartburn
- Shortness of breath

What Causes Scleroderma?

Scleroderma gets its name from two Greek words—*sklero*, meaning "hard," and *derma*, meaning "skin." However, it can affect not only the skin, but also other sites in the body, including the lungs, esophagus, and kidneys.

In scleroderma, the immune system attacks and damages cells that produce *collagen*, the substance that makes skin elastic and supports other connective tissues (joints, ligaments, and the capsules that surround internal organs). Collagen is a protein normally made in small amounts by specialized cells, called *fibroblasts*, and deposited on the outside of cells to support and heal tissues. It's constantly being made and broken down. If you cut your finger, a clot forms and collagen is laid down along the injured area to fill in the gap and form a scar; scar formation is an essential part of the healing process. Eventually the collagen is broken down, and the scar may become smaller and skin becomes more normal in appearance. But in scleroderma, fibroblasts start overproducing collagen where there's no injury to be healed, laying down too much of it and replacing normal tissue. Scleroderma can be *localized*, affecting only the collagen-producing cells in the skin, or it can be *systemic*, affecting collagen-making cells and small blood vessels in other areas of the body, interfering with normal function of organs and tissues.

For example, the esophagus and intestines are less able to contract to move food along because lack of blood flow or collagen accumulation have affected nerves that control motility; lung cells can't swap carbon dioxide for oxygen because scar tissue has formed over the thin membrane where this exchange takes place. Systemic scleroderma can be widespread (*diffuse*) or *limited*, affecting just a few areas.

According to the Scleroderma Foundation, up to five thousand Americans a year are diagnosed with systemic scleroderma (including limited and diffuse disease), 80 percent of whom are women, and six thousand more with localized scleroderma affecting only the skin.

The vascular component of scleroderma causes tiny blood vessels in the fingers and other areas of the body to become narrowed. In the kidneys, this can lead to high blood pressure. In the hands, diminished blood supply makes the fingers extremely sensitive to cold, causing *Raynaud's phenomenon*, exaggerated, painful spasms of the blood vessels when exposed to cold (see pages 116 to 117). Raynaud's occurs in 95 percent of people with scleroderma and also appears alongside RA and lupus, and can occur in otherwise healthy women.

It's not known just what triggers the immune reaction that causes collagen production to run amok, says Maureen D. Mayes, MD, MPH, who heads the National Scleroderma Family Registry at the University of Texas Health Science Center in Houston. "In scleroderma, small blood vessels suddenly become 'leaky,' releasing white blood cells and inflammatory substances that activate fibroblasts, which start making too much collagen. What causes the blood vessel damage in the first place is still unknown."

Also unknown: just why some women develop localized scleroderma and why others suffer systemic disease, sometimes without any visible signs on the skin.

The presence of specific antibodies may provide clues as to which women develop certain complications. "There are probably a host of genetic factors, and potentially toxins or environmental factors that trigger a reaction in people who are genetically susceptible and prompt the appearance of certain antibodies, which are probably present long before there are any symptoms," remarks Virginia D. Steen, MD, professor of medicine at Georgetown University in Washington, D.C., who has studied the disease for twenty years. "For example, we see certain antibodies in Caucasian women who develop pulmonary hypertension, and another antibody in African-American women who develop pulmonary hypertension."

There are ethnic differences. African-American women are more likely to develop the disease than Caucasian women, and they develop it at an earlier age, says Dr. Steen. "The average age at diagnosis is forty, but in African-American women it tends to be earlier. Black women tend to have more diffuse disease and also have more skin pigment changes than Caucasians."

A 2002 study from Johns Hopkins and the University of Maryland also found that black women have a 60 percent greater risk of dying of scleroderma than white women of the same age with the disease.

There is a strong genetic vulnerability; a recent study led by Dr. Mayes found that scleroderma is twice as common in people with a family history of the disorder. However, the study found that the absolute risk for each family member is actually less than 1 percent.

Symptoms of Systemic Scleroderma

Some women experience joint pain and puffy hands as the first symptoms of scleroderma, but most often they develop extreme sensitivity to cold and Raynaud's phenomenon (see page 107).

Normally when we're exposed to the cold, the body tries to slow the loss of heat and preserve normal core temperature by sending less blood to arteries near the surface of the skin and moving more blood deep within the body. To divert blood flow, the tiny blood vessels near the skin's surface (*arterioles*) contract. Everyone has these spasms in blood vessels, causing the hands to feel cold and painful and appear blotchy red. But in Raynaud's the reaction is intensified, and the color changes are more profound—and distinctive. "A woman may notice her fingertips tingle and turn pale within a few minutes of cold exposure as blood vessels tighten and keep blood from entering her fingers. The fingers then turn a bluish color from the deoxygenated blood. Then, as the fingers warm up and blood vessels relax, they turn very red as blood rushes in. This can be extremely painful with exposure to even slight cold, including an air-conditioned room or the freezer section of grocery stores. Women often put up with it for long periods of time," remarks Dr. Mayes. "But some women may develop little pinpoint-type sores, also called *digital pits*, on their fingertips, because of decreased blood supply. They can be quite painful and take weeks to heal. In some cases, the skin on the fingers has already started to become thickened. It's usually at this point that a woman will see a doctor."

It's important to note that up to 5 percent of healthy women have Raynaud's without any other disease (*primary* Raynaud's). The disorder is classified as *secondary* Raynaud's when it occurs in people with autoimmune disease. Between 85 and 95 percent of women with scleroderma and mixed connective tissue disease, and a third of women with lupus, have Raynaud's.

In women with scleroderma, the inside of the blood vessel wall becomes fibrotic because of excess collagen deposits, and the thickening of skin in the surrounding area causes an increased demand for oxygen in the tissues. When cells lining the blood vessels are damaged, they produce a substance called *endothelin*, which acts as a potent vasoconstrictor, causing an increased tendency to spasm. Ulcers can occur as a complication of restricted blood flow. In severe or prolonged cases, the tips of the fingers may become shorter and the bone may even become damaged from lack of blood supply.

Raynaud's may appear along with puffy hands, but it's the skin thickening that's the primary symptom of scleroderma. Puffiness and skin thickening in the fingers is called *sclerodactyly* and usually starts from the middle joints out to the fingertips. The thickened skin isn't red or bumpy—it's smooth and shiny. The swelling and skin thickening can make the fingers feel stiff, because the joints don't bend normally. Fingers may enlarge so much that rings can't be removed. The skin covering the finger joints can become so tight and inelastic that the fingers do not extend and are forced to bend inward (*joint contracture*). In severe cases, they may eventually become "frozen" in this position.

Other skin problems include itching caused by inflammation; pigment changes (darker or lighter patches of skin); ulcerations due to poor circulation, injury, or tearing of tight skin at joints and pressure points; and red spots caused by widening of small blood vessels in the skin (*telangiectasias*), usually on the face and hands. There may be hair loss in areas of thickened skin, due to both excess collagen around hair follicles and reduced blood supply (hair loss on the scalp can occur, but it's more common in lupus). Later in the illness, tiny calcium deposits can form (*calcinosis*), which feel like firm bumps under the skin; these can become very painful and inflamed, and become infected.

In the esophagus, the movements that normally push food into the stomach (*peristalsis*) are decreased because of scarring of nerve tissue and lack of blood flow, so you may have an uncomfortable sensation of food sticking in the throat or chest. The valve that's supposed to keep acid in the stomach becomes weakened, allowing acid to back up or "reflux," leading to chronic heartburn and *gastroesophageal reflux disease* (*GERD*). Heartburn doesn't just happen after meals but can occur several times a day (especially when lying down at night).

This constellation of symptoms in limited systemic scleroderma has been referred to as CREST—an acronym for Calcinosis, Raynaud's, Esophageal problems, Sclerodactyly, and Telangiectasias. However catchy the acronym, it's an imprecise term. Not every woman will have all of the external symptoms with internal involvement limited to the esophagus. Some may have limited cutaneous scleroderma with damage in the intestines and lungs.

Excess collagen deposits can also limit contractions of the bowel needed to move food and waste along. As a result, bacteria begin to overgrow in the small intestine, which interferes with the absorption of nutrients and fat, which can cause diarrhea and weight loss. When the large intestine is affected, it can cause constipation.

Most of the time, the earliest signs of systemic scleroderma may be dismissed as a minor complaint. "Many women say they had symptoms for two or three or even four years and sought help from a physician, and were just dismissed," comments Dr. Mayes.

It's a different story with *diffuse scleroderma*. Symptoms may come on suddenly and often do not include Raynaud's. A woman may have swollen hands and feet; swollen and/or painful joints, extreme fatigue, a sudden, severe rise in blood pressure (due to blood vessel spasm in the kidney) which causes severe headaches, shortness of breath, a stroke, or even kidney failure. A woman may then have progression of thickened skin beyond the hand that spreads up over the arms, legs, and trunk over a short period.

Other organ involvement includes the small intestines and the lungs. In the lungs, excess collagen interferes with the normal exchange of carbon dioxide for oxygen across the thin membrane that separates the tiny capillaries and the air sacs (*alveoli*). It's not clear what triggers the process, but activated immune cells and damaged blood vessels play a role. There's also inflammation in the air sacs, called *alveolitis*, which leads to scarring (or *pulmonary fibrosis*) and breathing problems. Pulmonary fibrosis might also be linked to reflux; there's some speculation that microscopic particles of stomach acid could be inhaled when a patient lies down during sleep. The primary symptoms of lung involvement are a chronic cough and shortness of breath.

In rare cases, women may have a condition called *scleroderma sine sclerosis*, or scleroderma without skin thickening. "She will have Raynaud's phenomenon, but there's often a long period of time between the onset of Raynaud's and other problems, leading to a delay in diagnosis, because the most visible sign, thickening of the skin, is not present," says Dr. Mayes.

Occasionally, diffuse scleroderma can have a very rapid course, progressing quickly to affect the kidneys, lungs, heart, and other organs, and can even be fatal. Fortunately, this is uncommon; most women with scleroderma have a relatively normal lifespan.

In *localized* scleroderma, patches of thickened, pigmented skin are called *morphea*. Localized skin thickening can also appear as a band or line down the face or an arm or leg (*linear scleroderma*), which may extend deep into the skin and muscle. Around 20 percent of women with localized scleroderma may develop joint pain (sometimes before skin changes appear, causing confusion with rheumatoid arthritis). Localized scleroderma may be self-limiting, with symptoms subsiding after a few years.

Karen's story continues:
The third rheumatologist I saw took one look at my hands and said I had scleroderma. He said that some people don't test positive for the antibodies for scleroderma, and to this day I don't test positive. There were times this disease really consumed me. I would lie on the couch for fourteen to sixteen hours a day. I had no energy at all; it was an effort to get up and walk to the bathroom. And I had been a pretty high-energy person, so this was very disturbing. I would sleep ten or eleven hours a night and still wake up exhausted. Having a doctor to help me through it made all the difference. You need hope and good medical care.

Diagnosing Scleroderma

A diagnosis of scleroderma can often be made by a physical exam alone, but bloodwork and other diagnostic tests may be needed to assess the extent of the disease.

"Most of the symptoms, like swollen fingers or heartburn, are pretty common, and many women and their doctors may dismiss them. The skin thickening may also be very subtle in the beginning and is not easily detected," says Dr. Mayes. "The difficulty we have is in determining when this constellation of symptoms points to scleroderma."

While Raynaud's phenomenon is often the first sign of scleroderma, it can also occur on its own, and it's very common. "In the beginning, it's hard to distinguish between scleroderma and Raynaud's," says Dr. Mayes. "One of the major indications of secondary Raynaud's is the sores on the tips of the fingers. This does not occur in primary Raynaud's disease."

If a woman has Raynaud's along with the characteristic skin thickening and digital pits, a physical exam alone may lead to a diagnosis. But other tests may be needed to confirm a diagnosis of scleroderma.

Tests You May Need and What They Mean

Antinuclear antibody (**ANA**) tests will be positive in 85 percent of scleroderma patients (and in 99 percent of women with lupus). A woman with Raynaud's and a positive ANA but no other symptoms needs to be followed closely for six-month intervals over a period of two to five years. "If they are symptom free for five years, it's virtually certain that they never will develop scleroderma or lupus," remarks Dr. Mayes.

Other antibodies, such as *anticentromere antibodies* (associated with CREST and limited scleroderma) and *anti-Scl 70 antibodies* (*anti-topoisomerase antibodies*, associated with systemic sclerosis), can be helpful in making the diagnosis, but are not 100 percent specific.

A **complete blood count** (**CBC**) will be needed to see whether there is a low red cell count due to anemia (caused by internal bleeding) or a low white cell count. Serum creatinine will be tested to help assess kidney function.

X-rays are performed if a woman is experiencing chronic heartburn, to assess problems or damage to the gastrointestinal tract. There are several types of tests: A **barium swallow** involves drinking a small amount of liquid containing *barium* (which shows up white on the x-ray) to see whether there is scarring or an ulcer in the esophagus. An x-ray movie called a **cine esophagram** may be done to see if there's decreased motion in the esophagus, an ulcer in the lower end of the esophagus, or a stricture. In an **upper GI series**, ingested barium is followed as it moves through the stomach to the small intestine. A **small intestine transit study** measures the amount of time this takes and can indicate impaired bowel function.

If you have chronic heartburn, **endoscopy** may also be done to check for inflammation or ulcers. This test uses a small tube (*endoscope*) with a fiber-optic device passed through the mouth down into the esophagus and stomach, allowing the doctor to examine the lining.

Pulmonary function tests are usually done to assess potential damage to the lungs if a woman has shortness of breath or a dry cough but should also be done at the time of diagnosis of scleroderma. *Spirometry* involves breathing into a machine that measures lung volume and lung flow to establish a baseline. "This way if a woman does develop shortness of breath or a dry cough, we can look back on that test and determine whether there's been a change from that," says Dr. Mayes. Pulmonary function tests also include a *diffusion capacity test* to measure how efficiently carbon dioxide is being exchanged for oxygen across the pulmonary membrane. CAT scans can reveal scar tissue and inflammation in the lungs before it's apparent on chest x-rays.

Based on the results of these tests and a clinical examination of the skin, a diagnosis of limited or diffuse scleroderma can usually be made. A diagnosis of *undifferentiated connective tissue disease* (*UCTD*) or an *undifferentiated autoimmune syndrome* (*UAS*) is given when a woman does not fully meet the criteria for scleroderma (or lupus). Up to 20 percent of women with symptoms of scleroderma or lupus may fit this category.

Sclerodermalike Disorders

There are a number of disorders that can resemble scleroderma but are actually quite distinct.

Sclerodema causes thickened skin on the upper body (the face, neck, head, and shoulders), sometimes spreading down to the arms or trunk. The disorder can occur in people with long-term diabetes. Women usually will not have Raynaud's, ANAs, or organ involvement.

Eosinophilic fascitis (*EF*) occurs when white blood cells, *eosinophils* and *leukocytes*, attack tissues called *fascia*, which separate muscle from fat. This thin sheet of tissue becomes inflamed, swollen, and tender. The skin overlying the area becomes dimpled (like the skin of an orange) and the underlying tissue will feel hard. EF affects the arms, trunk, and legs but not usually the hands or face (there's little fascia in those areas). The onset of EF is rapid, with skin changes that may be followed in a few weeks by decreased range of motion in the central body, shoulders, and hips and contractures of the elbows and knees. Raynaud's is usually not present, and ANAs will be negative, but there will be marked increases in eosinophils in the blood and fascial tissue (seen on biopsy).

Chronic graft-versus-host disease (*GVHD*) can cause patches of thickened skin on the arms, trunk, and legs that look like localized scleroderma. GVHD can occur in bone marrow transplant patients but is not reported after organ transplantation. In marrow transplants, high-dose chemotherapy is first given to "kill" the host immune system by destroying the bone marrow, then a patient is given an infusion of marrow from a matched donor to reconstitute the immune system. However, even with the best matches, the donor marrow cells can react against the recipient and set off a barrage of toxic cytokines; this acute GVHD is treated with immunosuppressants. The reaction can be chronic in some marrow transplant patients. Immunosuppressants can control chronic GVHD, but may not cure it.

The Female Factor

Eighty percent of those diagnosed with localized and systemic scleroderma are women. But if female hormones play a role, it's only slight, says Dr. Mayes. "Scleroderma is different from lupus or rheumatoid arthritis. Pregnancy usually makes symptoms of RA better, but in some cases lupus can worsen. In systemic sclerosis, pregnancy is considered a high-risk period because the disease itself, and not hormones, can cause problems for some women."

One of the intriguing theories of why women are more prone to scleroderma (and other autoimmune diseases) has to do with the presence of fetal cells from a past pregnancy that remain in a woman's bloodstream for many years (see page 11). It may be that the combination of self and nonself antigens (some from the father, some from the mother) in fetal cells may contribute to a form of graft-versus-host disease.

Studies have found that women with scleroderma have twenty times the number of persistent fetal cells than other women who'd had children but

---

Scleroderma Clusters

One of the diseases that may occur with scleroderma is *mixed connective tissue disease (MCTD)*, a combination of scleroderma, lupus, and polymyositis. MCTD can begin as scleroderma, or start out as polymyositis or lupus. Other diseases that cluster with scleroderma include:

- Sjögren's syndrome
- Polymyositis
- Rheumatoid arthritis
- Lupus

---

didn't have scleroderma. A recent study of tissue specimens found evidence of male cells (of presumed fetal origin, which can be flagged with a special chemical to highlight the Y chromosome) in the spleen, lymph nodes, adrenal glands, and skin tissue of women with systemic sclerosis who had borne sons. The study, reported in 2001 in the journal *Arthritis & Rheumatism*, examined tissues taken at autopsy from women with scleroderma and compared them to women who had died of non-autoimmune related cases, using a special process to "light up" male cells under a high-powered microscope. All of the women had given birth to sons. While male cells were found in at least one organ of women with scleroderma, the researchers did not find any male cells in the women who died of non-autoimmune causes.

"However, there are many scleroderma patients who have never been pregnant (or are male) that are not explained by this theory. Microchimerism may just be an incidental finding, since it is seen in other diseases and not all scleroderma patients. It may be a risk factor, like genes," remarks Dr. Steen. "We have no strong candidate for what causes scleroderma, whether it's a virus or environmental toxin. In fact, scleroderma could be several diseases which occur differently in women, in younger people, or in midlife."

Karen's story continues:
At first I was put on penicillamine, but I started to develop kidney problems and still had the fatigue. So I was put on low-dose steroids. That

calmed the disease down initially. But then my skin turned hard all over my body. It turned hard on my chest, and I couldn't wear a bra. It turned hard on my stomach, my legs, my arms, and my face. When I tried to smile or raise my eyebrows my skin would pull and stretch—it was just terrible. You feel like you've been put into this nightmare and you have to find the inner resources to pull yourself out of it, to try to cope with it. I had almost alligator skin. My doctor finally put me on this drug that's used for transplant patients, cyclosporine. It helped dramatically. Within about three months, my skin was softening all over. I was on the drug for four or five years, when the disease was very active. I got really well on cyclosporine; I went back to work three days a week. The scarring in my esophagus didn't go away, and the stomach acid backed up, so I took acid-blocking drugs. I also had some kidney damage and developed high blood pressure. I took medication for that and I'm still on steroids. The skin on my hands is still very tight, and they are very curved. But I feel much better and I have a pretty active life again and have plenty of energy for my children.

Treating Scleroderma

While there's no cure for scleroderma, many of the problems created by the disease can be treated individually.

Raynaud's

Most importantly, if you smoke, quit immediately; nicotine is a potent *vasoconstrictor* and can make your Raynaud's worse.

The medications used most often to ease symptoms of Raynaud's are *vasodilators*, usually calcium channel blockers, which improve blood flow to the small blood vessels in the fingers (see page 116). These include *nifedipine* (*Procardia*), *diltiazem* (*Cardizem, Dilacor, Tiazac*), *felodipine* (*Plendil*), *nicardipine* (*Cardene*), and *amlodipine* (*Norvasc*).

"Frequently, scleroderma occurs in young women who are quite thin, and they will have blood pressures of 90/60 and you cannot lower their blood pressure any further. They are going to get dizzy and lightheaded," says Dr.

Mayes. "With most women you start at a low dose, and if they become light-headed or dizzy or develop headaches, you have to stop the drugs."

In such cases, the drug *pentoxifylline* (*Trental*), which helps blood flow more easily through narrow blood vessels, may be helpful. Or one might try drugs that prevent platelets from forming clots, such as *dipyridamole* (*Persantine*) or *clopidogrel bisulfate* (*Plavix*). These drugs do not lower blood pressure, but can cause an increased risk of bleeding and cannot be used in pregnancy. Doctors generally advise against using pentoxifylline while breastfeeding. Nitroglycerin patches can be used to improve circulation and heal finger ulcers.

A newer high blood pressure drug, *losartan* (*Cozaar*) may be useful in treating Raynaud's. One recent study among fifty-two patients with scleroderma and in women with primary Raynaud's found that losartan improved the frequency and severity of Raynaud's attacks after twelve weeks of treatment.

An alternative approach to treating Raynaud's is biofeedback, in which it's possible to learn to increase blood flow to the fingers (see page TK). Most important, if you smoke, quit immediately; nicotine is a potent vasoconstrictor and can make your Raynaud's worse.

Gastroesophageal Reflux Disease (GERD)

In GERD, the esophagus is being affected by a weakening of the valve that keeps acid in the stomach, allowing the acid to "reflux" into the esophagus. Drugs called *proton pump inhibitors* such as *omeprazole* (*Prilosec*), *pantoprazole* (*Protonix*), or *lansoprazole* (*Prevacid*) decrease acid production. A newer version called *esomeprazole* (*Nexium*) can heal irritation and erosions caused by acid. Other drugs like *cimetidine* (*Zantac, Tagamet*) or *nizatidine* (*Axid*) block formation of stomach acid. Prokinetic agents like *metoclopramide* (*Reglan*) may improve decreased motility of the esophagus or small intestine.

The diarrhea caused by bacterial overgrowth in the small intestine can sometimes be cleared up with a short course of antibiotics.

Also helpful: eating slowly, chewing food thoroughly, drinking plenty of water (alternating sips of water with bites of food can ease passage of food), not eating within two hours of going to bed, and sleeping with the head of your bed elevated.

Lung Problems

For women with alveolitis, low doses of the chemotherapy drug *cyclophos-phamide* (*Cytoxan*) may be given along with prednisone or other immuno-suppressants like methotrexate or azathioprine. Cytoxan alone is also being tested. Some cases of pulmonary fibrosis may be caused by breathing micro-scopic particles of stomach acid during sleep, and treating GERD may improve symptoms. *D-penicillamine* is used to treat progressive pulmonary fibrosis, along with home oxygen therapy in some cases.

Blood Pressure and Kidney Problems

Women with early diffuse scleroderma need to monitor their blood pressure to be aware of any increase, which is the first sign of serious kidney problems. If blood pressure begins to rise, a physician must be consulted immediately so *angiotensin-converting enzyme* (*ACE*) *inhibitors*, a lifesaving treatment, can be given. A partial list includes *benazepril* (*Lotensin*), *captopril* (*Capoten*), *enalapril* (*Vasotec*), and *ramipril* (*Altace*).

High blood pressure in the lungs (*pulmonary hypertension*) occurs in about 15 percent of scleroderma patients, as small blood vessels in the lungs become thickened and resistant to blood flow. Pulmonary hypertension is treated with oxygen and blood thinners. In severe cases, *epoprostenol* (*Flolan, prostacyclin*) may be given in continuous infusions, using a small portable pump. This drug is a form of *prostaglandin*, a substance that occurs naturally in the body and is involved in many biological functions. Epoprostenol relaxes blood vessels and increases the blood supply to the lungs. Studies are under way with oral and inhaled prostaglandin preparations to make therapy easier and less expensive.

A new agent, *bosentan* (*Tracleer*), is used for treating pulmonary hyperten-sion. Clinical trials showed improved breathing, exercise potential, and qual-ity of life. The drug also has effects on the endothelial cells lining blood vessels, blocking a receptor for a protein that acts as a vasoconstrictor (endothelin).

Skin Thickening

Skin thickening sometimes improves on its own, but so far no drugs have been shown to soften skin. Skin thickening has been traditionally treated with

D-penicillamine, but results have been disappointing. (However, the drug may have other benefits for women with scleroderma.) Moisturizers and lubricants must be used regularly to prevent fissures and infections. If ulcers become infected, topical or systemic antibiotics are used.

What's Next?

Iloprost (a synthetic version of prostacyclin) is a potential antifibrotic drug. It is given by intravenous infusion and has vasodilating and anticlotting effects but also may help heal endothelial cells and may prevent fibrotic changes in skin, says Dr. Mayes. The medication is currently used in Britain as a routine therapy for finger ulcers.

High-dose chemotherapy with stem cell rescue involves harvesting stem cells (the cells that grow into different kinds of cells, including white blood cells), purifying them and freezing them, and then destroying a patient's abnormal immune system with high doses of chemotherapy. After the chemotherapy, the stem cells are infused back into the patient to reconstitute the immune system with lymphocytes that will not be autoreactive.

Stem cell transplantation has a high mortality rate (20 percent) and is reserved for those people who have such severe disease that they're at high risk of dying within the next five years or those women with early and rapidly progressive diffuse skin disease, who within the first year or so of diagnosis have some lung disease and heart disease, says Dr. Mayes. "In surviving patients we do see an improvement in skin, at least a stabilization in lung disease, and possibly a stabilization in GI disease. But it's very hard to predict who will do well."

Clinical trials are ongoing at several centers, including Northwestern University, Wayne State University, and the Fred Hutchinson Cancer Center in Seattle.

Thalidomide, which affects rapidly growing cells, was used in the 1960s as a morning sickness remedy for pregnant women until it was linked to severe birth defects and taken off the market. In recent years, it returned to use as *Celgene*, a treatment for leprosy and some forms of cancer, and has shown promise against chronic graft-versus-host disease.

A study at Rockefeller University in New York City found that thalidomide helped heal finger and extremity ulcers among a small group of patients with scleroderma. A longer-term trial of thalidomide in a larger group of patients is now under way.

Anti-thymocyte globulin (*ATG*) and *mycophenolate mofetil* (*CellCept*), two immunosuppressive agents that target the T-cells that set off the process that activates collagen-producing cells, are being tested as a potential treatment. The drugs were tested in a pilot study among thirteen patients in Britain and appeared to be safe and have some benefits.

Tracking Your Symptoms

Unlike lupus, where there are scales to track disease activity by frequency of certain symptoms, in scleroderma no standard means exist for assessing increased disease activity and severity to determine when more aggressive treatment is needed. In February 2002, scleroderma specialists from around the world met in Italy to explore the issue. While the criteria for such a scleroderma activity index are still being developed, Dr. Mayes suggests that several red flags should prompt medical attention:

• **Increasing shortness of breath, muscle weakness, and leg swelling.** "Fatigue tends to be chronic; it will wax and wane. But if a woman can distinguish progressive muscle weakness from fatigue, I think that's a key symptom. Leg swelling can be a symptom of kidney or heart problems."

• **Increased blood pressure.** "During the first five years after a diagnosis, women should keep a careful watch on their blood pressure with weekly blood pressure readings using a home monitor. Their physician can give them instructions on what to do if blood pressure goes over a certain level," says Dr. Mayes.

• **Fingers that turn blue or pale in the cold and do *not* return to normal color.** "If a woman has a blue or pale finger that does not go back to pink when warmed, that stays cool and discolored for twenty-four hours, that's something that should prompt physician attention," warns Dr. Mayes. "In this case, we need to try to open up the blood vessels with medication. If caught early, and treated early, we may be able to avoid the development of finger ulcers or irreversible tissue loss."

• **Weight loss and diarrhea that lasts more than two to three days.** This can be a sign of bacterial overgrowth in the gut, which is treatable with a short course of antibiotics. Some women may need to be on intermittent antibiotics. Weight loss can also be caused by an esophageal stricture that interferes with swallowing. A stricture can be dilated using an endoscopic procedure.

Karen's story continues:

It affected me in so many ways. Your sexual life is affected, you have to make adjustments there. I had always wanted to have kids, but the doctors had advised us not to get pregnant because they really didn't know what the disease was going to do, and I didn't want to take any chances. So we decided to adopt a child. Then I got pregnant. But three months into the pregnancy I went into a hypertensive crisis and was in the intensive care unit for ten days. I almost lost my life and I lost the baby. But the adoption went through when all this was happening. And this child was really a lifeline. Even when I had to have dialysis, I had to shift my focus to taking care of this baby. Eventually I got off dialysis, my energy came back, and we decided to adopt a second child, and my two girls are my joy. Still, it's hard sometimes. When I look in the mirror, my face looks so different. This disease changes your whole self-concept. But I have learned to live with this disease; it's part of my life. I focus on the positive aspects of my life, what's important. My husband is an exceptional man, but there were times I thought he should bail out. But he said, "I don't take a vow lightly, and this is not something I'm going to run from." He has been my strength. I couldn't have made it without him.

How Scleroderma Can Affect You Over Your Lifetime

Scleroderma can affect not only a woman's appearance, but treatments can also affect menstruation and fertility and influence the decision whether to become pregnant.

Menstrual and Reproductive Effects

Scleroderma does not appear to flare premenstrually. However, women with scleroderma may have menstrual and ovulation irregularities, and some of the medications used to treat scleroderma, such as prednisone, may also lead to irregular cycles and decreased fertility.

"If a woman has a lot of GI involvement and has lost a fair amount of weight, that will affect ovulation and menstrual cycles. A certain amount of body fat is needed to convert the hormones for starting menstruation. You see amenorrhea in women with anorexia because of low estrogen. In scleroderma, if you've had a fair amount of weight loss and you've lost a great deal of body fat, you may have the same situation," remarks Dr. Mayes.

Birth control pills do not seem to affect scleroderma. Treatment with cyclophosphamide can cause sterility (it may be temporary in younger women) and trigger an early menopause.

Pregnancy

Like Karen, almost half of women with scleroderma have their first symptoms before age forty, and childbearing is an important issue.

Early studies reported a high incidence of miscarriages, premature births, and smaller-than-average babies among women with scleroderma. But a recent study led by Dr. Steen found that women with scleroderma are no more likely than healthy women to suffer these complications of pregnancy. The 1999 study, done at the University of Pittsburgh, surveyed 214 women with scleroderma, 167 women with rheumatoid arthritis, and 105 healthy women, and found that 12 to 13 percent of women in *all three groups* had pregnancies that ended in miscarriage. The incidence of premature births was 8 to 10 percent in all three groups (but in scleroderma patients, prematurity increased after the onset of the disease). Another prospective study following 59 women with scleroderma given high-risk prenatal care found no differences in miscarriage, fetal losses, or pregnancy-related problems and no increase in small, full-term births, compared to 48 healthy women used as a control group. "We did see a much higher percentage of preterm births, especially in women with early diffuse disease," remarks Dr. Steen. "Patients who had diffuse disease for a long time had a significantly greater risk of miscarriage than the other groups." The majority of patients had no change in their symptoms during pregnancy, but 34 percent experienced a worsening of Raynaud's, arthritis, and skin thickening.

"We encourage women to have an early consultation with their rheumatologist to assess the type and activity of their disease. We discourage women with early diffuse disease from becoming pregnant during that period, because of the risk of kidney problems," says Dr. Steen.

Dr. Mayes advises women newly diagnosed with scleroderma to wait two to three years to see how their illness develops; limited scleroderma may be less risky for a pregnancy than diffuse disease (although there's some increase in prematurity). The disease must be stable (with no signs of hypertension or lung problems) because most medications must be stopped before a woman tries to conceive.

While many women with scleroderma have uneventful pregnancies, they should be under the care of an obstetrician who specializes in high-risk pregnancies because of the risk of premature births. Blood pressure must be carefully monitored. High blood pressure, preeclampsia (severe high blood pressure with protein leakage from the kidneys, *proteinuria*), and even more serious kidney damage have been reported more often in women with scleroderma. Preeclampsia may arise in scleroderma because of thickening and narrowing of blood vessels in the placenta, which hampers delivery of oxygen and nutrients to the fetus and the removal of wastes. If untreated, it can progress to eclampsia, which can cause seizures and death. ACE inhibitors are not given during pregnancy, unless other medications fail to control high blood pressure. If a woman develops preeclampsia and her blood pressure doesn't respond to medication, cesarean delivery is required.

The most common symptoms of pregnancy—morning sickness in the early months, and heartburn as the pregnancy progresses—are more pronounced in women with scleroderma.

Menopause

The atrophy of vaginal tissues that occurs as estrogen levels drop in menopause can also occur independently in women with scleroderma and Sjögren's syndrome (see page 155).

"Perhaps 10 percent of women with scleroderma have true autoimmune Sjögren's syndrome. Probably 30 to 40 percent of women with scleroderma have overlapping symptoms with Sjögren's, but when their parotid glands are examined, they are fibrotic," says Dr. Steen. Antibody tests can be used to determine which women have Sjögren's.

In both cases, vaginal tissues may feel dry; there may be itching, burning, and irritation, as well as painful sex. If the problem is due to menopause, oral estrogen replacement or estrogen cream can help relieve vaginal dryness. (If you have an intact uterus you need to take progestin to protect against endometrial hyperplasia.)

Menopause itself doesn't seem to affect the course of scleroderma, but there's been little formal research into the use of hormone replacement in women with scleroderma. "I have no problem prescribing hormones for women who are experiencing hot flashes, because my data does not suggest there's a problem with taking hormones," says Dr. Steen.

Estrogen does carry the risk of blood clots, may not be advisable for women with vascular or clotting problems, and is not recommended for the secondary prevention of heart disease. So a woman needs to discuss the pros and cons with her physician. One study suggests a slightly increased risk of Raynaud's among women taking estrogen.

"One major question about menopause is whether taking calcium supplements increases the frequency of calcinosis. I don't think it has anything to do with it, but it's one of those issues that has not been resolved," remarks Dr. Steen. "In general, we have not seen an increased risk of osteoporosis in scleroderma patients as there is with rheumatoid arthritis."

Sexuality

In any chronic illness, there's a higher risk of depression. This can affect sexuality, as can a negative body image from the changes caused by scleroderma. The fatigue of scleroderma can interfere with having an active sex life, and vaginal dryness can cause some women to avoid sex altogether.

However, a recent study of 150 women at the University of Medicine and Dentistry of New Jersey Scleroderma Program found that the vast majority remained sexually active despite their disease. And the main causes of that inactivity could be helped, the researchers say. Less than 10 percent of the women said that scleroderma was the primary reason for their sexual inactivity.

The most common symptoms reported by the group that influenced sexual function were fatigue (60 percent), vaginal dryness (42 percent), body pain (40 percent), depression, and vaginal discomfort (38.3 percent). Among those women who reported decreased sexual function, the problems of vaginal dryness, vaginal discomfort, Raynaud's phenomenon, and depression were more common; more than 28 percent of the women reported depression.

The researchers found that decreased blood flow interfered with sexual sensation and vaginal lubrication, and are testing a long-acting Viagra-type drug to address the problem. "Viagra was originally developed as an antihypertensive, so it may have dual effects in scleroderma," remarks Dr. Mayes. "The problem with Viagra is that it's not long-acting and it causes nasal stuffiness and other side effects. But by using drugs in this category, we may be able to piggyback scleroderma treatment to deal with sexual dysfunction related to circulation problems as well as finger ulcers." If you're suffering depression along with sexual problems, a combination of counseling and medication can help.

Hand Function

The hands can be severely affected early in scleroderma. Skin thickening and contracture can cause loss of flexibility in the fingers, loss of wrist motion, and a decline in fine motor skills, such as writing. Women, particularly those with diffuse scleroderma, need to do range-of-motion exercises to help slow or avoid loss of motion. Such exercises include stretching the tiny joints of the fingers by using the palm of one hand to press down the back of the finger joints of the other hand, flexing and extending the wrist, and doing rotations, two to three times a day. Women are often sent to an occupational therapist to help with exercising.

"There are also some individuals who will have a true arthritis with joint inflammation that contributes to the hand and wrist decreased range of motion in scleroderma," says Dr. Mayes. "It's sometimes difficult to figure whether the pain and swelling in the hand are due to the general puffiness that goes along with scleroderma, or to true arthritis joint inflammation that's making the joint swollen."

The arthritis that can occur in scleroderma is treated with the same anti-inflammatories and arthritis drugs used to treat RA, like methotrexate. There may be a potential for gastric bleeding with some pain medications, so the COX-2 inhibitors (like Vioxx or Celebrex) are used.

Psoriasis

Psoriasis is a chronic, inflammatory skin disease diagnosed in 150,000 to 260,000 people each year. It affects about 2.6 percent of Caucasians (about seven million Americans) and is slightly more common in women than men (around a two-to-one ratio).

Psoriasis is frequently diagnosed in a woman's late twenties to mid-thirties, but it can develop at any time, from childhood to old age. In some cases, skin injury, infections, stress, and certain drugs may trigger psoriasis. Heredity may also play a role. One out of three women with psoriasis has a family history of the disease, says noted psoriasis researcher Mark Lebwohl, MD, professor and chairman of the department of dermatology at the Mount Sinai School of Medicine in New York City. "If one parent has it, the likelihood a woman may also develop psoriasis is around 10 percent. If both parents have it, there's a 30 to 50 percent risk," he says. "Different genes may cause psoriasis. What we call psoriasis is probably a group of very closely related disorders. But the genetic abnormalities lead to the same pathway. That's why there are different patterns, and why some treatments work for some people and not others."

No one knows exactly what causes psoriasis; specific autoantibodies have yet to be identified. "What we can say is that psoriasis is a disorder of the immune system in which T-lymphocytes are activated in response to some yet to be identified antigen, and then cytokines cause skin cells to multiply too quickly," explains Dr. Lebwohl. A normal skin cell matures around every twenty-eight days and is then shed from the skin's surface. "In psoriasis, skin cells can turn over every two to four days. There is inflammation in the skin as well."

Warning Signs of Psoriasis

- Red, scaly patches of skin topped by silvery scales that appear on the elbows, knees, scalp, and elsewhere; patches may be small, then increase in size and number
- Itching and scaling of the scalp
- Sudden eruptions of inflamed skin, with tiny pustules or weeping lesions
- Dramatic, extensive sloughing and inflammation of the skin

Psoriasis clusters with arthritis and with Crohn's disease. As many as 20 percent of women with psoriasis will develop *psoriatic arthritis*. Like RA, psoriatic arthritis causes inflammation and stiffness in the soft tissue around joints, often involving the fingers and toes, as well as the wrists, neck, lower back, knees, and ankles. In severe cases, psoriatic arthritis can cause joint destruction and disability.

Types of Psoriasis

There are several forms of psoriasis. The most common, *plaque psoriasis*, is characterized by red, inflamed patches of skin topped by a layer of silvery white scales. Other forms of psoriasis include the following:

- *Guttate*, characterized by small dotlike lesions
- *Pustular*, characterized by pustules over inflamed skin
- *Inverse*, characterized by intense inflammation and little scaling in body folds
- *Erythrodermic*, characterized by intense sloughing and inflammation of the skin

Plaques can be limited to a few patches on the elbows or knees, or may involve more extensive areas of the skin, including the scalp, nails, palms, soles, torso, genital area, and, in rare cases, the face. Plaques may be symmetrical, in the same place on the right and left sides of the body.

For most people, the disease tends to be mild, but in some cases it can be disabling and even deadly. "In the more severe forms of psoriasis, the erythrodermic and the pustular forms, some patients will literally develop plaques overnight. Generalized erythrodermic and pustular psoriasis can be life threatening because they can affect 90 to 100 percent of the body surface, and people lose the protective functions of the skin," says Dr. Lebwohl.

The skin is actually an organ that serves as the body's first defense against infection and helps regulate body temperature. But when large areas of skin are affected in severe psoriasis, these functions are lost. "People lose protein and nutrients through the skin. They lose fluid, so their blood pressure can fall. They lose heat, so they can have low body temperature or develop fevers. In rare cases, a bacterial infection can cause death," says Dr. Lebwohl. According to the National Psoriasis Foundation (NPF), as many as four hundred people die of complications related to psoriasis each year.

Because each form of psoriasis has a characteristic appearance, a physical examination by a dermatologist is all that's needed to make a diagnosis. However, the first signs of psoriasis may not cause concern, allowing plaques to become more extensive. "Some people with mild psoriasis will treat scaly patches with moisturizers and never mention it to their physician," remarks Dr. Lebwohl. "There's no marker of who's likely to get psoriasis. Women with Crohn's disease may be unaware of the increased risk, and psoriasis plaques may not be noticed by a gastroenterologist."

Treating Psoriasis

While you may have a spontaneous remission, in many cases psoriasis requires continuous treatment. There are many options that can control or even eradicate plaques. However, some cause birth defects and cannot be used if you're planning a pregnancy (see page 132 to 133).

Topical Treatments

For people with mild psoriasis, creams, ointments, and solutions such as *calcipotriene* (*Dovonex*) and *tazarotene* (*Tazorac*) can be used alone or, in more severe cases, combined with topical corticosteroids such as *halobetasol* (*Ultravate*), *diflorasone diacetate* (*Psorcon*), *fluticasone propionate* (*Cutivate*), and *mometasone* (*Elocon*) or systemic therapies like methotrexate.

Topical steroids cause atrophy and thinning of the skin and are typically used only for limited periods. But if medium- or high-potency steroids are combined or alternated with Dovonex, for example, their use can be extended. Both Tazorac and Dovonex can be irritating, especially on the face and places where skin rubs against skin, like the groin or the armpit. Combining Dovonex and Ultravate can extend a period of remission or improvement up to six months. A common regimen is to use Dovonex and Ultravate twice a day for two weeks, then apply Ultravate only on weekends (but not on the face or areas like the groin).

Dovonex can also be alternated with other "superpotent" topical steroids, such as *clobetasol* (*Temovate*) or Psorcon, which otherwise must be used for limited periods because of their thinning effects on skin. For example, for scalp psoriasis, a two-week cycle of Temovate scalp application solution twice a day is followed by a cycle of Dovonex solution twice a day on weekdays and Temovate twice a day on weekends. Dovonex also increases the effectiveness of systemic therapies, allowing lower doses to be used and reducing the number of treatments with PUVA (ultraviolet light combined with the light-sensitizing drug psoralen—see below).

Tazorac, a derivative of vitamin A, works best for women with thick, stable plaques, rather than inflamed patches or thin skin. It must be used sparingly, however, because it can cause irritation and redness on unaffected skin surrounding treated plaques. Using Tazorac at night and a topical steroid in the morning can minimize this problem. As with other vitamin A derivatives, it cannot be used during pregnancy.

Light Therapy

Women with psoriasis may undergo therapy that exposes affected areas to ultraviolet light B (UVB), with or without medications that sensitize the skin to UV.

Ultraviolet light has several wavelengths. Most of the solar radiation that penetrates the earth's atmosphere is ultraviolet A (UVA), which penetrates more deeply into the skin and causes wrinkling and other signs of sun damage. UVB is a shorter wavelength and is the chief culprit in sunburn. Both UVA and UVB have been implicated in skin cancer.

For some people, moderate exposure to natural sunlight can help psoriasis. More intense but controlled exposure to UVB produces more of the reaction in the skin that helps clear plaques. In PUVA, the light-sensitizing drug *psoralen* produces a greater reaction by the skin when a person is exposed to ultraviolet A. PUVA does carry an increased risk of skin cancer.

"Phototherapy UVB is *not* the same spectrum of light as sunlight. And it's given in graded fashion, starting with low doses and increasing gradually to try to avoid burns, and we often cover the face," explains Dr. Lebwohl. "Study after study shows there's no increase in skin cancers in people treated with

UVB for psoriasis. But PUVA is clearly carcinogenic. About one out of six PUVA-treated patients will develop a skin cancer during her lifetime—typically squamous cell carcinoma, which usually is easily cured. The more PUVA you get, the more likely you are to get skin cancers."

Systemic Therapies

Women with psoriasis may be put on oral medications, such as the immuno-suppressant *cyclosporine* (*Neoral, Sandimmune*), *methotrexate* (*Rheumatrex, Folex*), and derivatives of vitamin A called *retinoids*, including *acitretin* (*Soriatane*). However, all of these vitamin A therapies cause birth defects.

Soriatane promotes the normal growth of skin cells and speeds up shedding. It keeps working in the body after it is discontinued, so pregnancy must be avoided for two to three years after stopping the drug (see page 132). You can't donate blood for transfusion for two to three years during treatment and for up to three years afterwards, and women of childbearing potential shouldn't drink alcohol while on the drug and for two months after discontinuing it. Alcohol can convert the short-acting acitretin to a longer-acting form that can stay in the body sixty times longer, increasing the chances of side effects. It should also not be taken with vitamin A, either in multivitamins or separate supplements, because the accumulation of vitamin A in the body can cause problems with vision, skin, and bone loss. It also can't be combined with other retinoids, such as oral *isotretinoin* (*Accutane*) or topical *tretinoin* (*Retin-A*).

"Pustular psoriasis responds well to Accutane, which stays in the body for a much shorter period than acitretin; thirty-one days after you stop using it, it's out of your system. Accutane also works well with ultraviolet light. So as long as we know a woman is not planning on becoming pregnant (and for thirty-one days afterward) she can go on Accutane," says Dr. Lebwohl. "Methotrexate and cyclosporine are very effective for psoriasis. But they do have serious drawbacks. Cyclosporine can damage the kidney; methotrexate can damage the liver. They cannot be combined with acitretin, since it may increase the chance of liver problems with methotrexate and increase the effects of cyclosporine."

A recent multinational clinical trial among people with moderate to severe psoriasis plaques found that short (up to twelve-week) intermittent courses of cyclosporine improved both psoriasis plaques and the safety profile of the drug.

Alefacept (*Amevive*) is a newly approved "biological" therapy that causes a decline in the "memory" T-cells, which trigger psoriasis plaques by setting off inflammation and abnormally rapid growth of skin cells. A single course of treatment involves weekly intravenous or intramuscular injections for twelve weeks.

Clinical trials involving more than one thousand patients, led by Dr. Lebwohl, found that 28 percent of those who received one course of Amevive achieved a 75 percent or greater improvement of their psoriasis, and more than half had a 50 percent improvement. After a second twelve-week course of treatment, 40 percent of patients achieved a 75 percent or greater improvement of their disease, and 71 percent reached 50 percent improvement. Remissions lasted as long as eighteen months.

New Biological Treatments

A second drug expected to be approved shortly affects another process that causes psoriasis. *Efalizumab* (*Xanelim*) is a monoclonal antibody designed to block critical immune system processes that drive the accelerated skin-cell growth of psoriasis. It is given by self-administered injections every week for twelve weeks. In one clinical trial involving almost five hundred patients, 39 percent showed an improvement of 75 percent or greater after one course of treatment and after a second twelve-week course of treatment, an additional 21 percent had the same degree of improvement. The most common side effect was a flulike syndrome (headache, chills, and other symptoms) after the first dose.

Etanercept (*Enbrel*), used to treat rheumatoid arthritis, was approved early in 2002 for psoriatic arthritis. "Enbrel is almost a miracle for psoriatic arthritis and for psoriasis. In some patients psoriasis clears completely. On average, there's a 50 percent improvement with only a three-month course of treatment. I think as treatments go more long term, Enbrel will show better responses and bigger proportions of patients responding," comments Dr. Lebwohl.

A second arthritis drug, *infliximab* (*Remicade*), appears to be very effective for treating psoriatic arthritis and is being evaluated for treating psoriasis.

In RA and in psoriatic arthritis, the inflammatory molecule *tumor necrosis factor* (*TNF*) is produced in elevated levels, leading to bone and tissue damage in the joints. Enbrel and Remicade block TNF by binding to it, preventing it from triggering inflammation.

"Remicade works dramatically. But patients can develop reactions to it, and we need to work out a way of giving it for psoriasis," comments Dr. Lebwohl.

How Psoriasis Can Affect You Over Your Lifetime

Psoriasis doesn't flare premenstrually and may improve in some women during pregnancy. "A rare form of pustular psoriasis called *impetigo herpetiformis* occurs during pregnancy," cautions Dr. Lebwohl. "Women can develop pustules all over, starting out small but often growing larger so that they merge and cover larger areas."

Pregnancy and Breastfeeding

The biggest problem for women involves medications used to treat psoriasis, some of which cause birth defects. Soriatane and Accutane stay in the body for varying periods of time. With Soriatane (which is stored in fatty tissues), women must use two forms of birth control beginning a month before treatment is started and for two to three years after it ends. Accutane stays in the body for thirty-one days, so women must avoid pregnancy during treatment and for thirty-one days after stopping the drug.

Breastfeeding is not recommended while taking the drug and for two to three years after treatment is stopped. Methotrexate is also *teratogenic* (harmful to the fetus) and not recommended during pregnancy or breastfeeding.

"There's a tremendous amount of data among women who underwent organ transplants and were on cyclosporine during pregnancy. So it does appear to be very safe. The only side effect is a reduction in birth weight," comments Dr. Lebwohl.

PUVA is not approved for use during pregnancy. While there do not appear to be any PUVA-related birth defects, there is a slight risk of miscarriage. "It certainly merits discussion with the patient. PUVA does involve a drug that you take by mouth; it gets into your skin and requires activation by ultraviolet light. However, the fetus isn't exposed to ultraviolet light, so it should be safe," he adds. Some women develop a facial rash or discoloration called *melasma* during pregnancy when exposed to ultraviolet light. Called "the mask of pregnancy," melasma can also occur in pregnant women undergoing PUVA therapy, on the arms as well as the face.

Acitretin also may interfere with low-dose, progestin-only oral contraceptives (such as *Micronor*), so women are advised to use birth control pills containing both estrogen and progestin. Oral contraceptives may affect levels of cyclosporine.

Menopause and Beyond

Psoriasis doesn't seem to be affected by hormonal fluctuations, so it may or may not improve with menopause. There are no known interactions between psoriasis medications and the estrogens or progestins used in hormone replacement (although there has been no research in the area).

Psoriasis medications have not been studied in older adults. But it is known that older people are more likely to experience side effects, and medications can stay in the body longer than in younger people. "For example, methotrexate is excreted more slowly when you're older because your kidneys don't work as well. Methotrexate also increases the risk of high blood pressure in people over sixty-five. Cyclosporine directly raises blood pressure, as well," says Dr. Lebwohl. Older women should discuss all medications with their physician, including any unusual side effects they may be experiencing.

Alopecia Areata

Alopecia areata is an autoimmune skin disease that affects hair follicles, causing hair loss on the scalp and elsewhere on the body. The National Alopecia

---

Warning Signs of Alopecia

- One or more round bald patches on the scalp
- Loss of hair in the eyelashes or eyebrows
- Sudden or progressive loss of hair on the scalp or body

Areata Foundation (NAAF) estimates that over 4.5 million people in the U.S. are affected, many of them women.

What Causes Alopecia Areata?

We actually lose hair all the time; each day you may shed as many as 100 hairs as part of the normal growth cycle. Each hair on your head grows about a half-inch per month for an average of four to seven years, then enters a "resting" phase (or *telogen*) lasting two to three months. About 85 percent of the hair on your scalp is growing at any given moment; 15 percent of your hair is in the resting stage. At the end of the resting stage, the hair falls out and a new hair grows in its place.

In alopecia areata, hair follicles are attacked by T-cells, resulting in the arrest of the hair growth stage, explains Madeline Duvic, MD, interim chair of dermatology and director of the Alopecia Areata National Registry at the M. D. Anderson Cancer Center at the University of Texas in Houston. "The hair breaks off because of the inflammatory infiltrate, so you get a little stubble. But the hair follicles are still there—they are not destroyed or damaged," explains Dr. Duvic. "No one knows why the T-cells attack hair follicles, how long the attacks may last, or why they stop. But hair growth often resumes spontaneously."

According to the NAAF, the autoimmune attack causes hair follicles to go into a dormant state, where they become very small and produce barely visible hairs (or no hair) for months or even years. The scalp is the most commonly affected area, but any hair-bearing site can be affected alone or together with the scalp. Illness and stress may play a role, though most people with alopecia areata are otherwise healthy. "When there's a stressor like an illness, or a fever, or a loss of blood, that can synchronize your hair. And after you've been sick, your hair starts falling out, you lose the resting hairs that are synchronized; that's *telogen effluvium*, which is reversible and different from alopecia areata," says Dr. Duvic.

Alopecia areata occurs in men and women of all ages and races, but it often begins in childhood. Genes play a role; at least one out of five persons with alopecia areata has someone else in the family with the disorder. When the disease occurs before age thirty, it's more likely there's a family history. Alopecia areata often occurs in families whose members have asthma, allergies, eczema, or other autoimmune diseases such as thyroiditis, diabetes, rheumatoid arthritis, lupus, vitiligo, pernicious anemia, or Addison's disease.

Recent research indicates that some people may have genetic markers that both increase their susceptibility and influence the severity of the disease.

Symptoms of Alopecia Areata

Alopecia usually begins with one or two small, roundish bald spots that appear on the scalp, or with diffuse shedding of hair. Some people may lose eyelashes in one area of the eyelid or eyebrow hair. In some people, the nails develop stippling that looks as if a pin had made rows of tiny dents; in rare cases, the nails become severely distorted. Some people may have coexisting vitiligo, a loss of pigment in patches of the skin (the pigment melanin is present in hair root bulbs) or regrowth of white hair.

Some women develop only a few bare patches that regrow hair within a year. In others, extensive patchy loss occurs. When all scalp hair is lost, the condition is referred to as *alopecia totalis*; when hair is lost from the entire scalp and body, it's called *alopecia universalis*. (This does not cause scarring, which can occur in lupus.)

Alopecia areata does not appear to be influenced by hormones. "A lot of my patients say they get worse in the spring or the fall; there's a 30 percent incidence of allergy and atopy in alopecia areata patients. So it's possible that they're allergic and the pollens in spring or fall set the reaction," says Dr. Duvic.

Some women may have alopecia areata and not even know it because hair loss occurs in the back of the scalp. In some cases, hairdressers are the ones who spot it.

Diagnosing Alopecia Areata

While the coin-sized patches of baldness characteristic of alopecia areata are the key symptom, a dermatologist will take a medical history, including when the problem began, if there was any associated life stress, what kind of medications are being taken, what the hormonal status is, any unusual diet, and whether there's a family history of baldness.

A dermatologist will also examine the scalp carefully for any scarring caused by trauma, lupus, or a skin disorder, which can be confirmed with a scalp biopsy. In some cases, a few hairs will be examined under a microscope. If there's a root bulb at the end of a strand, it indicates a telogen hair. Hair lost during the growth phase has a clublike shape on its root end and can indicate a reaction to medication, among other things. Blood tests may also be done to see whether a woman has thyroid disease, a hormonal imbalance, lupus, or anemia.

"You have to rule out fungal infection of the scalp. If you don't see specific patches and there's a generalized loss, you look for an infection. Low iron may be a contributing factor in some patients. There's about a 30 percent incidence of thyroid problems in adults with alopecia areata; it can precede it or develop after it," says Dr. Duvic. "A biopsy is the most definite way to make a diagnosis. You will see lymphocytes around the root bulb of the follicle."

Treating Alopecia Areata

The choice of treatment depends mainly on a woman's age and the type of alopecia. Alopecia areata occurs in two forms: a mild patchy form where less than 50 percent of scalp hair is lost and an extensive form where greater than 90 percent of scalp hair is lost. These two forms of alopecia areata behave quite differently, and treatment depends on which form you have.

Current treatments do not affect the autoimmune process that underlies alopecia but are aimed at stimulating the hair follicle to grow hair again. Treatments need to be continued until the disease process turns itself off. Treatments are most effective in milder cases.

Cortisone Injections

In cases of mild, patchy alopecia areata, multiple injections of cortisone are done in and around bald patches and repeated once a month. If new hair growth occurs, it's usually visible within four weeks. Local cortisone injections do not prevent new patches from developing, but do kill T-cells locally. Other than the needle prick and a slight tingling afterward, there are few side effects. Occasionally, temporary depressions in the skin result from the local injections, but these *dells* usually fill in by themselves. Topical, over-the-counter steroids don't work with alopecia areata.

Topical Minoxidil

A solution of 5 percent topical minoxidil applied twice daily to the scalp and eyebrows may help regrow hair. If scalp hair regrows completely, treatment can be stopped. Over-the-counter, 2 percent topical minoxidil solution is not effective by itself in alopecia areata; response may improve if cortisone cream is applied 30 minutes after the minoxidil. Topical minoxidil does not lower blood pressure in people with normal blood pressure. Neither 2 percent nor 5 percent topical minoxidil solution is effective in treating women with 100 percent scalp hair loss.

"Some people respond beautifully to minoxidil. However, those people may have grown back hair anyway. Alopecia areata is a hard disease to evaluate because a lot of people regrow hair no matter what, and there's no way to predict who will regrow hair," says Dr. Duvic.

Topical minoxidil hasn't been studied among pregnant women, although animal studies suggest it may cause problems during pregnancy. It's also not known whether topical minoxidil passes into breast milk. However, limited tests have been conducted among older adults (up to age sixty-five) and it appears to work better in younger patients. People with low blood pressure need to be careful about using too much and over large areas.

Anthralin Cream or Ointment

Anthralin is a synthetic, tarlike substance that is used for psoriasis. It's applied to bare patches once daily and washed off after thirty to sixty minutes. Anthralin can be combined with minoxidil for an increased effect.

"Anthralin irritates the scalp; it attracts other T-cells and they kind of override the hair-specific autoimmune attack. And then probably the immune system tries to shut off that reaction and takes the alopecia away. That's how we think it works," explains Dr. Duvic.

If new hair growth occurs with anthralin, it will be visible in eight to twelve weeks. Side effects include irritation and temporary, brownish discoloration, which can be lessened by shortening treatment times. Care must be taken not to get anthralin in the eyes. Hands must be washed after applying.

Anthralin may be absorbed through the skin, but no studies of its effects on pregnancy (either in humans or animals) have been done, and it's not known whether it can pass into breast milk. No data are available on whether anthralin works differently in older women.

Systemic Cortisone

Cortisone pills are sometimes prescribed when there is extensive scalp hair loss. "If someone is going completely bald really quickly, and it's her first episode of alopecia areata, we try systemic steroids. Because if you can cut it off before it becomes established, then you might make a difference," says Dr. Duvic.

The main problem is that any regrown hair is likely to fall out when the cortisone pills are stopped. In addition, there are health risks, such as bone loss, high blood pressure, diabetes, ulcers, and cataracts (see page 34).

Topical Immunotherapy

A treatment widely used in Europe and Canada involves producing an allergic rash or allergic contact dermatitis by applying chemicals to the scalp. The resulting rash looks like poison ivy or poison oak. "It's believed that the rash stimulates the immune system in the area and triggers hair follicles to produce hair again," says Dr. Duvic.

Approximately 40 percent of patients treated with topical immunotherapy regrow scalp hair after about six months. However, the treatment must be continued to maintain hair regrowth. Topical immunotherapy is now undergoing clinical trials in the U.S.

Other topical remedies include *Luxiq*, a scalp mousse, and *Protopic* (*FK506*), neither of which has been subjected to clinical trials in alopecia areata. Protopic, which is approved for treating eczema, is an immunosuppressant agent that blocks cytokine release in the skin.

A Little Artifice Aids Appearance

Women with extensive hair loss often opt for wigs. Some newer, well-made wigs of synthetic or human hair have special suction caps that keep them firmly in place, even during active sports (another option is special double-sided tape, which can be purchased in beauty supply outlets). Cosmetic tattooing can be done on the eyebrow area and along the eyelids for an eyeliner effect.

Vitiligo

Vitiligo is caused by an immune attack on melanocytes, the skin cells that produce *melanin*, the pigment that gives skin its color. The result is white patches of skin, which may enlarge and increase in number. In some cases the condition may stabilize and then start up again.

Vitiligo affects 1 to 2 percent of Americans, and while it's less obvious in light-skinned people, it can be traumatic for African-Americans and other women of color. Half of women with vitiligo develop the disorder between the ages of ten and thirty, and it may be genetic in some cases. Vitiligo is also associated with other autoimmune disorders. As many as 30 percent of women with vitiligo develop thyroid disease. Women with vitiligo also have an increased risk of pernicious anemia or Addison's disease (page 183).

People with vitiligo must protect their skin from the sun; without the protection of melanin the affected patches of skin can become seriously sunburned. Women must use sunscreen with a sun protection factor (SPF) of at least 30 on exposed skin year-round (there are special sunblocks, like 60 SPF Total Block, designed for people with extreme sun sensitivity and those at high risk of skin cancer). Long sleeves and pants and wide-brimmed hats should be worn during long periods spent outdoors. Sun-protective clothing made from fabric that blocks out UV light is available from companies like Solumbra and Sun Solutions.

Treating Vitiligo

There's no cure for vitiligo, but there are treatments that help restore lost melanin. The mainstay of treatment is PUVA, which can effectively darken white skin patches, especially if vitiligo is extensive. If vitiligo patches are very limited, occasionally psoralen can be applied directly to the skin before ultraviolet A treatment. At least a year of twice-weekly PUVA treatments is needed to restore melanin production.

PUVA is 50 to 70 percent effective in restoring pigment to vitiligo patches on the face, trunk, upper arms, and legs. However, the hands and feet respond poorly to PUVA. PUVA is not approved for use in pregnant or nursing women (see pages 132 to 133). If patches are small, corticosteroid creams may help restore pigment. However, chronic use of steroids can result in thinning and atrophy of the skin.

Better treatments are under investigation. Researchers from Henry Ford Hospital in Detroit have been able to restore pigment in five patients through a series of exposures to a limited spectrum (narrow band) of ultraviolet B radiation. In a recent report in the *Journal of the American Academy of Dermatology*, the researchers said that two dark-skinned black patients achieved more than 75 percent repigmentation after an average of nineteen treatments given three times a week. Two other patients, both light-skinned Caucasians, achieved up to 40 and 50 percent repigmentation after forty-eight and forty-six treatments, respectively.

Another new treatment being tested involves applying a synthetic enzyme, *pseudocatalase*, to vitiligo patches after exposure to narrow-band ultraviolet B light.

6

More Than a Dry Spell— Sjögren's Syndrome

I started having dryness symptoms in my middle forties. I kept complaining about dry mouth to my dentist, but he didn't seem concerned about it. I had lots of cavities and I didn't realize then that lack of saliva can cause your teeth to deteriorate. I had dry mouth for three or four years, but it started to become much worse. I found I couldn't eat anything. I was totally without saliva and could hardly swallow. As it turned out, there was a saliva specialist at the university where I work. My husband urged me to see him, but I said, "Why should I see a saliva specialist? I don't have any saliva!" But my husband insisted, and I finally went. The specialist told me right away I probably had Sjögren's. I had never heard of it before. When he asked me about dry eyes and eye pain, until then I hadn't realized that the shooting pains in my eyes were from dry spots. I simply connected my dry mouth to my eyes.

EVELYN, FIFTY-TWO

Having Sjögren's syndrome is like wandering in a desert, thirsting for a cool drink of water. Sometimes you're so dry, nothing can slake your thirst or make your mouth feel moist. Your eyes feel gritty and painful, and after a while other parts of the body dry out too.

Sjögren's syndrome is actually the second most common autoimmune rheumatic disease after rheumatoid arthritis. The Sjögren's Syndrome Foundation (SSF) estimates that two to four million people may be affected, 90 percent

Warning Signs of Sjögren's

- Dry, scratchy eyes
- Chronic dry mouth
- Reduced salivary flow
- Burning oral mucous membranes
- Frequent cavities
- Dry vagina and painful intercourse
- Fatigue
- Neuropathy
- Lung inflammation

of whom are women. Sjögren's often accompanies other autoimmune disorders like rheumatoid arthritis or lupus (in this case, it's called *secondary Sjögren's*), but 50 percent of patients have Sjögren's that occurs on its own (*primary Sjögren's*).

What Causes Sjögren's Syndrome?

In Sjögren's, the disease process targets the body's moisture-producing glands and tissues: the *lacrimal* glands that produce tears (located within the upper and outer margins of the eye socket, and in the eyelid), the *salivary* glands that produce saliva (located under the tongue and jaw, and deep within the angle of the jaw in front of the ear), and the mucous membranes in the nose, vagina, and lungs. The moisture-producing glands are regulated by the autonomic nervous system that governs automatic functions like breathing and blood pressure. As these glands become damaged by activated immune cells, they may be less able to respond to signals from an area of the brain that handles sensory input and triggers production of tears or saliva (for example, your mouth watering at the sight or smell of food). At the same time, inflammatory molecules (*cytokines*) released by immune cells may lead to damage to nerves (and diminished production of neurotransmitters) that stimulate the salivary or tear glands. In addition, these activated immune cells don't undergo normal programmed cell death, so they accumulate to perpetuate the autoimmune response.

The dry eyes of Sjögren's are caused by low tear production because of the destruction of the lacrimal glands and dysfunction of the tiny glands behind the eyelashes that secrete oil that prevents tears from evaporating (*meibomian glands*).

Tears are actually made up of three layers: the *mucin* layer on the surface of the eye is made up of secretions from the cornea and glands scattered throughout the *conjunctiva* (the mucous membrane covering the lining of the eyelids and outside of the eyeball); the middle, *aqueous*, layer is largely made up of water and proteins from the lacrimal glands; the outer layer, called the *lipid* layer, is made up of fatty secretions from oil glands in the eyelids (*meibomian* glands). The mucin layer provides lubrication for the cornea; without it, dry spots develop and cause discomfort. The aqueous layer of tears provides key proteins that protect the eye against bacteria. The lipid layer of the tear film prevents excessive evaporation of tears; if the lipid layer is inadequate, the tear film evaporates. Every time you blink, your eyelids distribute the tear film over the surface of the eye and lubricate it; if there's not enough

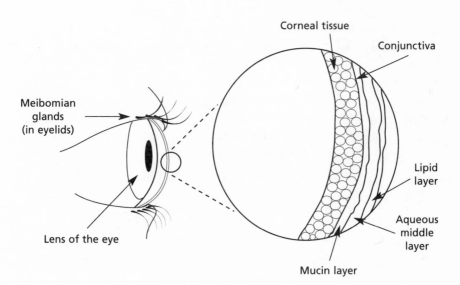

Tear Film Layers

tear film, the eyelid won't move as smoothly over the surface of the eye, caus-ing the gritty sensation that also characterizes Sjögren's. In fact, this evapora-tive problem is thought to contribute to two-thirds of all cases of dry eye, says David A. Sullivan, PhD, senior scientist at the Schepens Eye Research Institute in Boston. "It used to be thought that inadequate aqueous tears was the main problem in Sjögren's. But women with Sjögren's also have meibo-mian gland dysfunction and don't have enough oil in the tear film. So the tear film is unstable and evaporates."

The underlying cause of evaporative dry eye may be low levels of male hor-mones, or *androgens*, including testosterone. Androgens appear to play a key role in the function of the meibomian glands and also serve to dampen inflam-mation in the lacrimal glands, says Dr. Sullivan. While Sjögren's can emerge at any age, women typically develop the syndrome between ages forty-five and fifty-five, when androgens and estrogens decline.

In the case of mucous membranes and other tissues that produce moisture, cytokines may interfere with the normal passage of fluid onto the surface of those tissues, such as those in the vagina. Without moisture, these tissues become uncomfortably dry and ulcerated. Dry vagina and uncomfortable sex are common symptoms in Sjögren's. The disorder can also affect organs such as the lungs, kidneys, and liver, as well as blood vessels.

What triggers the autoimmune reaction in Sjögren's is unknown. Several genes are associated with Sjögren's, and the disorder tends to cluster in fami-lies. According to the SSF, around 12 percent of patients have one or more relatives (usually female) with Sjögren's.

It's possible that a viral infection or other injury may set off an immune reaction in genetically susceptible people. Some research suggests a role for *Epstein-Barr virus* (*EBV*). The virus lays dormant in the salivary glands for years and can be reactivated, perhaps during other viral infections. However, since most people have been exposed to EBV, the virus alone is not thought to be a trigger. EBV is also being studied for a possible role in other autoim-mune diseases, such as lupus.

Symptoms of Sjögren's

When you have Sjögren's, you'll typically have a gritty or burning sensation in the eyes, eyelids that stick together, mucus accumulation in the inner corners of the eyes (usually when you awaken), itching, sensitivity to light, blurred vision, and discomfort and difficulty reading or watching television (you may notice a "filmy" sensation that interferes with vision). Symptoms often worsen as the day goes on.

The symptoms of dry eye result from increased friction due to insufficient tears and evaporation of the tear film. In some cases, the eyelid may actually stick to the conjunctiva or corneal surface and can literally pull epithelial cells away from the surface, causing erosions. Dry eye, discomfort, inflammation, and defects in the surface layer of the conjunctiva and cornea are called *keratoconjunctivitis sicca* (*KCS*). Ironically, people with dry eyes may notice excessive tearing at first, as the eye compensates by producing more reflex tears (usually produced when there's a foreign body in the eye or other irritation). But women with Sjögren's are less able to produce reflex tears.

Similarly, saliva (actually a mixture of mucins, water, nutrient proteins, and growth factors) provides lubrication for the tongue, for speaking and swallowing, and for washing away bacteria and toxins from the surface of the teeth and mucous membranes. Loss of saliva is associated with increased amounts of cavities in the teeth (fillings may also loosen or break down more quickly) and oral yeast infections, and discomfort.

Dry mouth symptoms can include a burning sensation on the tongue or mucous membranes (*burning mouth syndrome*), problems with chewing or swallowing food (being unable to swallow dry foods like crackers without fluid), dry sticky oral surfaces, cracks in the tongue or corners of the mouth, problems with taste or smell, and a constant need to drink.

The *parotid glands* (the largest of the salivary glands, located above the angle of the jaw in front of the ear; also the glands affected by the mumps) may be enlarged or hardened. In fact, if you had mumps as a child and seemed to get it again as an adult, it's not mumps but may be a sign of Sjögren's. You may also have yeast infections in the mouth. There can be drying of the nasal passages (with crusting and nosebleeds) and throat hoarseness, as well as dry and irritated vaginal tissues.

A major symptom of Sjögren's is fatigue; in a recent survey, 77 percent of SSF members reported suffering fatigue. There may also be joint pain, fever, dry skin, allergic skin reactions, and sleep disturbances (waking up with dry mouth, drinking water, and then having to urinate more often), and gastrointestinal problems like constipation, all of which people may not associate with the disorder.

Sjögren's can also affect many systems in the body, including the nerves, kidneys, and lungs. It can cause peripheral nerve problems (*neuropathy*), lung inflammation (*interstitial pneumonitis*), and kidney dysfunction. Symptoms of lung problems in Sjögren's are shortness of breath and exercise intolerance.

Sjögren's symptoms can also mimic other conditions. The drying of tissues is often blamed on menopause; eye irritation may be attributed to conjunctivitis. Joint pain and fatigue may be blamed on lupus or rheumatoid arthritis, and nerve-related symptoms can be similar to multiple sclerosis. Not surprisingly, Sjögren's can be tricky to identify. A survey of SSF members found that 25 percent spent over five years trying to get an accurate diagnosis.

Women with Sjögren's also have an increased risk of lymphoma (malignancy of the lymph glands). So it's imperative to be carefully followed by an internist. Any lymph node lump in the neck, underarm, or groin should be investigated immediately. However, less than 10 percent of Sjögren's patients develop lymphoma.

Evelyn's story continues:

At the salivary dysfunction clinic, the first test I had was a "resting saliva" test. I sat for five minutes without swallowing and then spit into a little cup, and he looked at what I produced, which was a little blob of what looked like glue. He turned the cup upside down and it didn't move. Then he gave

---

Sjögren's Clusters

While dry eyes are a common symptom in autoimmune diseases, secondary Sjögren's frequently accompanies a number of diseases, including the following:

- Rheumatoid arthritis
- Systemic lupus erythematosus
- Hashimoto's thyroiditis
- Graves' disease
- Primary biliary cirrhosis
- Autoimmune hepatitis
- Multiple sclerosis
- Scleroderma
- Myasthenia gravis

---

me a stimulated saliva test, where you chew a little piece of wax to stimulate saliva production. As you chew you spit out what's in your mouth, and I didn't produce much of anything. Then he ran a series of blood tests, then sent me to an ophthalmologist, who confirmed the diagnosis. Getting a diagnosis was extremely helpful to me. I now do a fluoride treatment with my teeth every night, and I avoid eating foods with sugar. Without saliva, there's nothing to protect your teeth. That made a real difference. I've had a few cavities, but nothing like the kind of major dental work I had before.

Diagnosing Sjögren's Syndrome

As with Evelyn, it often takes years before a woman is properly diagnosed. Sometimes the symptoms are blamed on aging, says Ann Parke, MD, professor of medicine at the University of Connecticut Health Center in Farmington. "I have patients who come in and say they were perfectly fine until age forty or forty-five, and that's when they start to develop their complaints. But frequently they are not diagnosed for another ten years. To a certain extent we associate dry eyes, dry mouth, and dry vagina with aging, but I think a lot of people don't take these complaints seriously," says Dr. Parke. "The fatigue associated with Sjögren's also complicates things. Women go in to see their primary care physicians and say, 'I'm tired,' and they are labeled as having 'empty-nest syndrome' or being depressed. They are not asked the important questions: 'Do you have dry eye? Do you have dry mouth? Do you sleep OK?' It's a major problem."

Other causes of the symptoms associated with Sjögren's must also be ruled out, such as the drying effects of drugs, eye diseases or infection, the effects of allergies (and allergy medications), and lymphoma (malignancy of the lymph glands can sometimes involve the salivary glands). A workup should begin with a complete history and physical to assess the possibility of autoimmune, connective tissue, or glandular diseases. Your eyes, mouth, skin, and glands in your face and neck should also be carefully examined.

Tests You May Need and What They Mean

After an assessment of your symptoms, a number of blood tests can help confirm a diagnosis of Sjögren's. These include an *erythrocyte sedimentation rate*

(*ESR*, a general indication of inflammation, see page 27), as well as measuring levels of blood proteins called *immunoglobulins*. Elevated results are associated with Sjögren's and other related disorders. The specific antibody tests that are performed include the following.

Antinuclear antibodies (ANAs) are a group of antibodies that react against the components of a cell nucleus. ANAs are present in a variety of autoimmune diseases, including lupus, but about 70 percent of patients with Sjögren's will also have a positive ANA test (see page 27).

Rheumatoid factor (RF), an antibody associated with rheumatoid arthritis, is found in 60 to 70 percent of people with Sjögren's (see page 27).

Sjögren's syndrome–associated A antigen (SSA/Ro) and Sjögren's syndrome–associated B antigen (SSB/La) are antibodies against material in the nucleus of every cell. Seventy percent of people with Sjögren's have SSA/Ro antibodies (they are found in 50 percent of women with lupus), and 40 percent of Sjögren's patients have SSB/La antibodies (as do 15 to 20 percent of people with lupus).

Antithyroid antibody and thyroid stimulating hormone (TSH) levels will be checked. Autoimmune thyroid diseases can cluster with Sjögren's and share symptoms like dry skin and fatigue. Therefore tests will be done to measure antithyroid antibodies and assess thyroid function, including the level of TSH.

The **Schirmer test** is the simplest and most common eye test to assess tears and tear production. Small pieces of filter paper are placed between your eyeball and lower lid, and the amount of wetting produced within five minutes indicates the level of tear production.

A **slit-lamp examination** measures the amount of tears produced by the eye in its normal resting state. A lamp indirectly illuminates your eye to avoid producing reflex tears, and magnifies the surface so the normal layer of tears along the lower eyelid can be seen. The tear film may appear thickened with excessive debris. There may be inflammation of the conjunctiva.

Rose bengal staining determines the quality of the mucin layer of the tear film and its distribution over the surface of the eye. Rose bengal is a harmless vegetable dye. A single drop is administered after rinsing with a preservative-free tear preparation; reddish stain remains on the cells that have lost their mucin coating, a pattern of staining characteristic of keratoconjunctivitis sicca syndrome. Another dye called lissamine green can also be used. Other tests may be done to assess the tear film and the condition of the cornea.

A dentist or oral pathologist may measure your saliva production. As in Evelyn's case, this is done by stimulating saliva production using an acidic or sour substance, and then measuring the amount of saliva produced. In some cases, a salivary gland biopsy may be performed. The procedure involves making a small incision in the lower lip and removing five to ten tiny salivary glands, which are examined under a microscope for immune cell infiltration.

The combination of symptoms, positive antibody tests, and positive tests for dry eye and/or decreased salivary production, substantiate the diagnosis of Sjögren's. In most cases, a biopsy is not needed.

The Female Factor

While estrogen appears to play a role in some autoimmune diseases, androgen deficiency appears to be a more critical factor in dry eye. "Premenopausal women normally make about two-thirds of the amount of androgen that men do, and we have found that women with Sjögren's are androgen deficient. We have learned that androgens are important for optimal lacrimal and meibomian gland function," says Dr. Sullivan. "Androgens can significantly influence the nature of the lipids produced in the meibomian glands, and they appear to promote the formation of the tear film lipid layer, thereby enhancing tear film stability. Consequently, androgen deficiency may promote the development of dry eye."

Androgen deficiency can occur with aging, during menopause (peak years for Sjögren's), and with certain autoimmune diseases, like lupus. Androgens seem to dampen inflammation; studies indicate that dry eye improves in people given androgens, Dr. Sullivan adds. "In contrast, estrogen may worsen inflammation of the lacrimal glands, and may suppress meibomian gland function. If that's true, we would expect that when women go on hormone replacement therapy during menopause, there would be an increase in dry eye."

In fact, a 2001 study coauthored by Dr. Sullivan found just that. Researchers from the Schepens Eye Research Institute and Brigham and Women's Hospital in Boston looked at data from the Women's Health Study, which included 25,665 postmenopausal women, and found that almost 7 percent of women taking HRT reported dry eye syndrome (keratoconjunctivitis sicca, KCS). More than 9 percent of women using estrogen replacement therapy (ERT) alone had KCS. The longer a woman used hormones, the greater the risk; for each three years that women used HRT there was a 15 percent increase in the likelihood of being diagnosed with KCS or having severe symptoms. The study, which appeared in the *Journal of the American Medical Association*, was the first epidemiological link between postmenopausal hormone use and dry eye, but the study was limited since diagnostic tests were not done.

Evelyn's story continues:
The hardest thing for me is the social interactions. I always feel so self-conscious; I feel like everyone can see how dry I am. When I start a conversation with someone, and I don't have water with me, I can't have a conversation. It's impossible; I can't talk long without water. And it certainly affects eating. I have to have lots of liquid. At a cocktail party, I kind of ignore the food because I need to have something to drink and I can't juggle a plate and a glass. But I manage. I have it easier than people who also have arthritis or other painful syndromes. I have found ways to cope with the dryness. I have tried artificial saliva, and the sprays, but I can't stand the taste, and they are very short-acting. I took pilocarpine for two years, but it had a lot of side effects. The biggest way Sjögren's affects me is actually the fatigue. By nine o'clock at night, I just collapse.

Treating Sjögren's Syndrome

There are a variety of treatment options for Sjögren's syndrome.

Dry Eye

For some women, over-the-counter "artificial tears" can temporarily soothe dry eyes. However, these lubricating drops don't have lasting effects and, in severe cases, must be used frequently, increasing the risk of problems from preservatives, says Janine Smith, MD, deputy clinical director of the National Eye Institute (NEI). Ocular lubricant ointments can be helpful if used before bedtime but can blur vision, causing problems during the day.

There are preservative-free and preservative-releasing drops available, including *Refresh Tears* (multidose), *Bion Tears*, and *TheraTears*. "TheraTears has also been shown to increase production of mucin in a rabbit model," adds Dr. Smith. Some products provide the staying power of an ointment without blurring vision. "Lacrisert is a very tiny pellet, kind of like ointment in a pellet, that is placed between the eye and the lower lid, and it dissolves over a twenty-four-hour period. It's only effective in patients who have some tears, because it needs tears to dissolve," explains Dr. Smith. Several new gels have a consistency somewhere between eyedrops and ointment. GenTeal is a water-based gel and is among lubricants that contain "disappearing preservatives," which break down once the product is exposed to air.

Corticosteroid eyedrops (such as *Pred Forte* and *Pred Mild*) can also reduce inflammation. However, they can cause glaucoma and cataracts and are not safe to use for long periods. They are generally used as a short-term therapy for people who have not responded to other treatments. "If the eye is extremely inflamed, other measures won't work. If you can bring down the inflammation, other treatments may have a better chance of helping," says Dr. Smith.

Tiny silicone plugs (called *punctal plugs*) can be placed in your tear ducts near the corner of the eyes and can help tears stay around longer. "In women with Sjögren's who have very low tear flow, punctal plugs may make things worse. If you have no outflow of tears, as the tears evaporate, inflammatory proteins can concentrate on the surface of the eye and cause discomfort. So you need to use other measures to keep the surface of the eye lubricated and flushed," says Dr. Smith. In rare cases, the plugs can become contaminated and cause infections, and ducts may become damaged.

Special goggles for outdoor use decrease tear evaporation or slow it, adds Dr. Smith. Some goggles have special inserts or patches that increase the humidity around the eye. There are also plastic side shields for glasses and wraparound sunglasses. Humidifiers can make a big difference in the bedroom and elsewhere.

New therapies aimed at treating the underlying causes of dry eye are in the pipeline, including androgen eyedrops. "Animal data suggest that topical androgens may suppress lacrimal gland inflammation and correct the meibomian gland dysfunction in Sjögren's syndrome, aiding tear formation and production of a lasting tear film," explains Dr. Smith. "It's also thought that androgens have anti-inflammatory properties, and that there's a relative androgen deficiency locally in the eye that may allow inflammation to progress on the surface of the eye."

There are also receptors for androgens and estrogens in the eyelid, the conjunctiva, the cornea, the lacrimal gland, and even in the retinal pigment epithelium. "We're learning more about how complex the ocular surface is, and it's not something that you can just rewet with a lot of water. Really what's needed is something that will produce physiologic tears," comments Dr. Smith.

Tests are under way of an experimental eyedrop preparation (*INS365*) that acts on receptors in the eye (*P2Y2, purinergic receptors*) that regulate and stimulate secretion of tears and mucin. "It causes an increase in fluid on the surface of the eye. It's not tear fluid, but *transudate*, fluid that comes from underneath the conjunctiva that moves onto the surface of the eye. It results in an increase in tear volume on the surface of the eye by that mechanism. It's the only drug that works that way," says Dr. Smith. So far, the tests have not produced changes in outcomes.

The National Eye Institute at NIH and others have conducted a study of the anti-inflammatory drug cyclosporine in eyedrop form (*Restasis*). Restasis may prevent T-cell activation on the ocular surface and in the lacrimal gland. The drops, being studied in Sjögren's and in postmenopausal women with dry eye, increase tear production (seen in a Schirmer test). If approved by the FDA, Restasis would be the first therapy aimed at dampening the underlying inflammation of dry eye.

"Sjögren's probably needs to be attacked from several fronts. Androgens would attack evaporative dry eye and lacrimal gland inflammation. Theoretically, if you increase the tear flow, you will increase the clearance of pro-inflammatory cytokines," remarks Dr. Sullivan. "Using topical anti-inflammatory agents, such as cyclosporine, you can decrease some of the inflammation on the ocular surface that exists because of the disease. It's likely that some combination of therapies would be needed."

Dry Mouth

Salagen (*pilocarpine hydrochloride*) and *Evoxac* (*cevimeline*) are oral medications that stimulate saliva production, helping patients chew, swallow, speak, and even sleep more easily. Evoxac is also being studied for its effect on dry eyes. Salagen may have effects on dry eye, and some people using Salagen are using it in addition to other therapies.

A lozenge containing *interferon alpha* (*IFNα*) that may stimulate saliva production is also in clinical trials. IFNα may treat the secretory dysfunction in the salivary glands. In clinical trials, patients using the lozenge had more than twice the increase in saliva production as a placebo group. Researchers are also exploring possible gene therapy that would be delivered to the salivary glands and an implantable artificial salivary gland.

Dry Vagina

Vaginal moisturizers (such as *Replens, Vagisil Intimate Moisturizer,* and *KY Liquid*) can relieve dryness, itching, and burning, and a number of lubricants that can make sex more comfortable are available (see pages 155 to 156).

Systemic Therapies

NIH is also studying the effects of *dehydroepiandrosterone (DHEA)* in primary Sjögren's syndrome. DHEA has been used to treat women with lupus and has shown some effectiveness in Sjögren's patients. "The thought is the same as using the topical androgens, except oral androgens could affect the multiple systems involved in Sjögren's. It could decrease inflammation in the mouth, the eyes, the joints, and perhaps in the blood for some of the inflammatory markers of Sjögren's," adds Dr. Smith.

Drugs used to treat RA may also prove useful in Sjögren's syndrome, among them *etanercept (Enbrel)*, which blocks *tumor necrosis factor alpha (TNFα)*, a major promoter of inflammation. Studies have shown that Sjögren's patients have increased levels of TNFα in their salivary and lacrimal glands.

Evelyn's story continues:
You have to manage dry eyes and dry mouth to prevent other health problems. You should not just accept the fact that your eyes bother you. I make sure to keep my eyes moist, and I avoid certain environments that dry out my eyes—like air-conditioned stores, which are very dry—and I wear special sunglasses that have side panels so the wind doesn't dry my eyes. I'm careful about eating sugar and make sure to rinse my mouth or brush my teeth if I eat something sweet. I avoid eating any acidic foods, because they bother me—my tongue burns like crazy. Eventually this becomes part of you and you do things automatically.

How Sjögren's Can Affect You Over Your Lifetime

Sjögren's doesn't directly affect reproduction, but some of the antibodies associated with it can cause problems.

Pregnancy

Forty percent or more of women have antibodies to SSB/La, also associated with lupus. These antibodies to normal cellular components can be harmful to a growing fetus and can lead to cardiac, skin, or blood-related problems, which are all grouped under the term neonatal lupus. If you are pregnant and have Sjögren's, you need to have your serum (the clear part of the blood) tested for the presence and amount of these antibodies with a test called an ELISA (see page 60). If you are found to have antibodies to either Ro or La, you have a 2 percent chance of having a baby with neonatal lupus. The pregnancy is managed just as in women with lupus who have these antibodies (see pages 74 to 76 for information on neonatal lupus). Current information suggests that having a child with neonatal lupus does not increase the risk for lupus later in life.

Women with Sjögren's may also have *anticardiolipin antibodies* (*aCLs*), also detected by ELISA. These antibodies are related to *antiphospholipid syndrome*. The so-called lupus anticoagulant is another antiphospholipid antibody that may be detected in women with Sjögren's. These antibodies may predispose women to form clots in the placenta, hampering blood flow to the fetus, and are associated with recurrent miscarriages (most often during the late first trimester or second trimester). Women found to have these antibodies are prescribed blood thinners, such as aspirin or heparin. Pregnancies in women with Sjögren's found to have these antibodies are managed the same way as in women with antiphospholipid syndrome.

Gynecological Issues and Menopause

The major gynecological issue facing you with Sjögren's syndrome is vaginal dryness and painful intercourse. However, all vaginal dryness that occurs in women with Sjögren's is *not* related to the disease itself.

Vaginal lubrication does not come from moisture-producing glands but mostly from fluid that's passed from the bloodstream through the vaginal walls. "So dryness that occurs in Sjögren's may be due to autoimmune effects on the blood vessels and the circulation in the vaginal area," explains Lila E. Nachtigall, MD, professor of obstetrics and gynecology at the New York University School of Medicine. Other autoimmune diseases, such as lupus and diabetes, can affect circulation and vaginal secretions; the stress of any chronic illness may also reduce vaginal moisture.

Before menopause, estrogen helps stimulate the normal growth and development of vaginal cells, as well as vaginal secretions. As estrogen levels drop in the years before and after menopause, vaginal tissues gradually begin to thin and atrophy, producing fewer secretions (surgical menopause, removal of the ovaries, causes a more rapid onset of vaginal dryness). "Since Sjögren's is most often diagnosed in women age forty and over, some cases of vaginal dryness may be blamed on aging," remarks Dr. Nachtigall. Low estrogen levels occur during other times of life, such as during breastfeeding, and lead to vaginal dryness. Premature ovarian failure also causes dry eye and dry vagina (see page 192). Other causes must be ruled out before attributing the problem to Sjögren's.

You and your partner should be reassured that this is a physical problem and not related to any failure of sexual arousal, stresses Dr. Nachtigall. Lubricants can make sex more comfortable. These are different from "personal moisturizers." Lubricants are designed for use during sexual activity. "The ideal lubricant is odorless, tasteless, colorless, water soluble, and of a consistency that allows it to remain in the vagina. Never use oil-based products like petroleum jelly. They will interfere with the vagina's natural self-cleansing mechanism," she explains. Lubricants include *KY Jelly* and *Astroglide*.

Vaginal moisturizers are designed for regular use to relieve dryness and irritation and to attract liquid to the dry vaginal tissues. Moisturizers include *Replens* (containing pilocarpine, which adheres to vaginal tissues) and *Vagisil Intimate Moisturizer*. Both lubricants and moisturizers have an acidic pH that helps prevent vaginal infections and are nonhormonal.

Women with Sjögren's who have no other contraindications, such as a risk or history of blood clots or breast cancer, can safely use estrogen replacement therapy, says Dr. Nachtigall. "Although menopausal vaginal atrophy is somewhat worse in the Sjögren's patient, it responds to local estrogen therapy, either as cream or a slow-release estrogen ring. The ring releases a small continuous dose of estrogen to vaginal tissues and should be an excellent therapy for women with Sjögren's," she notes. Even women taking hormone replacement therapy may still need to apply estrogen cream to the vagina once or twice a week, she adds.

If you have an intact uterus, you'll also need progestin to protect against endometrial hyperplasia. But, again, estrogen replacement may make dry eyes worse. It's not known whether adding testosterone to HRT may alleviate this effect, says Dr. Sullivan. "The problem with taking androgens systemically are the side effects and the possibility that testosterone may actually be converted to estrogen by enzymes in various tissues. So we really don't know whether it will help."

Dry eye can be a component of menopause, so you need to mention it to your gynecologist. "I think it's very critical for women to recognize that Sjögren's can affect nearly every system in their body. Lung problems can cause shortness of breath; there may be nerve problems, which a woman may not connect to her Sjögren's," stresses Dr. Smith. "Women need to communicate to their physicians when they have problems or changes, because if they don't there's no hope of those problems being addressed."

7

Vanishing Hormones—Type 1 Diabetes, Premature Ovarian Failure, and Other Endocrine Problems

I had all the symptoms: the blurry vision, the enormous thirst, the ravenous appetite, and I would feel the deep, deep fatigue. But I didn't recognize them as diabetes. I was going through a divorce at the time and single motherhood, so not feeling "well" felt normal. So I missed the warning signs. Fortunately, I didn't have any damage. I had been diagnosed with another autoimmune disease, sarcoidosis, in 1973 and I was seeing a doctor every month to monitor my lungs for nodules. So the diabetes was found with a routine blood test. I didn't think about the symptoms or report them to the doctor until after he noticed the high glucose level and started asking me questions. It seemed so obvious after we got the blood test results, but it was so easy for me to overlook.
MARY KAY, FIFTY-FOUR

Type 1 Diabetes

Our bodies need fuel in order to run smoothly. We get that fuel from the carbohydrates and proteins we eat, which are converted to glucose and transported into cells by the hormone insulin. Normally the body keeps levels of blood glucose tightly regulated. But in diabetes that delicate balance is upset.

There are three forms of diabetes. *Type 1 diabetes*, or *insulin-dependent diabetes mellitus* (*IDDM*, once called *juvenile-onset diabetes*), is usually the result of an immune system attack on the insulin-producing cells in the pancreas that results in a shortage of insulin, so blood glucose becomes abnormally high, wreaking havoc on the body. *Type 2*, or *non-insulin-dependent diabetes mellitus* (*NIDDM*), is a strongly inherited metabolic disorder brought about by obesity and other risk factors that causes the body to gradually lose its ability to *use* insulin properly. Once termed *adult-onset diabetes*, an epidemic rise in obesity has increased the occurrence of type 2 diabetes among children. *Gestational diabetes* is a temporary form of diabetes that arises during late pregnancy, in which the body temporarily loses responsiveness to insulin. It usually resolves within days after delivery.

While type 1 diabetes affects women and men about equally, it often occurs with other autoimmune diseases common to women, including thyroid disease, celiac disease, pernicious anemia, Addison's disease, myasthenia gravis, and vitiligo.

The pancreas is part of the network of *endocrine glands* (including the thyroid, ovaries, and adrenal glands; see page 182) that secrete hormones directly into the bloodstream. As insulin-producing pancreatic cells are progressively destroyed by an autoimmune attack, the body produces less and less insulin and becomes less able to convert food into glucose and bring it into cells. As a result, glucose accumulates in the bloodstream. The blood vessel damage caused by high glucose leads to heart attacks, stroke, kidney disease, and blindness. High glucose can also cause nerve damage, poor circulation, and tissue death in the legs, leading to amputations.

According to the American Diabetes Association (ADA), approximately 800,000 Americans are affected by type 1 diabetes. But it can produce few or no symptoms in its early stage. The blurry vision and extreme thirst Mary Kay experienced only occur after blood glucose is greatly elevated. While type 1 diabetes can come on abruptly during childhood or adolescence, researchers now believe many middle-aged people thought to have type 2 diabetes actually have type 1 diabetes, but are misdiagnosed because they don't have a dramatic loss of insulin. Type 1 diabetes is more common in Caucasians, while type 2 is more prevalent in Latina, Native American, African-American, and Asian-American women.

Warning Signs of Type 1 Diabetes

- Unusual or excessive thirst
- Frequent desire to urinate
- Weight loss
- Fatigue, excessive tiredness
- Blurred vision
- Severe itching in the lower legs
- Chronic vaginal yeast infections

Women with diabetes are at greater risk than nondiabetic women for heart disease and stroke. It's already possible to use antibody tests to identify those at high risk of type 1 diabetes, so those women could be treated with drugs or other forms of therapy to prevent the disease. And there's a very real possibility that new technologies, such as cell transplants and gene therapy, may soon provide a cure for people with type 1 diabetes.

What Causes Type 1 Diabetes?

In type 1 diabetes, autoantibodies target the insulin-producing *islet* (or *beta*) cells in the pancreas, proteins made by beta cells that sit on the cell surface, and even insulin itself. Other types of islet cells in the pancreas escape unharmed. Autoantibodies may be present years before symptoms of type 1 diabetes appear. In fact, 70 percent of people with type 1 diabetes screened for the Diabetes Prevention Trial had one or more of the diabetes autoantibodies but no symptoms. As many as 70 to 80 percent of people newly diagnosed with type 1 diabetes have antibodies to islet cells; 80 to 95 percent have antibodies to a protein made by beta cells called *glutamic acid decarboxylase* (*GAD*); two-thirds have antibodies to *insulinoma antigen-2* (*IA-2*); and up to half have antibodies to insulin. Type 1 diabetes can come on gradually, but people with more antibodies may develop it more quickly.

"There are a number of autoantibodies involved, but insulin and GAD appear to be the early targets of the attack in type 1 diabetes. The beta cells are destroyed, but they may actually be innocent bystanders of an immune attack on a virus that invades those cells," remarks Noel Maclaren, MD, PhD, director of the Cornell Juvenile Diabetes Program at the New York Weill Cornell Medical Center. Among the suspects are viruses that fool the immune system.

You'll recall that some viruses and bacteria may have the same shape as cells in the body, a phenomenon called *molecular mimicry*. A small area of the GAD protein on beta cells looks almost identical to a protein called P2-C on the *Coxsackie virus* (one of the family of viruses that causes polio) and was identified by Dr. Maclaren and colleagues as a likely candidate for molecular mimicry. During an infection, T-cells target an invading virus and destroy it. But once the infection is over, T-cells on the prowl may see the GAD protein sitting on beta cells, think it's a virus, and attack. Because viruses must first invade cells, some scientists believe they may change something about the islet cells that provokes a T-cell attack. The Coxsackie virus, as well as viruses that cause meningitis, are known to cause diabetes in animals, says Dr. Maclaren.

Other immune system problems also contribute to type 1 diabetes—among them, not having enough natural killer T-cells (NKT cells) or the helper T-cells that tell the NKT cells which cells to target and which to ignore (together these are classified as *T-regulatory cells*, or *T-REGS*), says Dr. Maclaren. "This is a necessary defect in type 1 diabetes; you have to have it or you won't get the disease. But people with type 1 diabetes have family members with other autoimmune diseases, so we think this may be a more general defect, especially in diseases associated with type 1 diabetes, like vitiligo, pernicious anemia, and gonadal autoimmunity," says Dr. Maclaren. "There are also degrees to this defect. Some people have a more severe problem."

In type 1 diabetes (and other autoimmune diseases), another step in the instruction of killer T-cells also goes awry. T-cell receptors, which function kind of like TV antennae, need to pick up a signal from *antigen presenting cells* (*APCs*) to tell them which cells are foreign invaders and which aren't. The APCs display bits of antigens on their surface within special molecules, kind of like hot dogs in a bun, explains Denise Faustman, MD, PhD, who heads the immunobiology laboratory at Massachusetts General Hospital. If the antigens are not properly displayed, or if the presentation process is somehow incomplete, the T-cells never get the message to bypass the beta cells, says Dr. Faustman.

The foods we eat are also "foreign" proteins. The process of digestion breaks down these proteins so that they don't provoke an immune reaction when they're absorbed into the bloodstream. Some experts have suggested over the years that proteins in cow's milk fed to children during the early months of life (before their systems can process it properly) may provoke an immune reaction that leads to diabetes. But the evidence for this is weak. In *celiac disease*, an autoimmune disease that often clusters with type 1 diabetes, a protein in wheat called *gluten* triggers an attack on the lining of the intestine (see page 226). Some experts say this often can precede the development of type 1 diabetes and may be an early warning sign of risk.

No matter what triggers the attack, as beta cells are progressively killed off, the pancreas produces less and less insulin. Insulin is critical to keeping the body's cellular machinery running smoothly, fueling our cells. Think of insulin as a gas pump, and your cells as tiny cars. The "gas" is blood glucose, processed by the body from sugar in carbohydrates (all carbohydrates— whether donuts or fruits—are technically sugar). If the gas pump isn't working properly, cells don't get enough fuel and start to starve. The excess fuel in the pump backs up and spills over into the blood, and over time that high glucose can damage your blood vessels, your eyes, your kidneys, and your nerves. Insulin also helps the body store extra fuel as fat; to get badly needed fuel, the body taps into this reserve, and that's why people with type 1 diabetes lose weight.

In young children, the destruction of beta cells and the loss of insulin can be dramatic, but in adults (especially older adults) it can occur more gradually. By the time type 1 diabetes is diagnosed in adults, the majority of the insulin-producing cells have been destroyed. While there's no way at present to reverse that loss, researchers say it may one day be possible to regrow beta cells or trigger their regeneration with gene therapy.

As with other autoimmune diseases, there's a genetic component to diabetes. Although the disease can run in families, 85 percent of people who develop it have no family history of the disease (although family members may have other autoimmune diseases). The risk for people with a parent or sibling with type 1 diabetes is about 6 percent; the risk is 30 percent among identical twins. Even nonidentical twins or siblings have a greater risk of getting type 1 diabetes than people without a family history. More than a half-dozen genes are associated with the disease; some are more common among certain ethnic groups (like Scandinavians), making them more vulnerable to environmental triggers, like viruses.

Mary Kay's story continues:

I went into a diabetic coma a few months after I was diagnosed with diabetes in 1984. I think it was the result of a collision of medical events, including surgery that preceded it by six months, and an infection I developed afterward. The night before I went into the coma I had gotten the flu, and being newly diabetic I wasn't aware that dehydration and the flu are very dangerous for diabetics; it shoots your glucose level way, way up. So even though I had taken my insulin that day, because I was so sick I got dehydrated. I developed ketoacidosis and went into a coma in my sleep. Fortunately, I was staying with a friend at the time, who noticed that my breathing was irregular the next morning and that I wouldn't awaken. I was in a coma for nine days. If I had been home it might not have been noticed right away. I was a single mother with two small children; they were seven and nine at the time, and I don't think they would have known to call 911. They know now. In fact, in the months following that, they did become quite frightened, and if I tried to sleep in on a Saturday morning, they would shake me and say "Mom, are you all right?"

Symptoms and Complications of Type 1 Diabetes

In healthy people, the body carefully regulates the amount of glucose and insulin in the blood. When blood glucose becomes elevated (such as after eating), more insulin is produced to help remove it; when glucose falls, insulin secretion drops. In people with diabetes, the body isn't producing insulin, so glucose builds up in the blood instead of being transported into cells.

High blood sugar, *hyperglycemia*, causes intense thirst, dry mouth, and frequent urination. (Some of the excess glucose leaks into the urine, and the excess glucose causes the kidneys to produce more urine, which can result in dehydration.) Your doctor can detect glucose levels by dipping a specially treated paper into a urine sample. When cells don't get enough glucose, the body starts breaking down fat to use for energy, which produces weight loss.

As fats are broken down for energy by the liver, waste products called *ketones* are produced.

If ketones build up faster than they can be excreted in urine, they begin to accumulate in the bloodstream, causing the blood to become acidic. This is called *diabetic ketoacidosis*, and it can come on suddenly with life-threatening consequences. In addition to the classic signs of hyperglycemia, ketoacidosis produces a fruity-smelling breath, shortness of breath, dry mouth, loss of appetite, nausea and vomiting, muscle weakness, dry flushed skin, blurry vision, and sleepiness. In severe cases, ketoacidosis can cause coma. (Symptoms are similar to Addison's disease—see page 185.)

Ketoacidosis is usually brought on by a sharp drop in insulin (if you forget to take a dose of insulin), but it can also be brought on by illness or a major life stress (like a car accident), says Carol J. Levy, MD, an attending endocrinologist at the Cornell Diabetes Center and a clinical professor of medicine at the Weill Medical College of Cornell University. "When you're under stress, stress hormones tell the liver to release stored glucose. But these hormones also block the effects of insulin," she explains. If your insulin is low to begin with, a bout with the flu or extreme stress could bring on ketoacidosis, which requires immediate treatment with insulin and fluids. The risk of ketoacidosis is 50 percent higher in women, according to the ADA.

Sometimes diabetes can cause (or be associated with) menstrual irregularities, infertility, and pregnancy complications, and it is associated with premature ovarian failure and an earlier menopause.

High blood glucose can damage blood vessels in the eye, leading to leakage of fluid in the tiny blood vessels behind the retina. *Diabetic retinopathy* is the most common cause of blindness in people aged twenty to seventy-five. Often the first sign of a problem is a blurring of vision.

Diabetes also damages the blood vessels in the legs, impeding circulation and causing pain (*intermittent claudication*) while walking. Women are seventy-six times more likely than men to suffer damage to small blood vessels in their extremities (*peripheral vascular disease, PVD*).

As blood supply to nerves is diminished, the nerves are damaged and don't send out pain signals when there's an injury. So you may not feel a small cut, and it can become ulcerated. If diabetic ulcers go untreated, the tissue can die and become gangrenous, and the limb may need to be amputated.

As glucose accumulates in the bloodstream, it can damage large blood vessels, making it easier for fatty plaques to accumulate inside artery walls, narrowing key arteries, and impeding blood supply to the heart. If those plaques rupture and form blood clots, it can completely block an artery, leading to heart attack and stroke. If you have diabetes, you're three to four times more likely to suffer a heart attack and stroke than nondiabetics because you lose the protective effects of estrogen on cholesterol and blood vessel flexibility.

You're also at increased risk of bone loss and hip fracture, which studies suggest is partly due to a hormonal disruption and to lower levels of vitamin D and magnesium. You can also have an overactive *parathyroid gland* (see page 189), which causes the body to leach calcium from the bones. So you may need regular bone-density scans and possibly bone-building drugs.

Between 10 and 21 percent of women with diabetes develop kidney disease. Damage to kidney cells, *diabetic nephropathy*, is the most common reason for kidney dialysis (needed to help rid the body of waste products) or a kidney transplant.

Diabetes also causes skin problems, including fungal infections in the corners of the mouth and under the breasts and armpits. One of the common symptoms of diabetes is itching brought on by dry skin and poor circulation, especially in the lower legs. Women can develop a skin condition called *diabetic dermopathy*, which produces brown spots, especially on the legs. Atherosclerosis can also affect the skin when it narrows blood vessels in the legs, causing it to thin and feel cool; your toenails may thicken and become discolored and your toes may feel cold. You can also suffer chronic vaginal yeast infections, gum disease, and infections of the tiny glands in the eyelid (*styes*).

Diagnosing Type 1 Diabetes

Unlike other autoimmune diseases, it's not necessary to test for autoantibodies to diagnose type 1 diabetes. A complete medical history, the presence of clinical symptoms (especially extreme thirst, frequent urination, and weight loss), and high blood glucose are all that's usually needed to confirm a diagnosis.

However, since some people can develop a late-onset disease that looks very much like type 2 diabetes, autoantibody testing may help to diagnose those cases, since almost everyone who develops type 1 diabetes has one or more autoantibodies at the onset of the disease, says Dr. Maclaren. In addition, if experimental treatments are proven to halt or prevent the destruction of beta cells, testing people at high risk may help find the disease in its earliest stages. In fact, genetic testing of newborns at risk for type 1 diabetes is now being conducted at several centers around the country, along with monitoring for autoantibodies. Such autoantibodies may begin to appear in early childhood. Tests for autoantibodies to insulin and GAD are currently available in commercial laboratories. Dr. Maclaren also recommends close family members be tested for autoimmune diseases, including type 1 diabetes. "In fact, among first-degree relatives we may find a small percentage who are beginning to be type 1 diabetic themselves. But just by measuring their blood sugar we'd have never known," he says.

"If someone has the classic symptoms of diabetes and they're not overweight, chances are it's type 1. If someone is very overweight, has a strong family history of type 2 diabetes, and no other symptoms other than elevated glucose, chances are it's type 2. But autoantibody screening can help separate less clear-cut cases," says Dr. Levy. "I routinely test women for autoimmune thyroid disease. If a woman has fatigue, irregular bowel habits, and trouble with certain types of foods, and if she has another autoimmune endocrine disease, I will test for celiac disease and send her to a gastroenterologist for diagnosis. If she has classic symptoms of Addison's—a change or darkening in skin color, fatigue, increasing hypoglycemia—I immediately screen for adrenal insufficiency."

Tests You May Need and What They Mean

Fasting plasma glucose (FPG) is the preferred blood test for diagnosing type 1 diabetes. The day before the test, your doctor will ask you not to eat for eight to ten hours. The next morning, a sample of your blood will be taken and the glucose level measured. Normally, your glucose would be 110 milligrams per deciliter (mg/dl) of blood after not eating for that many hours. But if you have diabetes, your glucose will be 126 mg/dl or over. Levels in between are considered impaired fasting glucose and indicate a high risk of developing diabetes.

Postprandial glucose may be an earlier indication of impending diabetes than an FPG for most patients, says Dr. Maclaren. Postprandial glucose is the level seen two hours after eating. In this test you're given oral glucose after an overnight fast. If postprandial glucose is over 200, then you have diabetes. If it's between 140 and 200, you have impaired glucose tolerance.

Urinalysis (for ketones, protein, and sediment, like red or white blood cells) is also done. The presence of ketones in the urine can indicate the beginnings of ketoacidosis. (It can also just mean that you haven't eaten for a long time.) Protein in the urine and sediment are signs of kidney dysfunction.

Since one out of every one hundred people with type 1 diabetes will develop Graves' disease, and one in twenty will develop Hashimoto's thyroiditis, your doctor will likely order a test to measure **thyroid stimulating hormone** (TSH).

You and your immediate family also run a high risk (approximately one in twenty) of developing celiac disease. Many people with celiac are asymptomatic, and if the condition goes untreated it can lead to anemia, bone loss, and even cancer. Diagnosing it early can help prevent those problems.

Measuring the level of vitamin B$_{12}$ and folic acid in your blood helps to diagnose pernicious anemia. One in fifty adults with type 1 diabetes also develops pernicious anemia, an autoimmune disease in which the stomach is unable to absorb vitamin B$_{12}$; telltale symptoms include anemia and weakness. Testing for autoantibodies against the *parietal* cells in the stomach lining indicates autoimmune disease; low plasma B$_{12}$ indicates malabsorption.

Mary Kay's story continues:

The hardest thing about diabetes isn't choosing foods, but making yourself eat when you're not hungry and not always being able to eat when you are hungry. I mix two kinds of insulin in my morning injection, Humulin R and Humulin N; one is long-acting and the other is short-acting. You need to eat breakfast, and I was never a breakfast eater; and you need to eat approximately four hours after your first injection. My appetite has always been zero first thing in the morning, and it sort of grows during the day. Everyone thinks it must be hard or painful to give yourself shots, because we all remember those painful immunizations we got as kids. But it's really not like that at all. In fact, I don't really feel the injections; they have these itty-bitty fine needles now. I think the most difficult part is balancing diet and insulin. You don't just get to eat when you're hungry anymore; you eat when you have to. The most difficult part for me is the constant paying attention to eating. I mean, diabetes makes you eat a healthy diet. And you can certainly lead a normal life with it. But my schedule is so irregular and I travel so much that I really have to plan well. It means never going anywhere without candy bars or fruit in your purse, in case your blood sugar gets too low, and never getting caught without food. And always making sure if you've taken your insulin shot, to eat within four hours. It's been almost twenty years, and after that amount of time I can tell when my glucose is low. I can feel the symptoms of hypoglycemia before it really gets bad. For me, it feels very much like a hot flash. And I have such a rapid metabolism, I never seem to get enough calories.

Treating Type 1 Diabetes

The goal of treatment in type 1 diabetes is to keep blood sugar levels normal, or as close to normal as possible. Replacement insulin is needed to achieve that tight control, along with a well-managed diet, regular exercise, and avoidance of obesity. The *Diabetes Control and Complications Trial* (*DCCT*), a major clinical trial involving 1,441 men and women, showed that tight control can help slow the development and progression of complications of diabetes, especially diabetic retinopathy.

Replacing Insulin

How much insulin you need depends on your glucose level, and that requires testing blood glucose throughout the day (see page 169). After you eat, the body normally releases just enough insulin to process glucose; with a schedule of insulin injections timed before meals, you can mimic the normal release of insulin. As Mary Kay does, some women use a combination of long- and short-acting insulins. If a woman is eating three meals a day (and one or two snacks), she might use a short-acting insulin just before each meal, and inter-mediate- or long-acting insulin once or twice a day to maintain a basic-level (*basal*) insulin. Some women wear insulin pumps that can be programmed to release different doses of insulin at different times of the day. "The only issue for some women is body image; you have to wear a pump twenty-four hours a day, seven days a week, and some women don't feel comfortable with that," says Dr. Levy. Insulin pumps are also useful in pregnancy, when blood sugars can be erratic, she adds.

Your body may respond better to a particular type of insulin, or a combi-nation of insulin preparations, says Dr. Levy. The most commonly used are human insulins produced by genetic engineering, which act just like natural insulin. Some are faster-acting than others. For example, a rapid-acting human insulin (*human lispro*) goes to work within five to fifteen minutes, while regu-lar insulin (*Humulin R*) takes up to an hour to begin working. (There's also a rapid-acting synthetic insulin, or insulin analogue, *lispro*). Fast-acting insulins last around four hours in the body. In contrast, an intermediate-acting insulin (*human Lente*) reaches the blood within three to four hours and takes a longer time to be absorbed (up to eighteen hours). Long-acting insulin (*human Ultralente*) takes six to ten hours to reach the bloodstream and can be effective for up to twenty hours. "If a woman is eating a lowfat diet, which many women do, she'll do much better with short-acting insulins or insulin analogues in combination with a new insulin called *glargine* (*Lantus*). How-ever, if you go out to dinner and eat higher-fat items, like pizza, then these insulins don't work as well," says Dr. Levy. Taking several injections of fast-acting insulin can give you more flexibility in planning meals (you can take a little extra to cover a second helping of pasta, for example).

You can mix insulins yourself or buy premixed preparations, depending on the regimen you choose. Insulin therapy is a highly individualized process that should be worked out with a specially trained health care provider, such as a certified diabetes educator. A diabetes educator can also help you learn to give yourself injections and learn to use an insulin pump. An inhaled form of insulin is also being tested. (An indispensable reference to help you manage insulin treatment is the *American Diabetes Association Complete Guide to Dia-betes*; see Appendix B for more information.)

Pregnancy and oral estrogens can also affect blood glucose and the amount of insulin you need, so you may need more frequent glucose testing if you've just begun taking oral contraceptives or hormone replacement. Illness and stress can also affect glucose, requiring adjustments in insulin.

You need to match the amount of insulin you take with the amount of food you eat (which raises glucose) and the amount of exercise you get (which lowers glucose). But even if you ate the same amount of food each day and exercised the same amount daily, your need for insulin could still fluctuate, so self-monitoring of glucose is vital.

Glucose Self-Monitoring

If your goal is keeping glucose levels as close to normal as possible, you may need to test up to five times a day. The standard times to self-test are before breakfast, lunch, and dinner (and before eating a larger snack), one to two hours after eating, and before bedtime. According to new guidelines set by the ADA, acceptable blood glucose ranges are 80 to 120 milligrams per deciliter of blood (mg/dl) before meals, and 100 to 140 mg/dl before bedtime. People without diabetes generally have a glucose level of less than 110 mg/dl before meals, and under 120 mg/dl before going to bed, but you may not be able to achieve those levels.

Glucose home monitoring is usually done with a disposable pinlike device; you prick a finger to produce a drop of blood and apply it to a specially treated piece of paper or to a handheld glucose meter. A newly approved device (*GlucoWatch*) is worn like a wristwatch and senses the amount of glucose in the skin; another is a continuous monitoring device (*MiniMed Continuous Glucose Monitoring System*). However you test, you should keep track of the results in a small book. The patterns you see (for example, a rise in glucose after eating certain foods, or during the premenstrual period) can help you make adjustments in your insulin intake.

The 2002 ADA Diabetes Diet Guidelines

In the past, women with diabetes were told to avoid sugary foods because they would send blood glucose soaring. But new dietary guidelines from the American Diabetes Association (ADA) say it's OK to have sweets occasionally—as long as your blood sugar levels are well controlled.

According to the guidelines, issued in January 2002, it's not so important what kind of carbohydrates you eat, but that you keep an eye on your total carbohydrate intake. However, you are advised to

- eat more nutritious carbohydrates, like fruits, vegetables, and whole grains;
- limit saturated fat to under 10 percent of daily calories;
- restrict cholesterol to less than 300 milligrams a day;
- limit sodium to 2,400 milligrams a day;
- cut back on trans-fats; and
- eat more fiber.

"I let my patients eat what they want as long as they can appropriately cover it with insulin and exercise," remarks Dr. Levy. "As long as you eat a health-ful diet, there are no limitations if you don't have problems with weight or cholesterol. But you really need to be careful to balance your carbohydrate intake."

People with type 1 diabetes may process protein faster, but because most of us eat 50 percent more protein than we need (15 to 20 percent of daily calories), you won't suffer protein deficiency. If you follow a vegetarian diet, be sure to include plant proteins (like beans, nuts, sweet potatoes, and avo-cado) to avoid deficiency.

Calorie-free sweeteners approved by the FDA—such as saccharine (Sweet'n Low, Sugar Twin), aspartame (Nutrasweet), and sucralose (Splenda)—can safely be used by people with diabetes. But the ADA advises staying away from fructose (often used to sweeten soft drinks).

Alcohol can cause both high and low blood sugar, depending on the amount that's consumed and whether it's taken with food. It can also raise blood pressure. But moderate alcohol consumption is not harmful, so follow the standard recommendation for women of one or fewer drinks per day (one drink is 12 ounces of beer, 5 ounces of wine, or 1.5 ounces of spirits).

The ADA guidelines stress that regular exercise is as important as diet to maintain normal blood sugar. In fact, moderate exercise can lower blood sugar to the extent that you may even need less insulin. Exercise can also help raise HDL cholesterol and lower blood pressure, which can lessen the risk of car-diovascular complications, notes Dr. Levy.

The DCCT showed that people who received intensive diabetes care had significantly less diabetic retinopathy, neuropathy, and other complications over a six-year period. Intensive diabetes care means a solid education in controlling glucose; balancing diet, exercise, and insulin; and the support of an active health care team (including a diabetes nurse specialist, a dietitian, and a physician) to provide regular followup.

Your care team can also help you reduce the risk of heart attack and stroke. Your goals are to keep blood pressure below 130 mm Hg systolic and less than 80 mm Hg (the resting rate) and maintain total cholesterol under 200 mg/dl (with HDL above 50 mg/dl).

Women who develop high blood pressure or kidney disease will need medications to control those conditions, such as angiotensin-converting enzyme (ACE) inhibitors. If retinopathy develops, there are treatments to coagulate leaky blood vessels and prevent vision loss with laser therapy.

Avoiding Hypoglycemia

The one time sugar *does* come in handy is during an episode of *hypoglycemia*, or low blood glucose. This can occur if you don't take enough insulin, skip a meal or a snack, eat a meal unusually late, or drink alcohol on an empty stomach. You can also suffer low blood sugar if you exercise too vigorously (it can even occur during sex). Even if you're doing everything right, you can still have an episode of hypoglycemia, since the body may not always use insulin consistently; hypoglycemia is also more common during pregnancy. Warning signs can occur at any time, even waking you up from a sound sleep (sometimes you may have a nightmare, due to the effects of low blood sugar on the brain). Symptoms include:

- Shakiness
- Dizziness
- Sweating
- Feeling faint
- Rapid heartbeat
- Headache
- Hunger
- Chills

- Clammy, pale skin
- Confusion, difficulty concentrating
- Sleepiness
- Clumsy or jerky movements
- Sudden mood changes, like sadness or anxiety

The first thing to do when those symptoms hit is to test your glucose—hypoglycemia is generally considered to be a glucose level of 50 mg/dl or under, but some women can have symptoms with slightly higher levels. If glucose is low, eat something containing sugar. It's a good idea to carry things like hard candy to help raise glucose quickly if needed; you can also carry glucose tablets, available in most drugstores. Something as simple as a half-cup of orange juice or a handful of raisins (both of which contain 10 to 15 grams of carbohydrates) can raise your blood sugar and head off a more serious reaction, such as seizures or loss of consciousness. After you've eaten, wait fifteen to twenty minutes and then retest. Sometimes, you may need a second snack to get your blood glucose back to where it should be. Even if you don't have your test kit with you, treat hypoglycemia immediately.

After you've had diabetes for a number of years, it's not unusual to lose the ability to feel the early warning signs, and you may suffer from more severe

---

Type 1 Diabetes Clusters

There's a high risk of thyroid disease in type 1 diabetes, and it can also occur in the autoimmune polyglandular syndrome type 2 (page 188). Diseases that cluster with type 1 diabetes include:

- Thyroid disease
- Celiac disease
- Alopecia areata
- Premature ovarian failure
- Addison's disease
- Myasthenia gravis
- Pernicious anemia
- Vitiligo

---

episodes. *Hypoglycemia unawareness* can also occur during pregnancy. This is another reason why testing is crucial.

Mary Kay's story continues:
I was diagnosed with thyroid disease a couple of years ago during a routine wellness exam, and I have been taking a very low dose of Synthroid ever since. My doctor said it was "borderline" hypothyroidism. There was no history of diabetes in my family or other autoimmune diseases; no arthritis, no thyroid disease. When they were searching for the cause of my lung nodules in 1984, I was tested for lupus and for rheumatoid arthritis, and all those tests were negative. But here I am with thyroid disease and diabetes. And my brother has the same lung nodules I had, so it's possible that there is some genetic component . . . but he hasn't had a diagnosis of sarcoid. And they only found the lung nodules by accident with a routine x-ray. He was also diagnosed with gout, and that's a form of arthritis. So there could be something.

What's Next?

Researchers are hard at work to make the insulin-food-exercise juggling act of type 1 diabetes a thing of the past. Tests are being conducted in humans and animals of gene therapy, immune-based therapies, vaccines, and islet cell transplants, and many researchers say a true cure may be possible.

Transplants of islet cells have met with some success. A study of seventeen patients in Canada who underwent islet cell transplantation found that the benefits seem long-lasting. A report in the July 2002 journal *Diabetes* said more than half of the patients do not need insulin injections an average two years after the treatment. The downside is a lifetime of immunosuppressant drugs. But researchers from Harvard Medical School say they may be able to help people *regrow* islet cells—and even get rid of the immune cells that attack the pancreas. Working with lab mice bred to have type 1 diabetes (non-obese diabetic or NOD mice), the researchers first made the attacking T-cells self-destruct by exposing them to the inflammatory agent *tumor necrosis factor alpha* (*TNFα*), they then coaxed the remaining T-cells into growing normally, so they would not attack the islet cells. Once the enemy was gone, the remaining cells started to grow again, and no further immune attacks took place.

"The surprising thing was that the treatment was fairly short, 40 days, and it totally eliminated the autoimmune disease for the life of the animals," remarks Dr. Denise Faustman, who headed the study. "Humans have the same defects in T-cells that cause them to attack islet cells, so the treatment would be the same. The only thing we don't know is if humans have similar regenerative potential. But we now have a therapy that works in established autoimmunity."

Dr. Maclaren's team at Cornell is investigating another potential therapy that would stimulate underactive regulatory T-cells. "There's a deep sea sponge off the coast of Japan that has a lipid compound called *alpha-galactosylceramide* that strongly stimulates NKT cells. And so far three groups have reported that giving this compound to NOD mice can prevent diabetes," he explains. Human trials of the sea sponge extract are being planned.

An insulin-based vaccine is also under investigation, aimed at directly preventing the attack on insulin-producing cells. "We found that insulin is an important early target in type 1 diabetes in women and in the NOD mice. In mice, the attack on beta cells is directed at insulin, and by reeducating immune cells to make a nondestructive response to insulin, we can completely prevent beta cell destruction," says Dr. Maclaren. "In our studies, after we gave the mice the insulin-based vaccine, we virtually eliminated diabetes for life. If we had not treated them, 85 percent of the female mice would have developed diabetes and died of it." Dr. Maclaren hopes to test the vaccine in women newly diagnosed with type 1 diabetes to see whether the destruction of beta cells can be halted.

Another promising new treatment involves coaxing stem cells into becoming insulin-producing beta cells. The experiment, done with embryonic stem cells (which are known for their ability to transform into almost every cell type), might provide a better strategy for growing beta cells than merely transplanting normal beta cells. Scientists are also experimenting with transplanting beta cells from genetically modified pigs engineered so the cells would not be rejected. Potential gene therapy would infuse into the pancreas cells that lack genetic defects that lead to type 1 diabetes.

An experimental drug called *DiaPep277* is in clinical trials in humans and has been shown to halt the progression of type 1 diabetes, prevent destruction of beta cells, and reduce the need for insulin in a small group of newly diagnosed patients. Researchers from Hadassah Hebrew University Medical School and the Weizmann Institute of Science in Israel tested the drug in a ten-month randomized trial among thirty-five men, half of whom received injections of a placebo and half of whom received DiaPep277. The drug seemed to "reeducate" the immune system, halting attacks on beta cells. It did not suppress the entire system, as existing therapies do. It's not yet known if the drug will work as well in women, and clinical trials are continuing.

How Type 1 Diabetes Affects You Over Your Lifetime

Many women with type 1 diabetes were diagnosed during their teenage years, and there's an interaction between the disease and hormonal factors during the reproductive years.

Menstruation and Fertility

Women diagnosed with type 1 diabetes in adolescence often get their periods late (at age 13.5, versus the average age of 12.5), and more than a third have menstrual irregularities. These problems can include the absence of periods (*amenorrhea*) due to anovulation, scanty periods (*oligomenorrhea*), and more frequent menstrual cycles (*polymenorrhea*) with less time in between periods.

The fluctuating levels of hormones that underlie these problems can make it harder to control blood glucose. Some studies suggest that high progesterone may affect the action of insulin within cells, causing a slight insulin resistance and raising blood glucose. At the same time, elevated estrogen levels may improve the action of insulin, so blood glucose may be lower than normal when estrogen is high or "unopposed" by progesterone.

The high levels of both estrogen and progesterone during the premenstrual period can wreak havoc with blood glucose. "Women with diabetes who have this problem typically complain that their blood glucose is elevated during the week before they get their period, then after they get their period, their sugars come crashing down," says Dr. Levy. "Or, some women will tell me their sugars are crazy at certain times of the month and they can't figure out why. So I will have them chart their glucose in relation to their cycles, which is very helpful. It enables us to tailor the insulin regimen to different times in the menstrual cycle."

For example, if you have regular menstrual cycles, your insulin dose may be increased the week before your period. Once you get your period, the dose may be cut back. "Some women don't have predictable cycles, so they don't know when they are going to get those glucose highs and lows. And other women have pretty severe fluctuations in spite of everything. Those women, we put on birth control pills to stabilize their cycle, to make things more predictable," says Dr. Levy.

Monophasic birth control pills (which do not change the hormone levels during the 21 days you take the pill) may help minimize changes in blood glucose. Women who have high blood pressure or peripheral vascular disease or who smoke should not take the pill. Progesterone can cause elevations in glucose, and pills containing newer forms, such as *gestodene, desogestrel, norgestrel*, and *norgestimate*, can make a huge difference, says Dr. Levy. "The risks with birth control pills are in the amount of estrogen, which can increase the risk of blood clots in some women, and the newer pills have a much lower estrogen dose." Some newer progestins may also have less clotting risk.

If you seem to have lower than usual blood sugar right before your period, discuss with your doctor the advisability of gradually reducing the dose premenstrually. And you may want to up your carbohydrate intake (but go for the healthier carbs, like fresh vegetables). Cut back on alcohol, chocolate, and caffeine; they can affect blood glucose as well as mood. Stick with your meal plans and eat at regular intervals, since large blood glucose swings can affect mood, exacerbating PMS.

If you have type 1 diabetes, you may have menstrual irregularities, which may make it harder to predict when you'll get your period, possibly interfering with your ability to become pregnant. A study in the August 2001 issue of *Diabetes* by researchers at the University of Pittsburgh comparing 143 women with type 1 diabetes to 186 nondiabetic women found that almost 46 percent of women with type 1 diabetes had menstrual irregularities before age thirty. In women who don't ovulate or menstruate, estrogen is produced but not progesterone (which triggers shedding of the menstrual lining each month). The *Diabetes* study found that, on average, women with type 1 diabetes have a 17 percent decrease in the number of their reproductive years.

"Women with type 1 diabetes have more anovulatory cycles, but the reasons for this are not well understood," comments Mary Loeken, PhD, senior investigator in the Research Division at the Joslin Diabetes Center in Boston and an assistant professor of medicine at Harvard Medical School. "One of the things we do know is that you need to have a certain amount of fat mass in order to cycle appropriately. Just as athletes who overtrain and lose too much body fat stop cycling, women with type 1 diabetes may lack sufficient fat, especially if the disease is not well controlled. One of the hormones secreted by fat is leptin. It's associated with weight gain, but it's also required for menstruation. There are leptin receptors in the brain, and this may trigger the release of neurotransmitters that control the hypothalamus and the pituitary, and in turn the ovaries."

You also need a certain amount of body fat to maintain a pregnancy, adds Dr. Loeken. "So leptin production is nature's way of ensuring that the mother will be nutritionally able to support the pregnancy. In addition, ovarian hormones are also needed to build up the lining of the uterus. If a woman's glucose is out of control, she may have enough body fat to ovulate and conceive, but not enough for normal hormone production, so the embryo will not implant in the uterus. It may die before it's implanted. Women with type 1 diabetes may have unrecognized early miscarriages."

If you have menstrual irregularities, a home ovulation test kit can be helpful, as can taking basal (morning) body temperature, which is normally 98.6 degrees and may rise as much as 1.5 degrees at ovulation.

Pregnancy and Lactation

Diabetes can lead to a number of complications during pregnancy, including a higher risk of *preeclampsia* (high blood pressure) and *toxemia*, a disorder characterized by high blood pressure, protein in the urine, headaches, and fluid retention (*edema*).

Pregnancy may increase the need for insulin and for more frequent glucose testing. "Once you become pregnant, there are a lot of changes in the energy requirements, not just for the mother but for the developing embryo, which, because it's growing so rapidly, consumes a lot of glucose. So the mother needs to be able to provide enough fuel," explains Dr. Loeken. "The body also reacts to hormones produced during pregnancy by very rapidly increasing the production of adrenal steroid hormones, mostly cortisol. Those hormones interfere with the action of insulin. They increase glucose output by the liver, change fat composition of the body, and mobilize fat for energy."

However, you need to get your glucose under tight control if you're even thinking about becoming pregnant, says Dr. Loeken. "The formation of major organ structures takes place about the time a woman misses her period and first suspects she's pregnant. If a woman's glucose levels go too high, those organ systems may be formed in an abnormal way and the baby develops a congenital malformation. A woman doesn't usually have her first obstetrics appointment until around eleven weeks, and by then a malformation may have already occurred. So it's important to discuss with your doctor your plans to become pregnant so you can maintain tight glucose control from the start."

While developmental problems can arise in the second or third trimester, birth defects are less likely to occur because the organ systems are already formed. Congenital abnormalities can occur in as many as 6 to 12 percent of babies born to women with diabetes. Potential problems can include abnormalities of the heart, kidney, and central nervous system.

Keeping tight control of blood glucose and carefully monitoring the baby's growth can prevent these problems and others, including having a large baby (*macrosomia*, which can lead to a cesarean section) and lung problems. "If the mother is hyperglycemic, glucose is delivered to the fetus at a high concentration and the baby's pancreas responds by producing insulin. Insulin acts like a growth factor in a fetus. So you get growth of the long bones, you get a lot of glycogen storage in the liver and fat deposition, you get a big baby," explains Dr. Loeken. "Insulin also interferes with fetal adrenal steroids that stimulate lung maturation. So high insulin can hamper maturation of the baby's lungs, and the baby can suffer from respiratory distress syndrome."

Because of the genetic component of type 1 diabetes, a child has a greater risk of developing diabetes some time in his or her life if either parent is affected. However, for reasons we don't understand, the risk is six times less if the mother has diabetes than if the father does.

Breastfeeding can lead to low blood sugar. Your glucose levels drop as your baby takes in your milk, and you could have more frequent episodes of hypoglycemia. You may need to take in extra calories and drink a beverage before and right after you nurse, and you should monitor your glucose more frequently to adjust your insulin dose.

Pregnant women with type 1 diabetes have an increased risk of gum inflammation (*periodontitis*) and periodontal disease, and the damage can be more severe. So get regular dental care.

An important note here about gestational diabetes (GD): This temporary, type 2–like form of diabetes, which develops during pregnancy, is *not* an autoimmune disease and usually resolves itself after delivery. However, in a small percentage of cases, what appears to be GD may actually be the onset of type 1. "Because we screen every woman for gestational diabetes, sometimes it may actually unmask type 1 diabetes and we can treat a woman before she gets into trouble," remarks Dr. Levy. "If your diabetes doesn't go away after you deliver, you're not overweight, and you don't have a strong family history of diabetes, we have to consider whether this is actually early type 1 diabetes."

> Mary Kay's story continues:
> *I started taking estrogen replacement therapy in my mid-forties. I was having very, very strong premenopausal symptoms. I am Irish, and thin, and my mom has been on estrogen for a long time to prevent osteoporosis. So when I started having menopausal symptoms, I didn't feel it was dangerous for me to take estrogen—actually, the opposite. For the first month I was on estrogen, I doubled my daily blood testing to see if taking estrogen would affect my glucose level or increase my need for insulin. It didn't, in my case. But I was also switching from one kind of insulin to a more human insulin, so that may have made a difference. My gynecologist never told me to increase my daily testing, even though she knew I was diabetic. I knew about gestational diabetes, how high estrogen affects glucose, and it just made sense to me that taking estrogen could affect my need for insulin. I had no idea that diabetes could bring on menopause early. My gynecologist never mentioned it. But my mother went through menopause in her fifties, and I was in my forties, so I guess I was about six years earlier than my mother.*

Menopause and Beyond

Just when you thought you'd gotten the hang of controlling those monthly blood glucose swings, you start to approach menopause and things are thrown out of kilter again. Perimenopause can occur any time after age thirty-five, and, far from being a long decline in estrogen, this transition period can be a hormonal roller-coaster ride, with irregular periods and months where you don't ovulate at all. Increases in hormones can boost blood sugar; decreases can send it plummeting. Low-dose birth control pills can help regulate your cycle.

Recent studies suggest that women with diabetes undergo an earlier menopause, sometimes by six to seven years. An August 2001 study in *Diabetes* found that women with diabetes went through menopause at an average age of 41.6, compared to their nondiabetic counterparts, whose average age at menopause was closer to 50. "There's just something about type 1 that totally disrupts the regulatory cycle for menses, and some women develop a condition called *hypothalamic amenorrhea*. No one knows why type 1 women develop it, but the pituitary gland just shuts off. We're unsure of the reasons for this, but it might be dependent on blood sugar control," remarks Dr. Levy. "We will measure estrogen and follicle stimulating hormone (FSH) in women who have trouble getting pregnant or whose periods stop. If estrogen levels are low and FSH is high, you've gone through menopause."

During this period, episodes of hypoglycemia may become more frequent and more severe. Low blood sugar can disrupt your sleep, along with hot flashes. In fact, menopausal symptoms can be confused with low (or high) blood sugar, especially moodiness and inability to concentrate or short-term memory loss.

You'll need to test glucose more frequently during the menopausal transition. Loss of estrogen after menopause can decrease the body's sensitivity to insulin, requiring adjustments in your insulin dose. Estrogen loss can also increase your risk of osteoporosis; a recent study in *Diabetes Care* found that women with type 1 diabetes were more than twelve times more likely to report hip fractures compared to nondiabetics. For women with osteoporosis, the new once-a-week formulations of *alendronate* (*Fosamax*) or *risedronate* (*Actonel*) can make these drugs easier to take. You're also at increased risk of high blood pressure and high cholesterol—both risk factors for heart disease—and those problems may need to be treated separately with appropriate medications.

Dr. Levy believes there's no reason why women with type 1 diabetes who don't have significant risk factors for cardiovascular disease can't take low-dose estrogen for menopausal symptoms, as long as it's taken with progestin to prevent overgrowth of the uterine lining. Combination hormone replacement therapy (HRT) with estrogen and progestin can help combat the effects of hormone loss on glucose levels and make them easier to regulate. "It is true that diabetic women have a higher risk of cardiovascular disease, but in studies that suggest estrogen can worsen coronary disease, the risk in nondiabetic women appears to be due to blood clotting, and it may well be the type of estrogen," she comments. "In my clinical experience, I have seen type 1 diabetes improve with HRT." Dr. Levy believes there's no reason why women with type 1 diabetes who don't have risk factors for cardiovascular disease can't take low-dose estrogen for menopausal symptoms, as long as it's taken with progestin to prevent overgrowth of the uterine lining. Hormone replacement therapy (HRT) with estrogen and progestin can help combat the effects of hormone loss on glucose levels and make them easier to regulate. "It is true that diabetic women have a higher risk of cardiovascular disease, but in studies that suggest estrogen can worsen coronary disease, the risk in nondiabetic women appears to be due to blood clotting and it may well be the type of estrogen," she comments. "In my clinical experience, I have seen type 1 diabetes improve with HRT." Recent studies show that HRT can not only increase the risk of heart disease and stroke, but that progestin may also increase the risk of breast cancer (see page 45). These are important issues to discuss with your physician.

The combination of diabetes and menopause can also affect your sex life. Reduced circulation to the genital area may make it harder to lubricate during arousal and more difficult to achieve orgasms. The normal decline in testosterone can also lower your sex drive. Again, some form of hormone therapy may help (see HRT, pages 44 to 45).

Autoimmune diseases that affect other components of the endocrine system in women include *Addison's disease (adrenal insufficiency), hypoparathyroidism,* and *premature autoimmune ovarian failure* (or premature menopause). Ovarian failure can also occur as part of an *autoimmune polyglandular syndrome* and in connective tissue diseases such as lupus. Ovarian autoimmune disease itself has only recently been recognized as a single entity.

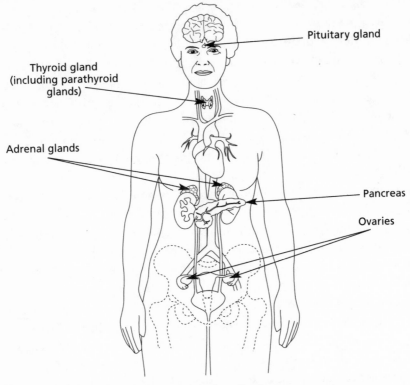

Pituitary gland

Thyroid gland
(including parathyroid
glands)

Adrenal glands

Pancreas

Ovaries

The Endocrine System

The ductless glands of the endocrine system—the thyroid, pancreas, pituitary, and adrenal glands—secrete hormones that affect almost every body function, including reproduction. You may not think of the ovaries as endocrine glands, but sex hormones (estrogen and androgens) are actually steroid hormones that regulate not only reproduction but many other functions in the body. For example, estrogen is needed to maintain bone density.

The endocrine glands also aid our responses to internal or external stimuli. The adrenal glands secrete certain "stress" hormones (like *adrenaline*, also known as *epinephrine*) to assist us in the primitive *fight-or-flight* syndrome by increasing heart rate and breathing, and pushing more blood into the muscles. Endocrine cells can also be found in other organs (like *gastric cells* in the stomach).

Warning Signs of Autoimmune Endocrine Disorders

- Weight loss, fatigue, muscle weakness, brown patches on the skin, low blood pressure (Addison's disease)
- Hot flashes, irregular or stopped periods, infertility (premature ovarian failure)
- Numbness or tingling in the extremities, muscle cramps, anxiety, depression (hypoparathyroidism)

Like the thyroid, other endocrine organs are regulated in a feedback loop by the hypothalamus, an area in the brain that makes *releasing hormones.* These releasing hormones send a signal to the pituitary, which in turn sends out a chemical messenger to stimulate other endocrine glands. In the case of the ovaries, one chemical messenger is *follicle stimulating hormone (FSH),* which stimulates the *follicles* to secrete estrogen and to produce an egg each month. Not surprisingly, when one of the endocrine glands isn't working right, it can throw off the entire system.

But endocrine disorders don't usually come on dramatically; they develop gradually over a period of years, and you may not even pay much attention. The diagnosis usually involves blood tests for hormone deficiency, and the treatment is replacing the lost hormone (or hormones).

Addison's Disease

Of nonthyroid autoimmune endocrine disorders, Addison's disease—the autoimmune destruction of the adrenal glands—is the most common among women, typically occurring during the twenties and thirties. In half of those women Addison's occurs as an isolated disorder, and in the other half it occurs as part of a *polyglandular endocrine disorder* (see page 188) or along with other autoimmune diseases.

The two triangular-shaped adrenal glands, which sit atop the kidneys, are actually two organs in one. The outer region, called the *adrenal cortex*, secretes steroid hormones like *cortisol* (also called *hydrocortisone*), which affects metabolism (how we use food and tap into stored energy) and suppresses inflammation in the body; *aldosterone*, which regulates the amount of salt excreted by the kidneys (helping to maintain blood pressure and blood volume); and small amounts of male hormones, or *androgens*. (The hydrocortisone produced by the adrenal glands is a naturally occurring form of corticosteroid drugs used to dampen inflammation in autoimmune disease.)

The amount of steroid hormones secreted by the adrenal cortex is regulated by a feedback loop with the hypothalamus and the pituitary gland. On a chemical signal (a releasing factor) from the hypothalamus, the pituitary sends out *adrenocorticotropic hormone* (*ACTH*), which directly stimulates the adrenal cortex. ACTH is actually produced in a twenty-four-hour cycle, peaking around six o'clock in the morning and falling slowly during the day to hit its lowest level around midnight. If levels of hydrocortisone get too high, it inhibits ACTH production and slows secretion of hydrocortisone. Emotional stress or injury can stimulate the release of ACTH and hydrocortisone, which the body needs to bounce back from stress.

The inner region of the adrenal gland, called the *medulla*, is linked to the *sympathetic nervous system* and reacts to emotional and physical stresses by secreting hormones like *epinephrine* and *norepinephrine* (also called *noradrenaline*).

What Causes Addison's?

In Addison's disease, autoantibodies attack the steroid-producing cells of the adrenal cortex, causing inflammation and fibrosis that prevent hormone secretion, and eventually completely destroy the cortex. *Adrenocortical autoantibodies* can target cells that produce specific hormones (autoantibodies can also block ACTH).

There's a genetic component to Addison's (most often in women with adrenal disease associated with autoimmune polyglandular syndrome), but less than a third of women with Addison's have a family history of the disease. Genes associated with Addison's (like DR3) are also linked to Graves' disease and other autoimmune diseases. It's mainly a disease of reproductive-age women but "we don't know what precisely predisposes women to Addison's disease," remarks Paul W. Ladenson, MD, professor and director of the division of endocrinology at Johns Hopkins. "It appears that a variety of genes may be involved, some of which may be gender related, but that does not explain why adrenal insufficiency is more common in women."

Symptoms of Addison's Disease

When the adrenal glands are not working properly, it can cause low blood pressure, often in the form of *postural hypotension* (or *orthostatic hypotension*), where you feel faint as blood pressure suddenly drops when you go from lying down to sitting up, or from sitting to standing. "Addison's disease can present with very nonspecific complaints, such as fatigue or loss of appetite, which makes it hard to recognize," comments Dr. Ladenson. "But almost everyone with this disease has lost weight, whereas most people who have similar symptoms for other reasons have not."

Very often a woman may have a minor illness (like stomach flu) or a physical stress, become extremely dehydrated, and have an episode of low blood pressure that lands them in an emergency room, says Dr. Ladenson. "It's not unusual for a woman to have a history of emergency room visits before an alert physician notices a pattern and picks up on the possibility of Addison's. Laboratory abnormalities, such as low urinary sodium, high potassium, and high calcium, are clues that would prompt a good physician to look for adrenal insufficiency."

In an acute adrenal crisis there can be fever, low blood pressure, abdominal pain, and even delirium. Chronic symptoms include loss of appetite, weight loss, fatigue, nausea, diarrhea, abdominal pain, anemia, and orthostatic hypotension. A darkening of the skin and mucous membranes may also occur. "The hardest part of making the diagnosis is to think of the possibility of Addison's disease, because the laboratory testing for it is very straightforward," comments Dr. Ladenson.

Diagnosing Addison's

A number of laboratory tests will be run to determine whether your symptoms are due to adrenal insufficiency. The adrenal glands produce salt-retaining hormones (aldosterone), glucocorticoids (cortisol), and weak androgens. Your cortisol level will be measured before and after administration of synthetic ACTH, and imaging of the adrenal glands may also be done to rule out tumors.

However, an intravenous infusion of 100 milligrams of hydrocortisone is usually given immediately when an adrenal crisis is suspected, and followed with 100 milligrams every eight hours until the crisis has passed or the diagnosis of Addison's is confirmed.

Tests You May Need and What They Mean

Adrenocorticotropic hormone (ACTH) is elevated in Addison's. Normally, the ACTH level at midnight should be half of that in the morning (20 to 100 picograms per milliliter of blood [pg/ml]).

Cortisol is measured before an injection or intravenous infusion of synthetic ACTH, *cosyntropin* (*Cortrosyn*). Then cortisol is measured thirty minutes and an hour later, explains Dr. Ladenson. Cortisol levels that fail to rise to more than 20 micrograms per deciliter of blood (mcg/dl) with administration of ACTH confirm the diagnosis of adrenal insufficiency.

Blood urea nitrogen (BUN), the amount of nitrogen in the blood in the form of urea, a normal waste product (a measure of kidney function), is elevated in people with low blood pressure. The normal BUN level is 7 to 18 mg/dl.

Urine testing to measure sodium, potassium, and calcium, is often done. Sodium is decreased during episodes of low blood pressure (*hyponatremia*). High potassium or *hyperkalemia* (Addison's) compromises the kidney's ability to excrete potassium. Calcium can also be elevated (*hypercalcemia*) in Addison's disease.

Blood tests may also reveal high levels of *eosinophils*, a type of white blood cell associated with inflammation and allergies. Low red blood cell counts (*anemia*) are common in women with Addison's. Thyroid stimulating hormone (TSH) may also be measured.

Adrenocortical autoantibodies in the blood can indicate adrenal gland autoimmunity, but hormone deficiency is needed to diagnose adrenal insufficiency.

Treating Addison's Disease

The treatment of Addison's involves replacing the glucocorticoid adrenal hormone with *prednisone, hydrocortisone* (*Hydrocortone, Cortef*), or *cortisone acetate*, and *mineral corticoid* with *fludrocortisone* (*Florinef*).

"We try to administer synthetic adrenal hormones in a way that approximates the natural pattern of adrenal steroid secretion. Since cortisol is highest in the early morning and lowest late at night, patients will take a larger dose of hydrocortisone or cortisone acetate in the morning and a smaller dose in the afternoon," explains Dr. Ladenson. For example, many patients take 20 milligrams of hydrocortisone in the morning, and 10 milligrams in the afternoon. Mineral corticoid therapy is given as a single dose of fludrocortisone.

"Our ability to assess adrenal replacement in the laboratory is limited, so we generally monitor patients' clinical responses. Have symptoms like weight loss, nausea, or loss of appetite gone away? And are there symptoms of excessive replacement, such as weight gain, easy bruising, depressed mood, or muscle weakness?" says Dr. Ladenson. Fludrocortisone therapy is monitored by assessing blood pressure standing and lying down, and measuring serum potassium and plasma renin.

Women need to adjust their doses of hydrocortisone during the third trimester of pregnancy. And if they have an illness accompanied by fever, fludrocortisone may need to be decreased during the premenstrual period, since it can exacerbate fluid retention. Corticosteroids may also increase blood glucose levels. You'll be advised to take in more salt (especially if you work out regularly and perspire) to guard against low sodium, since adequate sodium levels are needed to maintain normal blood pressure. It's a good idea to wear a MedicAlert bracelet or necklace so that proper care can be given in an emergency.

How Addison's Disease Can Affect You Over Your Lifetime

Like other autoimmune diseases, Addison's affects women during the various stages of their lives.

Endocrine Clusters (Autoimmune Polyglandular Syndromes)

Autoimmune endocrine disorders tend to cluster together, affecting several glands, sometimes with years separating the onset of each disease. There are three types of autoimmune polyglandular syndromes (APS). Type 1 APS is more common in childhood and affects both sexes equally. Type 2 APS is more common in women and occurs between ages twenty and forty, says Dr. Ladenson, usually with Addison's presenting first, and type 1 diabetes (or thyroid disease) occurring later. In type 3 APS, autoimmune thyroid disease is accompanied by two other autoimmune diseases, but a woman does not develop Addison's disease.

Type 1 APS
- Hypoparathyroidism
- Adrenal insufficiency (Addison's disease)
- Chronic yeast infections of the skin or nails
- Malabsorption problems
- Alopecia totalis (or universalis)
- Vitiligo
- Sjögren's syndrome
- Chronic autoimmune hepatitis
- Pituitary insufficiency (*hypophysitis*)
- Gonadal autoimmunity
- Type 1 diabetes (less commonly)

Type 2 APS
- Adrenal insufficiency
- Thyroiditis
- Type 1 diabetes
- Alopecia
- Pernicious anemia
- Myasthenia gravis

Type 3 APS
- Thyroiditis
- Myasthenia gravis (or another nonendocrine autoimmune disease)

Menstruation and Pregnancy

Women with Addison's disease often have menstrual irregularities or premature ovarian failure (see page 191). Oral contraceptives can be used to regulate the menstrual cycle, and hormone replacement therapy (HRT) can be used for menopausal symptoms, as there are no cross reactions with estrogen, says Dr. Ladenson. Fluid retention during the premenstrual period may worsen with fludrocortisone, so the dose may be decreased for a few days before menstruation.

In general, women don't need to increase glucocorticoid medication during the first two trimesters. "However, labor and delivery are a physical stress, and glucocorticoid coverage may need to be increased at the time of delivery," says Dr. Ladenson. "We also switch women from oral medication to injectable corticosteroids."

While drugs like prednisone are generally considered safe during pregnancy, fludrocortisone should be used cautiously; too much may cause a baby to be born with an underactive adrenal gland. Fludrocortisone and drugs like prednisone can pass into breast milk and may cause growth problems, so women with Addison's are usually advised not to breastfeed.

Hypoparathyroidism

The tiny parathyroid glands, nestled behind the thyroid gland, produce parathyroid hormone, which, along with vitamin D and *calcitonin* (a hormone secreted by cells in the thyroid gland), regulate the amount of calcium in the body.

In *autoimmune hypoparathyroidism*, autoantibodies attack the four pea-sized glands, destroying hormone-producing tissue. Dr. Noel Maclaren's group at Cornell reported that autoantibodies against the calcium-sensing receptor of the parathyroid glands (which sense how much calcium is available to the body) are frequently observed in this disease. Calcium is not only needed to maintain bone mass, but is also required for muscle contractions. Having too little parathyroid hormone (PTH) leads to tingling and numbness in the hands and feet, muscle cramps, fatigue, irregular heartbeat, depression, and anxiety. It also causes a condition known as *tetany*, a heightened excitability of nerves that causes uncontrollable, painful spasms in the face, hands, and feet; spasms of the larynx; and sometimes seizures. Hypoparathyroidism can occur in women with autoimmune hypothyroidism, or as part of type 1 autoimmune polyglandular syndrome. It's diagnosed by measuring parathyroid hormone in the blood. (In *hyperparathyroidism*, too much calcium is removed from the bones and accumulates in the blood, causing excessive thirst and urine output, kidney stones, confusion, seizures, and even coma. It's more common in women, and is often caused by a benign parathyroid tumor.)

An underactive parathyroid is treated with oral calcium and vitamin D, sometimes in a form called *1,25-dihydroxyvitamin D (Calcitriol)*, to help absorb the calcium. "Because of the lack of parathyroid hormone, the kidney can't convert native vitamin D to its more active form as readily, and very large doses are needed, as high as 50,000 International Units, while the U.S. daily requirement is 400 units for healthy people," comments Dr. Ladenson. "Calcitriol is very potent and easily absorbed by the body. Dosing has to be done carefully, because the toxic range is narrow. However, if you overtreat, you need only withhold a dose or two of Calcitriol, whereas toxicity caused by large doses of native vitamin D can take weeks to go away." Calcitriol is usually taken in capsule form (it's also available by injection).

You need a certain blood level of vitamin D to become pregnant. But the dose must be carefully regulated in pregnancy; taking too much vitamin D can cause the baby to be more sensitive to vitamin D and lead to problems with the parathyroid gland and a heart defect. Only small amounts of Calcitriol pass into breast milk; it has not been reported to cause problems in nursing babies.

An injectable version of parathyroid hormone *teriparatide (Forteo)* has been approved for rebuilding bone in osteoporosis, and might have some utility in hypoparathyroidism in a more easily used form, says Dr. Ladenson.

I was absolutely shocked to find out that I was in menopause at age thirty-two. Really shocked. We had been trying to have a baby for a couple of years, and finally went to see an infertility specialist. After he did some tests, he told me the reason I couldn't get pregnant was premature ovarian failure. For some reason, he said, my body had destroyed the eggs in my ovaries. It was really hard to believe—I mean, I didn't have any hot flashes, or anything like that. I thought you went through menopause because your ovaries started to shut down and that only happened when you got older. I cried for days. I know a lot of women have infertility problems. But this was like my body stole something from me . . . it really hurt to think I couldn't have a child. But there wasn't anything we could do about it, so right away we decided to adopt. Now I have a wonderful two-year-old daughter from China. I'm taking hormones and I feel OK otherwise. But I admit I feel different from the other mothers I know, since they're mostly my age and none of them is quote "menopausal" yet.

CELIA, THIRTY-FIVE

Autoimmune Premature Ovarian Failure

Premature ovarian failure (POF), the onset of menopause before age forty, occurs in 1 to 1.2 percent of women, affecting between two and five million women. While some cases of POF have a genetic cause (such as *Turner's syndrome*), or are due to chemotherapy or trauma, recent studies suggest that many cases of premature menopause may actually be due to an autoimmune attack on the ovarian follicles and the eggs (*oocytes*) they contain.

Two-thirds of women are affected between ages twenty-six to thirty-four, and 30 to 40 percent may have a family history of POF. Approximately 15 percent of women with POF have other autoimmune endocrine diseases, most commonly thyroid disease, Addison's disease, type 1 diabetes, and autoimmune polyglandular syndromes (as many as 15 percent of women with type 1 APS have ovarian failure). One percent of women with rheumatoid arthritis experience POF, and it's also associated with vitiligo, lupus, myasthenia gravis, and Crohn's disease.

Some ethnic differences have been noted; a recent study published by Judith Luborksy, PhD, director of Reproductive Immunology at the Rush-Presbyterian Medical Center in Chicago, found that POF affects 1 percent of Caucasian women, 1.4 percent of African-Americans and Latinas, 0.5 percent of Chinese women, and only 0.1 percent of Japanese women. Other studies have found that most women with POF did not menstruate at a later age. Most had their first period at the usual age, 12.5, and initially had otherwise normal menstrual cycles and normal fertility, notes Dr. Luborsky.

While the causes may be different, the symptoms of autoimmune and nonautoimmune POF are the same as in a normal menopause, with hot flashes, thinned and dry vaginal tissues (atrophic vaginitis), painful sex, infertility, bone loss, and an increased risk of cardiovascular disease caused by estrogen deprivation. As with other endocrine disorders, the treatment is replacing the lost hormones, in this case hormone replacement therapy (HRT) with estrogen and progesterone to protect the heart, bones, genital and urinary tract tissues, and the nervous system.

Autoimmune POF is not identified by the traditional test for ovarian function, says Dr. Luborsky. The tests include blood levels of *follicle stimulating hormone* (*FSH*) made by the pituitary gland, and estrogen (made by the ovaries). As ovarian function declines, estrogen decreases and FSH increases. To be diagnosed with premature menopause (or menopause), FSH must be above 40 International Units per liter of blood (IU/L). (This is true for all types of POF and natural menopause.) Blood levels of estrogen and other ovarian hormones, such as progesterone, reflect the activity of a group of follicles in the ovary. The total number of active follicles decreases with age or as a result of autoimmune disease or other trauma. "If you measure hormones in individual ovarian follicles during the declining phase, before menstruation ceases completely, you get a different picture than from measuring hormones in the blood. Maturing follicles in older women may be healthy, but they don't seem to be going through follicular development and ovulation at the same rate as in younger women. The follicles produce normal amounts of hormones, but because there are less of them in older women, the amount of hormones we see in the bloodstream is less," Dr. Luborsky explains. "However, in patients with anti-ovarian autoantibodies there is more variability in the levels of hormone in the follicles. For instance, in some women with ovarian autoantibodies the follicular cells make huge amounts of progesterone, others may make very little. A lot of these women have functional follicles, but they don't look as normal as in women who are just getting older," she observes. However, the changes in the menstrual cycle, the shortening or lengthening of cycles, and changes in bleeding patterns that occur with a normal menopause, also occur in women with autoimmune ovarian failure.

The primary cause of autoimmune POF is believed to be destruction of ovarian follicles and oocytes by ovary specific autoantibodies. Research indicates that around half of women with POF who have no other coexisting autoimmune disease have *anti-ovarian antibodies*. About 4 to 12 percent of women with autoimmune polyglandular syndromes involving Addison's disease, and additional autoimmune disease of endocrine glands, have POF. The autoantibodies associated with those disorders (*steroid cell antibodies*) may also have an effect against the hormone-producing tissue of the ovaries and also react against specific steroid hormone–producing enzymes that are common to the ovary and adrenal gland.

Diagnosis of autoimmune POF depends on measuring autoantibodies to the ovary. "Not all women with premature menopause have an autoimmune disease. If you are having symptoms of an early menopause, you should consider getting tested so you know what's going on," advises Dr. Luborsky. Tests are available to detect anti-ovarian autoantibodies; you can ask your doctor to send a blood sample to the company that has licensed the tests (ReproMedix of Woburn, Massachusetts. For information log onto www .ReproMedix.com). A workup for autoimmune POF may also include blood tests for other nonspecific autoimmune markers, such as an elevated SED rate, antinuclear antibodies, and rheumatoid factor, as well as levels of thyroid stimulating hormone (TSH), elevated blood glucose, and the diagnostic tests for Addison's disease (see page 186). Accurate diagnosis of autoimmune POF can help rule out other causes of POF, such as stress (which may be reversible).

Infertility (ovarian function but an inability to become pregnant) may be an early sign of autoimmune POF. "We believe there is a group of women with this autoimmune disease, who have autoantibodies and go through a period of infertility as they progress to a total ovarian failure. The success of infertility treatments may depend on where a woman is in this progression," explains Dr. Luborsky. Women labeled as having "unexplained infertility" (no tubal blockages or other physical problems that prevent pregnancy) may actually have autoimmune infertility. "A significant proportion of these women have anti-ovarian autoantibodies, and this is independent of the hormones typically used to determine ovarian function. Which means you can't use FSH to diagnose ovarian autoimmunity in women with unexplained infertility," remarks Dr. Luborsky.

In fact, many cases of POF are diagnosed at infertility clinics. In some women with autoimmune POF, follicular function may spontaneously resume, and a pregnancy can occur. However, if a woman with POF wants to become pregnant, aggressive treatment can be tried with hormones to stimulate ovarian follicles to produce multiple eggs, followed by *in-vitro fertilization* (*IVF*), but the success rate so far is low.

Testing for anti-ovarian autoantibodies may help identify women more likely to succeed with IVF. "Our studies found that women who became pregnant with IVF had a lower frequency of antiovarian antibodies compared to the women who did not succeed with IVF," comments Dr. Luborsky. "Women found to have anti-ovarian antibodies may be candidates for future immune-based therapy. A few studies indicate immune suppression may result in a return of normal periods and pregnancy, although this treatment is somewhat controversial," she notes. The consequences of POF go beyond infertility. "If you're in your twenties or thirties and you're having hot flashes, you need to know if you're entering menopause early and take appropriate precautions. For example, your risk for osteoporosis is going to be much, much higher," warns Dr. Luborsky. Without replacement estrogen, atrophy of vaginal tissue can make sex uncomfortable and lead to frequent urinary tract and yeast infections. "Make sure you talk to your gynecologist if you are not comfortable discussing menopausal symptoms with a rheumatologist or other specialist," she adds.

8

Tough to Digest—Inflammatory Bowel Disease (Crohn's Disease and Ulcerative Colitis), Celiac Disease, and Pernicious Anemia

I was diagnosed with Crohn's when I was twenty. But, looking back, I'd had symptoms ever since I was a child. I would have these strange periods of a week or two where I would have fevers, abdominal pain, and such fatigue and exhaustion that I couldn't move. But my pediatrician used to tell my parents "She's just trying to get out of going to school. Don't take it seriously." And then during stressful times, I would get really sick. Like during exams or the week of my high school graduation. It took a long time to figure out what was wrong with me. I was going to lots of doctors. I was going to a gynecologist, I was seeing my family doctor, and they were all saying different things. One said I was developing an ulcer and I should reduce the stress in my life, and I needed to take acid reducers. My gynecologist said I had ovarian cysts and that's what was causing the pain. I was told I had irritable bowel syndrome . . . I was put on antibiotics . . . but no matter what they did, nothing helped. When I was at my sickest, I dropped around twenty pounds. I was also having fevers and night sweats, which are all classic symptoms of Crohn's during a flare. But it still took a long time to be diagnosed. And that only happened because I was so sick my gynecologist decided to admit me to the hospital to find out what was wrong. Once I was put in the hospital, they ran some CAT scans and barium tests and

they found the Crohn's. But that was only after the pain and inflam-
mation were so bad, and my small intestine became so inflamed that it
burst through my bladder. So I had to have a whole section of my intes-
tines removed. If they had caught it early, maybe I could have just had
medication and been fine.

JANINE, TWENTY-SIX

As Janine found out, diagnosing *inflammatory bowel disease* (*IBD*) is rarely quick or simple. The two types of IBD—*Crohn's disease* and *ulcerative colitis*—are often mistaken for each other, and their early symptoms of diarrhea and cramping are frequently confused with a non-autoimmune problem called *irritable bowel syndrome* (*IBS*). Sometimes they occur together. (However, IBS and IBD are not the same, even though the abbreviations are similar.) In Crohn's disease and ulcerative colitis, it's as if something is eating at you, destroying the parts of your body needed to extract vital nutrition from food and protect you from bacteria in the gut. Both are technically "foreign" antigens, and for our intestines to be tolerant of food and protect against invasion by bacteria, the thin mucosal lining must have a tightly regulated immune system. In IBD and celiac disease (another autoimmune disease that affects the intestines), this system fails, disrupting normal digestion.

The process of digestion can be likened to an assembly line, with the various parts of the digestive system moving food along on a conveyor belt powered by smooth muscle tissue. Food is first chopped up into manageable pieces as we chew, moistened by saliva (which also contains enzymes that begin to break down carbohydrates) and, after a minute or two, is loaded onto the conveyor belt with each swallow. The muscles in the esophagus contract (this is called *peristalsis*) to push food down into the stomach, where it's mixed with acid and digestive juices produced by the stomach lining (which help break down proteins). Your stomach continuously churns as it breaks down and mixes food into a semiliquid consistency, and after two to four hours sends it into the many loops of the small intestine.

This part of the conveyor belt has three sections: the *duodenum* (the part that connects directly to the stomach), the *jejunum* (the section just below it), and the *ileum* (which connects to the *colon*, or large intestine). In the duodenum, liver enzymes and bile salts (produced by the gallbladder) break down

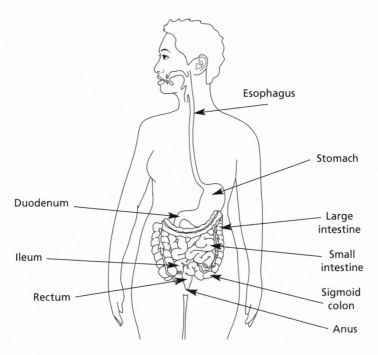

Esophagus

Stomach

Duodenum

Large intestine

Ileum

Small intestine

Rectum

Sigmoid colon

Anus

The Digestive System

fats, and digestive juices from the pancreas continue the breakdown of carbohydrates and proteins. The final breakdown of food is carried out by glands in the lining of the small intestine, and nutrients are extracted by frondlike projections from the inner lining called *villi*; the layer of cells just beneath the lining helps nutrients pass into the bloodstream.

This process takes anywhere from one to four hours. Finally, the conveyor moves food into the colon. Here, the lining has indentations called *crypts*, which extract most of the water. The solid waste that's left over is moved out of the body as feces. This is actually the longest part of the process, taking anywhere from ten hours to a couple of days.

The inflammation of IBD speeds up the passage of food, so the intestines empty more frequently, causing diarrhea. Because your body doesn't get enough time to absorb food properly, calories pass out of the system before you can use them, so you start to lose weight.

Inflammation also breaks down the thin layer of cells lining the intestines (*epithelial cells*). This one-cell-thick sheet of cells, and the layer of mucin they produce to lubricate and shield them from digestive chemicals, serves as the only barrier against bacteria and toxins in the bowel; without it, we'd be overwhelmed by massive infections. Some T-cells are found in the epithelial layer, but the immune system of the intestines only allows a certain amount of other white blood cells into the gut to take care of viruses or excess bacteria (we need a certain amount of bacteria for normal functioning, and they must constantly be kept in a delicate balance). Immune cells in the gut must be programmed for tolerance of food antigens and to react against anything else foreign. As inflammation breaks down the lining of the intestine, the normal immune function of the gut breaks down as well, leading to overgrowth of bacteria and infections.

The erosion of the intestinal lining causes ulcerations or cracks (*fissures*) that can bleed. The disease also triggers overgrowth of smooth muscle cells in the intestine wall, which thickens the wall and narrows the opening through which food passes. In some cases, the narrowing is so severe it blocks food from moving along (*strictures*). Inflammation can also spread outside the bowel wall, penetrating to an adjacent area of the intestine, sometimes causing sections of bowel to stick together (*adhesions*).

Crohn's disease typically affects the lower part of your small intestine (the *terminal ileum*), but can produce inflammation and ulcerations along any part of the digestive conveyor belt, from the mouth to the anus (as well as nearby tissues) and can cause symptoms in other parts of the body (see page 204). The terms *ileitis* or *proctitis*, refer to inflammation in the rectal area. In ulcerative colitis (UC), inflammation usually occurs only in the lower colon and in the rectum, but may spread to the entire colon.

IBD is actually the second most common chronic inflammatory disorder, next to rheumatoid arthritis. Crohn's and ulcerative colitis commonly occur between ages twelve and twenty-eight, and spikes again after age fifty. Opinions are divided as to whether women are more prone to Crohn's disease; some studies show women are two to three times more likely to develop it. Crohn's is a lifelong, chronic disease, but new treatments have made lengthy remissions possible; UC can be cured with surgery to remove the affected area of bowel.

Warning Signs of Inflammatory Bowel Disease

- Chronic diarrhea
- Abdominal pain
- Nausea and vomiting
- Fever
- Fatigue
- Night sweats
- Weight loss
- Mouth ulcers, ulcerations in the perianal area (Crohn's disease)
- Joint pain
- Clubbed fingernails

Crohn's Disease

Crohn's disease seems to stem from a combination of genetic and environmental causes, especially bacterial infections. Around 5 to 10 percent of people with Crohn's have a close family member with inflammatory bowel disease. If you have a parent or sibling with IBD, your chances of developing it are increased. "With one affected parent the risk is 3 to 7 percent; with two affected parents it goes up to 33 percent for the child," remarks Sunanda V. Kane, MD, a gastroenterologist and assistant professor of surgery at the University of Chicago School of Medicine. Crohn's is also more common in Caucasians and among people of Jewish descent.

What Causes Crohn's Disease?

Scientists at three U.S. universities and in Europe have identified the first genetic abnormality that increases susceptibility to Crohn's disease. The gene involves a protein called NOD2, which helps immune cells called *macrophages* target bacterial invaders by recognizing a key component of its cell membrane. Macrophages, the Pac-Man-like cells of the immune system, engulf and break down bacteria they encounter, then display crumbs of their meal on their surface as a signal to other immune cells to join in the fight. This signal also helps the other immune cells "remember" their prey. In flawed forms of the NOD2 gene, a small portion of the protein is missing, making it less effective in recognizing the bacteria. How this triggers the inflammation of Crohn's disease isn't clear. The scientists, writing in the May 31, 2001, *Nature*, speculate that if macrophages are less efficient in sensing bacteria initially, then the other immune cells that are eventually activated and react to the bacteria may cause an exaggerated, prolonged inflammatory response. About 15 percent of people with Crohn's disease have a damaged form of the NOD2 gene. Having one copy of a defective NOD2 gene may double the risk of developing Crohn's; having two copies could increase risk fifteen to twenty times.

While NOD2 is likely to be only one of several genes that increase risk, the finding gives an important clue as to how bacteria, even those that normally live in the gut, could contribute to Crohn's disease. For example, *Escherichia coli* (*E. coli*) bacteria are normally present in the intestines, but if you eat or drink food or water contaminated by fecal matter, certain strains of E. coli can cause a diarrheal infection. People with Crohn's are often infected with the bacteria. French researchers reported in 2002 that E. coli infection causes cells lining the intestine to produce molecules called MICA, which activate natural killer T-cells. The T-cells then release a chemical signal that causes inflammation. One theory of how inflammatory bowel disease develops is that bacteria may constantly stimulate the mucosal lining of the intestines and the resulting activation of immune cells and production of inflammatory cytokines (like *tumor necrosis factor alpha, TNFα*) lead to chronic inflammation that eventually breaks down these tissues. So a big surge in MICA molecules in the intestines due to an E. coli infection could set off an immune response that causes Crohn's disease. Or, people with a defective NOD2 gene may be genetically "programmed" to mount a prolonged immune response to the infection, causing chronic inflammation of the intestines that leads to Crohn's. It may also be that toxins produced by E. coli (or other bacteria) could also damage the intestinal lining.

Molecular mimicry could also play a role. There may be similarities between the structure of part of the E. coli bacteria and part of the colon cells. In lab experiments, anticolon antibodies, found in the blood of people with Crohn's and ulcerative colitis, react against colon cells *and* E. coli.

Another bacterium linked to Crohn's is *mycobacterium paratuberculosis,* which has been found in biopsies of intestinal tissue from Crohn's patients. Crohn's has been confused with intestinal tuberculosis, and one of the drugs used to treat TB is *paraminosalicylic acid,* an aspirinlike drug closely related to *5-aminosalicylic acid,* a component of *sulfasalazine (Azulfidine),* which is used to treat Crohn's disease.

There are also suspect viruses, including the measles virus. Several recent studies have linked exposure early in life (or prenatal exposure) to the measles virus with an increased risk of developing Crohn's. Measles virus is a type of virus that infects cells and can stay dormant in the body for years. In theory, the virus could infect cells lining the intestine and be reactivated at some point, causing an abnormal immune response.

Smoking is a major risk factor for Crohn's but, ironically, seems to be protective in ulcerative colitis. "One of the theories is that in ulcerative colitis, nicotine may stimulate mucin production, and mucin acts as a barrier to help prevent bacteria in the gut from invading the intestinal wall and stimulating the immune system. In Crohn's disease it seems to be the opposite—mucin production is reduced," explains Lloyd Mayer, MD, professor and director of the Center for Immunobiology at the Mount Sinai School of Medicine in New York City. "However, we don't know whether it's the nicotine or whether it's something else in cigarette smoke that's causing this effect. But we try to get all of our Crohn's patients to quit smoking."

I think I must have had this my whole life . . . I remember when I was in second grade, I was in a gifted class, and when we would have tests I would have severe stomach pains. I would be doubled over; I was in the bathroom all the time. But when my parents took me to a doctor, they were told I had a "spastic colon," a "nervous stomach." That's what I was told all my life. I've been living on diarrhea medicines since I was a kid. At times the pain would be so bad I thought I had appendicitis. It was only after I had my second child in 1990 that my doctor said, "I think it's time you got this checked out." I went to a gastroenterologist, who did a colonoscopy—and that's how I found out I had Crohn's. But there had been other signs. In 1985 I suddenly started bleeding vaginally. I went to my gynecologist and found that I had an ulcer in the vagina that was bleeding. He tried cauterizing it, but no matter what he did nothing worked. Then one night I started to hemorrhage. The ulcer had exposed an artery and they had to tie it off. That was in 1985. It kept happening. I must have had around ten to twelve different surgeries for vaginal ulcers. They would seem to heal, then a month or two later another one would open. They lasered them . . . twice they used placental tissue for a graft . . . but it wasn't really that successful. They thought maybe it was Behcet's disease, but I didn't meet all the criteria for that. Then, as suddenly as it started it just seemed to go away . . . years later, after I developed another one and it was biopsied, we confirmed that they were Crohn's ulcers.

LAURA, FORTY-SIX

Symptoms of Crohn's Disease

Crohn's can develop gradually over a period of years before you have obvious symptoms. Even when there are some symptoms, you may have thought you were simply prone to diarrhea. In some cases, however, Crohn's can come on suddenly.

The most common symptoms are frequent bowel movements, diarrhea, and abdominal pain, often in the lower right side of the abdomen. In contrast to ulcerative colitis, in which the pain may be intermittent and relieved by a bowel movement (see page 219), if you have Crohn's disease, pain will be more constant and will worsen after you eat. The diarrhea is accompanied by a sense of urgency, and may come on at night. Abdominal pain after eating is also a symptom of *diverticulitis,* the formation of tiny inflamed sacs in the lining of the intestine (usually the lower part of the colon). Diarrhea and abdominal pain are also symptoms of celiac disease, where an autoimmune attack on the bowel leads to an inability to digest gluten in wheat (see pages 226 to 237).

It's not uncommon for women with Crohn's to be initially diagnosed with irritable bowel syndrome (IBS) because of the shared symptoms of chronic diarrhea and abdominal pain after meals, remarks Christine Frissora, MD, an assistant professor of medicine at the Weill Medical College of Cornell University. Adding to the confusion, there's an increased incidence of irritable bowel syndrome (IBS) among women with Crohn's.

"IBS has been called a 'spastic colon,' but we think it may be caused by a loss of synchronization between the small and large intestines. Instead of working in concert with each other, one of the intestines may have a stronger reaction to a food or stressful event, and that can cause altered emptying of the bowel," explains Dr. Frissora. "To be diagnosed with IBS, you must have had abdominal discomfort that's relieved by defecation, associated with a change in stool consistency and frequency, or mucus in the stool and bloating. About a third of women have a diarrhea-predominant form of IBS, a third have more constipation with their IBS, and the remaining third alternate between the two. However, in Crohn's disease, in addition to such bowel dysfunction, you have associated symptoms of inflammation."

Those symptoms include fever, fatigue, and weight loss due to malabsorption, she adds. If your fever is low-grade (up to 100.4 degrees), you may not even be aware you're running a temperature. You may feel lethargic and irritable, but not feverish. If your Crohn's is flaring or severe, you can run a high fever (up to 104 degrees), with night sweats. *Diverticulitis* also causes fever, abdominal tenderness, and strictures.

Crohn's can cause sores or ulcerations anywhere in the digestive tract or where there are mucous membranes, including the mouth. These include *aphthous ulcers*, tiny shallow sores that often occur between the gum and the lower lip, or along the base of the tongue. While canker sores last a week or two, Crohn's ulcers can last for months. Some women, like Laura, may develop ulcers in the area between the vagina and rectum, or around the vagina itself. Bleeding may be serious and persistent, leading to anemia. In some cases, a *fistula* (an abnormal, tunnel-like opening) can occur between the rectal and vaginal areas or between the bowel and the skin near the anus. (Fistulas can also occur internally between adjacent areas of the bowel.)

"Recurrent oral and genital ulcers also occur in a rare inflammatory condition called *Behcet's disease*, which is thought to be autoimmune," notes Dr. Frissora. (Behcet's disease is more common in Mediterranean countries and in Japan, where it's a major cause of blindness.) Other symptoms it shares with Crohn's are eye inflammation and raised, red bumps called *erythema nodosum*, often on the shins and ankles (which can also be a sign of increased disease activity in IBD).

Because the intestinal tract isn't absorbing nutrients properly, you may have deficiencies of vitamin B_{12}, calcium, vitamin D, and protein. Malabsorption causes you to lose weight, and unexplained weight loss is another key symptom of Crohn's (and ulcerative colitis).

Sores, cracks (*fissures*) in the anal area, and rectal bleeding can occur in Crohn's, as well as hemorrhoids, skin tags in the anal area, or cauliflower-shaped mounds of thickened tissue; the skin tags and areas of thickened skin can both resemble hemorrhoids. There may be pain in the perianal area, abnormal discharge of mucus and pus (if there's an internal rectal abscess), or discharge of pus and fecal material due to false openings in the rectum called *sinus tracts*.

In up to 30 percent of women, Crohn's can also cause symptoms in other areas of the body, most commonly joint pain. Between 10 to 20 percent of people with IBD have inflammatory joint disease in their extremities, with the joint pain accompanying (or following) bowel inflammation. In fact, IBD may be causing your arthritis without producing bowel symptoms, possibly by the migration of immune cells related to inflammation to the joint lining (*synovium*). Unlike rheumatoid arthritis (which can cluster with Crohn's), the joint pain associated with IBD is not usually symmetrical and doesn't usually produce changes seen on x-rays. Treating your Crohn's usually results in an improvement of joint problems. (Some of the same medications used to treat rheumatoid arthritis are also used to treat Crohn's.)

Women with Crohn's can also develop kidney stones, gallstones, or liver disease. An autoimmune liver disorder, *primary sclerosing cholangitis* (*PSC*), the blockage of bile ducts by scar tissue, occurs in a small percentage of women with Crohn's (though it's more common in ulcerative colitis). Fifteen percent of women may have skin rashes, including erythema nodosum, usually on the legs. You may also experience eye inflammation (*uveitis*) or pain, light sensitivity, blurred vision, and dry eye.

Women with Crohn's may already have bone loss when they first present to a physician, remarks Dr. Kane. "Crohn's disease in itself can cause osteoporosis, due to inflammatory cytokines and malabsorption of calcium and vitamin D. Many Crohn's patients have also avoided dairy products because it makes their diarrhea worse, so they don't get enough calcium to begin with," she says. "Bone mass studies in IBD patients have found that anywhere from a third to 60 percent will have low bone mass, without any other kinds of risk factors." (Steroids and other medications used to treat Crohn's can cause or worsen bone loss, as well.)

A child or adolescent with Crohn's may have growth problems or delayed puberty. Menstrual periods and fertility may be normal, but you may find yourself avoiding sex because of pain in the anal or genital area.

Diagnosing Crohn's Disease

The diagnosis of Crohn's disease is made on the basis of symptoms and findings of diagnostic tests. Blood tests can pick up systemic inflammation, anemia, vitamin deficiencies, and other problems related to Crohn's, but sigmoidoscopy and a barium x-ray of the colon (and sometimes an intestinal biopsy) will reveal the classic inflammation and ulcerations.

The *Crohn's Disease Endoscopic Activity Index of Severity (CDEAIS)* measures the percentage of affected areas of mucosal surface in six segments of the intestines (the ileum, right and left colon, transverse and sigmoid colon, and the rectum), but the index doesn't really correlate to the severity of disease activity. A series of diagnostic tests, including stool analysis (to detect bleeding and other causes of inflammation, such as parasites or bacteria), may be needed to confirm the diagnosis and assess the extent of the Crohn's, says Dr. Mayer.

"Crohn's disease involves all of the layers of the bowel, and a lot of times the inflammation never hits the surface. So if you do a sigmoidoscopy or a barium study you may not see any changes in the mucosa," he remarks. "If you just do a CT scan, all you might see is a thickening of the bowel. But if it's just in a short segment, a single CT may not be able to pick it up. So we often need to do a combination of tests to see what's going on in Crohn's."

Tests You May Need and What They Mean

Flexible sigmoidoscopy uses a lighted, flexible fiber-optic scope inserted through the rectum to examine the lower areas of the *sigmoid* colon. The inner lining of the colon can be seen clearly through the scope. If you have Crohn's disease, your doctor may see patches of red, inflamed tissue, ulcerations, and fistulas (which makes the diagnosis more likely, especially if it's a rectal-vaginal fistula). Most cases of Crohn's involve both the small and large intestine; 15 percent of cases may involve only the colon (and can be mistaken for ulcerative colitis). However, in Crohn's there may be "skip areas" where patches of diseased bowel occur next to areas of normal tissue and the rectum is usually not affected.

Sigmoidoscopy can be done in a physician's office without much discomfort (some people may need a mild tranquilizer). The only preparation you'll need is a mild enema with tap water to cleanse the colon one or two hours before the test. A more thorough examination of the entire colon can be done with *colonoscopy*, a similar fiber-optic procedure (see below).

A **barium x-ray** (barium enema) is an x-ray of the colon using barium, a contrast agent that shows up as white on the x-ray. It's usually done if you have symptoms but a sigmoidoscopy is negative or inconclusive. You'll be asked to drink a solution to clean out the colon and take a mild enema an hour or two before the test. Just before the x-ray, a small amount of barium is infused into the colon through the rectum. The contrast agent will coat the inside of the colon (which will look like a white tube on the x-ray). In Crohn's, the normally rounded hills and valleys in the surface of the colon are flattened, and there may be tiny ulcerations or fissures. Diverticula show up as protrusions on the outer surface. The test is performed in a radiology facility.

An **upper GI series** uses barium and x-rays to examine the small intestine, the terminal ileum, and the beginning of the colon. There's no prep involved; you simply don't eat anything after midnight the night before so food is less likely to be present in the ileum. On the morning of the test, you drink a small amount of liquid barium (it's chalky, but comes in several flavors). It takes about two hours for the barium to pass through the loops of the small intestine and reach the colon. In Crohn's, the normal pattern of the intestinal lining (including the villi) is often distorted or lost, and there may be narrowing of the opening inside the intestines (the *lumen*). Additional x-rays may be taken using a compression paddle on the abdomen to separate adjoining loops of bowel, so the end portions of the ileum can be seen clearly (this is similar to the way compression is used when you get a mammogram, so that the tissues of the breast are more visible on x-ray).

Colonoscopy involves a more detailed examination of the entire colon using a very flexible fiber-optic endoscope (*endo* means "inside"). Because the scope must pass through all the pretzel-like loops and curves of the colon, sedation is used to make the procedure more comfortable. The fiber-optic scope used for the procedure magnifies the image of the colon's inner lining up to ten times its normal size so it can be thoroughly examined. Photographs and videotapes can even be made during the procedure by mounting a small camera on the viewing end of the scope. The scope is hollow, so a biopsy device can be passed through it.

You'll be asked to eat a liquid diet for the forty-eight hours before the test (with only clear liquids during the preceding twenty-four hours) to minimize the chances of any fecal residue in the colon. In Crohn's disease, colonoscopy may reveal patterns of inflammation (the characteristic "skip" pattern), ulcerations or other lesions, and loss of the normal folds in the inner surface (those folds are needed to thoroughly extract moisture and nutrients). The scope can reveal polyps, and biopsies can be taken. The biopsy may reveal *granulomas*, a microscopic granular-like lesion caused by an influx of inflammatory cells, seen in up to 10 percent of people with Crohn's. Ulcerations may bleed (and blood may be present in a stool sample). The lining of the colon can also take on a cobblestone-like texture in Crohn's.

Colonoscopy is an extremely valuable test, but it needs to be done by a qualified gastroenterologist. It's only performed when adequate information can't be obtained from other diagnostic tests, or if cancer or polyps are suspected, because inflammation can make the colon more prone to injury during the procedure.

Gastroscopy involves the examination of the lining of the esophagus, stomach, and the uppermost portion of the small intestine (duodenum) with a thinner fiber-optic scope. Crohn's disease can cause inflammation and ulceration of these areas, and the test can help distinguish between Crohn's and ulcerative colitis. Sedation is usually given to reduce discomfort and quiet your gag reflex as the scope is passed down the throat.

Computed tomography (CT) scans can help detect abnormalities in the intestinal mucosa and other areas in Crohn's. Radioactive dyes may also be used to assess the extent of inflammation. Other imaging techniques, like *transabdominal ultrasound* or *magnetic resonance imaging* (*MRI*), may also provide useful information.

Complete blood count (CBC) can reveal iron deficiency anemia due to bleeding, vitamin B_{12} deficiency due to malabsorption, or depletion of red blood cells. You may also have a low platelet count (*thrombocytopenia*), a high platelet count (*thrombocytosis*), or a high white blood cell count, a sign of inflammation.

C-Reactive protein (CRP) is a marker of inflammation found in the blood that will be elevated in Crohn's.

Erythrocyte sedimentation rate (SED rate) will be elevated because of inflammation (see page 27) in Crohn's, but CRP is more helpful in determining disease activity.

Tests to measure **antibodies associated with Crohn's disease** can be useful for separating Crohn's from ulcerative colitis and other disorders. They include antibodies against baker's yeast (*anti-Saccharomyces cerevisiae*), present in 50 to 70 percent of Crohn's patients (but only 6 to 14 percent of people with UC). Antibodies to *pancreatic antigens* (*PABs*), a protein in pancreatic secretions, are seen in 31 percent of Crohn's patients (and only 4 percent of people with UC). Testing for these antibodies is not yet routine, but may be useful in some cases.

Janine's story continues:
Two years after my surgery I was put on sulfasalazine. First they got me into remission with steroids, then they tapered me off the prednisone and put me on Pentasa, and I've been doing really well with it. I have not let my disease interfere with my life, apart from watching what I eat. I have been active in support groups and on the Internet. I think that getting to know other people with inflammatory bowel disease helps tremendously. You need that emotional support.

Treating Crohn's Disease

The treatment for your Crohn's depends on how much of the bowel is involved and how severe the disease is (for example, if you have fistulas) and any other complications you may have. The goal is to control inflammation; relieve symptoms like abdominal pain, diarrhea, and rectal bleeding; and correct any nutritional deficiencies. Treatment may include medications, surgery, nutritional supplements, or a combination.

You can experience long periods of remission—sometimes years without any symptoms—with proper treatment. But there's no cure for Crohn's, and it can recur periodically. Unfortunately, there's no way to predict when this may happen. Although it can be controlled, Crohn's is a chronic disease, and you'll need regular medical visits, periodic diagnostic tests in the event of a recurrence, and sometimes a change in your medication.

Sulfasalazine (Azulfidine) had been the most common drug for treating Crohn's. It contains a sulfa preparation (*sulfapyridine*) that has antibiotic properties. Sulfasalazine also contains *mesalamine*, an aspirinlike substance that helps control inflammation and is used to treat mild to moderate Crohn's (see box on page 212). Sulfasalazine is also helpful in treating flares of Crohn's colitis and ileitis. Side effects include nausea, vomiting, heartburn, diarrhea, appetite loss, and headache. If you've had allergic reactions to other sulfa drugs, you may have a rash in reaction to sulfasalazine; in this case, the drug may be stopped. It can also interfere with the absorption of digoxin and folic acid. Your doctor will continue the medication until symptoms go away. Once you're in remission, you'll be put on a maintenance dose. Sulfasalazine can safely be used during pregnancy (see page 216).

5-aminosalicylic acid (5-ASA) *agents* are aspirinlike drugs that also contain mesalamine, and have largely replaced sulfasalazine. The 5-ASA agents include *olsalazine sodium* (*Dipentum*) and *mesalamine* (*Pentasa, Asacol*).

"These are coated capsules with pure 5-ASA that are delivered either to the small bowel or to the terminal ileum into the early part of the colon; or, if it's the distal colon, Asacol is delivered to that area. Pentasa is delivered to the small bowel," explains Dr. Mayer. "The 5-ASA compounds usually are the first drugs that we prescribe, and we often add antibiotics because there is some component of bacterial overgrowth."

Immunosuppressants are used to treat moderate to severe Crohn's disease. The most commonly prescribed are *6-mercaptopurine* (*6-MP*) and *azathioprine* (*Imuran*), a chemical cousin to 6-MP. Immunosuppressive agents work by blocking the immune reaction that contributes to inflammation. It may take three to four months for 6-MP to show benefits.

These drugs can cause fever, bone marrow suppression, and, in some cases, pancreatitis. While taking these drugs you'll need careful monitoring of your blood counts and liver function tests. Immunosuppressant drugs may also cause side effects like nausea, vomiting, and diarrhea, and may lower your resistance to infection.

Corticosteroids (glucocorticoids) are also used to treat moderate to severe disease, as well as severe or fulminant Crohn's. Among the most commonly prescribed are *prednisone* (*Deltasone, Orasone*) and *prednisolone* (*Prelone*).

Although your doctor may try to avoid the use of corticosteroids because of side effects (like a fatty liver) and the risk of osteoporosis, these drugs may enhance the effects of immunosuppressive drugs. When used in combination with immunosuppressants, the dose of steroids can be lowered. While steroids are very effective in bringing about a remission, nearly half of women may become dependent on them and need to be tapered off the drug. (For more details on corticosteroids, see pages 34 to 35.)

Infliximab (Remicade) was the first treatment specifically approved for Crohn's. Remicade blocks the inflammatory cytokine *tumor necrosis factor alpha* (*TNFα*), which damages tissue in Crohn's, rheumatoid arthritis, and other autoimmune diseases. It's a monoclonal antibody that targets the TNF molecule, binds to it, and removes it from the bloodstream before it reaches the intestines, preventing further inflammation.

Remicade is given intravenously to treat moderate to severe Crohn's, and to those who don't respond to sulfasalazine, 5-ASA agents, or immunosuppressive agents; it's also approved to treat people with fistulas and to induce and maintain remissions of Crohn's. Side effects include an increased risk of serious infection, and a lupuslike syndrome. It is used in combination with 6-MP, azathioprine, or a 5-ASA compound.

Remicade should be avoided during pregnancy (see pages 216 to 217). Levels of C-reactive protein, a marker of inflammation in the blood, are used to determine whether a patient is in remission.

Long-term therapy may provide prolonged remissions for some women. The ACCENT I (A Crohn's disease Clinical trial Evaluating infliximab in a New long-term Treatment regimen) trial reported in 2001 that maintenance therapy (infusions every eight weeks for a year) produced prolonged remissions in more than half of 573 patients with moderate to severe Crohn's, compared to a single treatment. The ACCENT II trial is testing Remicade's ability to heal and close fistulas.

"We are giving Remicade every two to three months, depending on the patient. And if they are not on 6-MP or Imuran, I will put them on either of the two drugs, and hopefully that will keep them in remission," says Dr. Mayer. "I think Remicade is going to change the natural history of Crohn's disease. It is the only drug we have that produces mucosal healing, does away with inflammation, and changes the natural history of the disease. One of the big problems of Crohn's is that patients get scarring, stenosis, obstructions, and fistulas, and this drug just shuts all that down."

Budesonide (Entocort EC) capsules were approved in 2001 for mild to moderate Crohn's disease involving certain sections of the small and large intestines. Entocort is a steroid that's released in the intestine, where it works locally and topically to decrease inflammation, avoiding many of the side effects of systemic corticosteroids.

Clinical trials among 651 men and women with active Crohn's disease found that the drug significantly improved symptoms. The most common side effects include headache, respiratory infection, and nausea. In comparison with prednisolone, fewer patients on Entocort experienced facial swelling and acne.

Antibiotics are used to treat bacterial overgrowth (and resulting inflammation) in the small intestine caused by fistulas, strictures, or prior surgery. Commonly prescribed antibiotics include *ampicillin, sulfonamide, cephalosporin, tetracycline, ciprofloxacin (Cipro)*, and *metronidazole (Flagyl)*.

Antidiarrheal agents can be used to relieve the cramps and diarrhea of Crohn's. These include *diphenoxylate (Lomotil)* and *loperamide (Imodium)*. In severe cases you may become dehydrated, so you'll need plenty of fluids (such as Gatorade) to replenish electrolytes.

Cholestyramine (Questran) is a cholesterol-lowering agent that can be helpful in controlling diarrhea. Patients with IBD affecting the end portion of the ileum (or who have had surgery) may not be absorbing bile salts in the area, which causes the colon to secrete fluid and electrolytes, leading to watery diarrhea.

Nutritional supplements, either oral supplements or injections, may be recommended in people who have deficiencies of vitamin B_{12} or vitamins D, A, or K. The anemia caused by malabsorption of vitamin B_{12} in the ileum is treated by monthly B_{12} injections.

In severe disease with considerable weight loss, special high-calorie liquid products are sometimes used to boost nutrition. A small number of patients with severely inflamed intestines, or who cannot absorb enough nutrition from food, may need temporary feeding by vein.

Women with Crohn's also need to watch their diet, avoiding foods that irritate the bowel, such as spicy foods or high-fiber foods.

Disease Activity in Crohn's

The following classifications have been developed by the American College of Gastroenterology (ACG) and are used to help determine or adjust treatment.

- *Mild to moderate disease*: You are able to eat normally without pain, abdominal tenderness, painful intestinal masses (or obstruction), fever, or dehydration.
- *Moderate to severe disease*: You have failed treatments for mild to moderate disease, or you have prominent symptoms like fever, weight loss (more than 10 percent of your body weight), abdominal pain and tenderness, periodic nausea or vomiting (without bowel obstructions), or anemia.
- *Severe (or fulminant) disease*: Symptoms persist despite treatment with corticosteroids or other immunosuppressant drugs, or you present to your doctor with high fever, persistent vomiting, abdominal tenderness, severe weight loss, evidence of an abscess or obstruction.
- *Remission*: This is defined as the absence of symptoms or signs of inflammation. It includes women who have undergone acute treatment or surgery.

Surgery

If symptoms don't respond to drugs, or there are repeated blockages or bleeding in the intestine, surgery may be the next step. While surgery to remove a damaged section of intestine can help Crohn's disease, it doesn't cure it. Unfortunately, inflammation tends to recur right next to the resected area of intestine.

In severe cases where Crohn's has damaged the large intestine, some women may need to have their entire colon removed. The procedure, called *colectomy*, brings the end of the ileum to the surface of the lower right side of the abdomen, with an opening the size of a quarter (*stoma*), to allow waste to exit into an external pouch (which is emptied as needed). In some cases, women can avoid a colectomy, having only the diseased section of intestine removed and the two ends reconnected (*anastomosis*), with no stoma or bag needed. However, this procedure has a higher risk of disease recurrence. (Smoking also increases the risk of recurrence after surgery.)

Mesalamine, 6-MP, and Imuran are all being tested to see whether they can prevent recurrences after surgery. If your Crohn's is severe, you need to discuss the pros and cons of surgery with your physician.

Small bowel transplants may hold better hope. According to the Crohn's & Colitis Foundation of America (CCFA), more than 450 patients (most of them children) around the world have received transplants of a small section of healthy intestine from a donor to reverse intestinal failure. The procedure is no longer considered experimental, and it's hoped that it will be used in more adults. As with any transplant, lifelong immunosuppressant treatment is needed.

What's Next?

Researchers continue to look for more effective treatments for Crohn's, including other "smart bomb"type drugs that target specific inflammatory processes.

The first of a new class of drugs, called *alpha 4 integrin inhibitors*, is designed to prevent white blood cells from latching onto receptors in inflamed tissues. A randomized, placebo-controlled clinical trial of the drug, *natalizumab (Antegren)*, reported in 2001, showed a major reduction in disease activity in patients treated with the drug. *Interleukin 10 (IL-10)* is a cytokine that suppresses (rather than produces) inflammation, and studies are under way into a synthetic form of IL-10 for treating Crohn's disease. *Interleukin 12 (IL-12)* is an inflammatory cytokine, and the target of another new drug. "The anti-interleukin 12 agent we are testing appears to produce results as dramatic as Remicade," remarks Dr. Mayer. "The nice thing about these agents is that they are targeting different aspects of the abnormal immune response in the gut, so it may be possible to shut down these different pathways."

Antibiotics are now used to treat the bacterial infections that often accompany Crohn's disease, but some research suggests that they might also be useful as a primary treatment for active Crohn's disease and for fistulas.

A preliminary clinical trial of *medroxyprogesterone acetate*, a version of progesterone that's similar to cortisol but with less steroid-type side effects, induced remissions in a majority of patients. Larger, randomized trials are planned.

Thalidomide (*Thalidomid*) has been used with some success in Crohn's and is being tested in ulcerative colitis (see page 223). And the use of stem cell transplants to treat severe Crohn's is also being investigated.

Zinc supplementation may even hold promise. Scientists say harmful oxygen molecules called *free radicals* (produced during infections and periods of stress, among other things) may contribute to inflammation in Crohn's. Zinc removes free radicals from the bloodstream, and supplements of the mineral may help reduce inflammation.

Janine's story continues:
I always had worse symptoms around my periods . . . I would have increased bowel activity, going to the bathroom a lot more during that time of the month. I went on birth control pills for other reasons—I actually was having ovarian cysts and they were concerned about that. But after I started on them I didn't fluctuate, even on my off week. My doctor was kind of reluctant to put me on the pill, so he put me on a low-dose pill because he thought maybe the hormones would cause my Crohn's to flare. But I've never had a problem with it. The only non-GI symptoms my doctor ever asks about are

---

Crohn's Disease Clusters

If, like Janine's, your gastroenterologist is mainly focused on GI symptoms, you need to be aware of the other diseases that can cluster with Crohn's.

Ankylosing spondylitis is an inflammatory disease that affects the spine and nearby structures and progresses to a fusing of the bones of the spine (*ankylosis*). It mostly affects men, but can occur in women with Crohn's. Symptoms can include stiffness and pain in the spine, neck, shoulder, and hips.

Other autoimmune diseases that can cluster with Crohn's include:

• Rheumatoid arthritis
• Thyroid disease
• Primary sclerosing cholangitis

---

joint pain. But we never discussed my susceptibility to other autoimmune diseases. And I'm not sure if it's just because he's a gastroenterologist and he's not thinking about it because he's only interested in my Crohn's. But aside from arthritis concerns, they don't monitor me for thyroid or anything else.

How Crohn's Disease Can Affect You Over Your Lifetime

Crohn's can create special problems for women. Ulcerations and pain in the perineal area can cause painful sex (leading some women to avoid sexual contact), and some may develop a negative body image. "Women worry about having children, being attractive to the opposite sex, feeling that they are somehow ugly, and scarred, that they will be alone in their lives with this diagnosis," comments Dr. Kane. "There are also intimacy issues and worries about sexual performance. Crohn's disease can be a very disfiguring disease, especially when we are talking about deep ulcers and fistulas, around the perianal area and in the vagina."

Other issues that can interfere with relationships include diarrhea, sleep disturbances, and fatigue. Women may also have more problems with fecal incontinence, before and after surgery for Crohn's, or after injury to the anal sphincter during childbirth.

Menstruation

If inflammatory bowel disease begins during childhood or adolescence it may lead to a delayed puberty, and women may get their first menstrual period later than usual.

There are also reports that women experience more severe symptoms around the time of their menstrual periods. There are no clinical studies of premenstrual flares, but a survey of women with irritable bowel and inflammatory bowel disease done at the University of Chicago found that women with IBD seemed to have more symptoms of PMS. "They polled a group of healthy women, and then compared that to a group of women with inflammatory bowel disease and a group with irritable bowel. The healthy women had premenstrual symptoms, and the group with ulcerative colitis and IBS had the same symptoms but in higher percentages. Of the women with Crohn's disease, 100 percent had premenstrual symptoms," remarks Dr. Kane.

Fertility and Pregnancy

Fertility seems to be unaffected when Crohn's disease is inactive, but if your disease is active you may have some trouble getting pregnant. There are also reports that fertility may be decreased if you've had surgery for Crohn's.

"Two-thirds of women with inactive disease at the time they conceive will do just fine, but perhaps a third may get worse," says Dr. Kane. "Among women who have active disease at the time of conception, one-third will stay the same, one-third will have worsened disease activity, and one-third will actually get better. We simply don't know which group a woman will fall into, even if it's a second or third pregnancy." Women with severe, active disease of the terminal ileum may have a harder time with pregnancy, she adds.

The goal is to maintain a remission during pregnancy, and most treatments do not pose a risk. So you need to stick with medication. Sulfasalazine can cause nausea, which may worsen morning sickness in the first trimester and may exacerbate heartburn in the later part of pregnancy. "Sulfasalazine does not carry a risk of fetal malformation. It does cross the placenta, but is only minimally found in breast milk. Sulfasalazine does interfere with folic acid metabolism, so we give women an extra milligram of folic acid a day," says Dr. Kane. Folic acid protects against neural tube defects. "Mesalamine, our first-line medication for both ulcerative colitis and Crohn's, is a topical anti-inflammatory, and we have not seen any increased risk in pregnant women." The dose of prednisone should be reduced in nursing mothers, if possible.

Ulcerations in the genital area are a concern seldom discussed. "I have seen a patient who developed a rectovaginal fistula after an episiotomy. What happens is the rectal tissue is inflamed, it doesn't heal, and a tract starts forming between the vagina and rectum. For women with IBD, episiotomy should not be taken lightly," adds Dr. Frissora.

Although Remicade is contraindicated during pregnancy, a recent study of 59 women who became pregnant while taking the drug showed rates of miscarriages and other complications were no higher than in healthy women. Immunosuppressants like azathioprine and 6-MP should be avoided during pregnancy.

Crohn's may worsen during the first trimester and after delivery, but this may be because women go off their medications in order to breastfeed, remarks Dr. Kane. IBD may also occur for the first time during pregnancy, or in the postpartum period.

While the course of pregnancy and delivery is usually not affected in most women with Crohn's disease, you need to have a thorough discussion with your doctors before you start trying to conceive. If you're taking Remicade, you'll need a six-month washout period (see page 210). Colonoscopy and x-ray procedures should be avoided, particularly during the first trimester; sigmoidoscopy can be done to track disease activity, however.

Inflammatory bowel disease is not "inherited" in the same way as a disease like cystic fibrosis (in which inheriting two copies of a defective gene, one from each parent, means you will develop the disease). There are likely several genes involved. Still, not enough is known to predict how many children of women with IBD will be *predisposed* to Crohn's (or ulcerative colitis).

Menopause and Beyond

Crohn's disease that develops in midlife and beyond seems to affect more women than men. Women with Crohn's who have severe menopausal symptoms can consider hormone replacement therapy, says Dr. Kane. "The risks and benefits are the same as for other women."

Osteoporosis is a major concern for all women after menopause, and especially so for women with Crohn's. "Since Crohn's causes osteoporosis, we encourage weightbearing exercise and tell women to take calcium. Some women may need bone-building drugs, depending on how severe the bone loss is," adds Dr. Kane.

Perhaps 15 percent of patients with inflammatory bowel disease first develop symptoms after age sixty-five. Although the symptoms and course of the disease are similar to that in younger patients, there's slightly more colon involvement when Crohn's affects older people. Conditions that can mimic IBD in older age include diverticular disease, colitis caused by medications (especially nonsteroidal anti-inflammatory drugs), infections, cancer, and other diseases. However, medical and treatment options are not different from those for younger women.

> Janine's story continues:
> *I had started to have severe back pain, and I was lucky to find a really smart orthopedist, who looked beyond just the bones. This doctor really looked at my history. He sees a forty-six-year-old woman who had a hysterectomy, who has Crohn's disease, who took prednisone for many years, who is not on estrogen, who has a small frame and is suffering severe back pain. He said it could be osteoporosis and asked me when my last bone density screening was, and I hadn't had one yet. I was first put on Fosamax, but it irritated my esophagus, so I was put on Evista. But after years of prednisone the osteoporosis is pretty severe. Now they think about it as soon as they put you on steroids. But years ago they didn't. And if any woman is on steroids and her doctor doesn't mention her bones, she should make sure she's being protected.*

Ulcerative Colitis

In contrast to Crohn's, ulcerative colitis affects only the top layers of the lining of the colon and the rectum, producing inflammation and ulcerations. But the effects of inflammation are the same: the colon empties frequently, causing diarrhea. UC can be difficult to diagnose because the symptoms are similar to irritable bowel syndrome and to Crohn's. It develops most often between ages fifteen and forty (although children and older people can have it, too). The incidence of UC may be 20 percent higher in men, and it seems to run in families.

What Causes Ulcerative Colitis?

Many of the same theories as to what causes Crohn's disease also apply to ulcerative colitis (see pages 199 to 201). It seems likely that in vulnerable people, a reaction to a virus or a bacterium causes ongoing inflammation. Those bacteria could be among those normally found in the gut. Although emotional stress and sensitivities to certain types of food may trigger symptoms, they do not cause the disease itself.

Multiple genes are also likely to be involved in ulcerative colitis. It does tend to run in families; as many as 20 percent of patients have a close relative with ulcerative colitis or, less often, Crohn's disease. But again, genes tell only part of the story.

Symptoms of Ulcerative Colitis

The most common symptoms of UC are abdominal pain and bloody diarrhea. You may also experience fatigue, weight loss and loss of appetite, dehydration, and rectal bleeding.

One of the first signs that you may have UC is stools that are looser and softer than usual, often with blood mixed in. You may also feel an intense urge to defecate (called *tenesmus*), and this may result in the accidental passage of a small amount of stool, soiling your underwear. This is due to inflammation of the rectum, usually present at the onset of UC and one of the signs that distinguishes it from Crohn's. Moving your bowels relieves this urge only temporarily, another key sign of UC. You can experience this problem during the night, causing sleep disturbances. Crampy, abdominal pain is also common (caused by inflammation in other areas of the bowel). Half of women with UC have only mild symptoms; that's common if the disease is confined to the lower (*sigmoid*) colon and the rectum.

When inflammation is confined to the rectum, it's called *ulcerative proctitis*. This may only produce blood and mucus in the stool, and tenesmus. If your disease is more severe and involves large areas of the colon, the symptoms will be more severe and likely to include anemia (from bleeding), weakness, fever, and weight loss.

Because of its inflammatory component, ulcerative colitis may also cause arthritis, eye inflammation, fatty deposits in the liver, and liver disease such as chronic hepatitis, cirrhosis, and primary sclerosing cholangitis (a disease more common in men). *Ankylosing spondylitis*, a form of inflammatory arthritis affecting the lower back and spine, affects 2 to 6 percent of patients with ulcerative colitis, causing low-back pain, morning stiffness, and sometimes a stooped posture. You may also experience skin rashes, anemia, and kidney stones. Large, circular ulcers called *pyoderma gangrenosa* that eat away at the skin and soft tissues can occur in UC (and, less commonly, in Crohn's). As with Crohn's, osteoporosis is a frequent complication. Many of the inflammatory symptoms subside when UC is treated.

Diagnosing Ulcerative Colitis

Ulcerative colitis is also a clinical diagnosis, requiring a thorough physical exam and two key diagnostic tests: sigmoidoscopy and a barium enema. In some cases, colonoscopy is needed to determine the extent of the disease. (For details, refer back to pages 206 to 207.)

Tests You May Need and What They Mean

Sigmoidoscopy can often easily distinguish ulcerative colitis from Crohn's; UC is not patchy, and there will be continuous areas of inflammation and ulcerations. In ulcerative proctitis, there will be a clear separation between red, inflamed tissue and normal bowel above it.

During periods of remission, ulcerations in the lining of the colon may heal to such an extent that the colon will appear close to normal during sigmoidoscopy or a barium x-ray.

Disease Activity in Ulcerative Colitis

The following classifications have been developed by the American College of Gastroenterology (ACG) and are used to help determine or adjust treatment.

- *Mild disease*: Patients have four or fewer bowel movements a day, with or without small amounts of blood present, no systemic signs of toxicity (such as fever or anemia), and a normal SED rate.
- *Moderate disease*: Patients have four or more bowel movements a day (usually bloody), with only minimal signs of toxicity.
- *Severe disease*: Patients have six or more bloody bowel movements a day and fever, anemia, rapid heartbeat (*tachycardia*), or an elevated SED rate.

A **stool sample** can reveal bleeding or infection in the colon or rectum. Since rectal bleeding or blood in the stool can also be a sign of colon cancer, further tests may be needed (such as colonoscopy with a biopsy).

A **complete blood count** (**CBC**, see page 28) can pick up anemia, which can be a sign of bleeding in the colon or rectum. A high white blood cell count is a sign of inflammation.

Erythrocyte sedimentation rate (**SED rate**) will be normal in mild to moderate UC, and elevated in severe disease. (For a complete explanation of a SED rate, see page 27.)

Treating Ulcerative Colitis

Unless your disease is very severe, it's likely you'll be given medication. In many cases, medications can bring about long periods of remission, from months to years, where the mucosal lining of the colon heals and virtually returns to normal. Unfortunately, your symptoms are likely to return eventually. If the disease is severe, you may need to have the entire colon removed.

In cases of severe symptoms, such as extensive bleeding or diarrhea causing dehydration, you may need to be hospitalized. In that event, you'll be given medications to stop the diarrhea and bleeding and replace lost fluids and electrolytes. If the colon is severely inflamed you may need a special diet or intravenous feeding.

Ulcerative colitis is a chronic disease (the only cure is radical surgery) that requires long-term medical care, and you need to be followed by a gastroenterologist.

Aminosalicylates are given orally or rectally (or both) to suppress inflammation in the rectum and colon. Oral medications include sulfasalazine and 5-aminosalicylic acid (5-ASA, mesalamine, olsalazine), which are generally used in mild to moderate ulcerative colitis, and as maintenance therapy. In cases of extensive but mild disease, only oral sulfasalazine or 5-ASA medications are used. If disease is moderate and extensive, azathioprine or 6-MP may be added.

Side effects of oral 5-ASA drugs include nausea, vomiting, heartburn, diarrhea, and headache (see page 209 for more about sulfasalazine and 5-ASA drugs). Topical 5-ASA agents in suppository form or suspension enemas

(*Rowasa*) can cause hemorrhoids, itching, and allergic reactions (rashes) in some people. They can also stain your clothing.

Corticosteroids include prednisone, **methylprednisolone (Medrol, Depo-Medrol)**. They can be given orally, intravenously, through an enema, or in suppository form, depending on where the inflammation is located. These medications are used in UC patients with moderate to severe disease. Systemic corticosteroids carry a risk of osteoporosis and can cause side effects like weight gain, acne, facial hair, mood swings, high blood pressure, diabetes, and an increased risk of infection.

Immunosuppressants used to treat ulcerative colitis include azathioprine (Imuran), 6-mercaptopurine (6-MP), and cyclosporine (Neoral). These drugs dampen immune activity and keep immune cells from provoking inflammation. They are usually given orally to patients who have not responded to aminosalicylates or corticosteroids. Azathioprine or 6-MP may also be used in combination with corticosteroids (they also allow lower doses to be used) in moderate and extensive disease. It can take up to three months before benefits are seen with these drugs. Intravenous cyclosporine may be given for severe disease.

"The first-line therapy is the 5-ASA drugs. If the disease involves only the rectum or the rectum and the sigmoid colon, we use topical agents such as 5-ASA enema or, in some cases, like cortisone enemas. And that can control distal disease. For mild disease, usually the oral 5-ASAs are effective," remarks Dr. Mayer. "For flares, steroids are used a little more often, but we try to avoid their use, or use them only for very short periods." As with Crohn's disease, other drugs may be given to relieve pain, diarrhea, or infection (see pages 209 to 211).

Surgery

If the disease cannot be controlled with medication, or if there's extensive bleeding, rupture, or the threat of colon cancer, surgery may be recommended (see page 212).

Until recently, radical surgery to remove the entire colon and rectum (colectomy), with an ileostomy and an external bag to collect solid waste, had been the only "cure" for ulcerative colitis. However, newer surgical techniques allow for the colon to be removed without the need for an ileostomy.

The *ileoanal anastomosis* (commonly called a *pull-through operation*) preserves part of the rectum and allows patients to have normal bowel movements. In this procedure, the diseased part of the colon and the inside of the rectum are removed, leaving the outer muscles of the rectum intact. The ileum is attached to the inside of the rectum and the anus, creating a pouch that stores waste, which is passed in the usual manner. Inflammation of the pouch and more frequent, watery bowel movements are possible complications.

The type of surgery depends on the severity and extent of the disease; you need to get as much information as possible to make an informed decision.

What's Next?

A number of new treatment approaches for ulcerative colitis are now in clinical trials. "There are epithelial growth factors that are being tested; they may speed healing of the colon lining and prevent infiltration of inflammatory cells," says Dr. Mayer.

Another experimental drug being used is an antibody to a molecule dubbed *alpha4beta7* that has been shown to contribute to inflammation in IBD. Preliminary clinical trials involving 28 patients found the drug *LDP-20* induced remissions in 40 percent of patients, compared to those on a placebo. Further clinical trials are under way in ulcerative colitis and in Crohn's.

A once-banned drug may have new use in fighting IBD. Thalidomide was given as an antinausea drug to pregnant women and caused catastrophic birth defects; it was banned in the 1960s. But in recent years, it has been tested against ulcerative colitis, Crohn's, and other diseases. A small study among men at the Cedars-Sinai Medical Center in Los Angeles found that about half the patients showed a reduction in disease activity. Side effects include sedation, numbness, and dry skin.

Tests are also being conducted of other forms of thalidomide called *selective cytokine inhibitory drugs*, which inhibit an enzyme that spurs production of tumor necrosis factor. These drugs seem to be more potent at dampening inflammation than thalidomide, and animal tests have not shown any birth defects.

It's an odd occurrence that smoking seems to be protective in ulcerative colitis, so nicotine is being studied as a potential therapy. In one early study, some patients given nicotine patches or enemas showed improved symptoms.

"Again, we don't know that nicotine is what seems to be protective in ulcerative colitis, and we do not recommend that patients start smoking or use nicotine patches," stresses Dr. Mayer.

Your Risk of Colon Cancer

About 5 percent of people with UC develop colorectal cancer, and the risk increases the longer you have UC and with the extent and location of the disease. For example, if the entire colon is involved, your risk of cancer may be as high as thirty-two times the norm; if UC involves only the lower colon and rectum, your risks are not higher than normal.

Ulcerative colitis can lead to precancerous changes called *dysplasia* in the cells lining the colon. Signs of *dysplasia* can be picked up during colonoscopy and biopsy. Guidelines for colon cancer screening (endorsed by the American Cancer Society, the American College of Gastroenterology, the American Society of Colon and Rectal Surgeons, and the Crohn's & Colitis Foundation of America) advise that people who have had IBD throughout their colon for at least eight years, and those who have had IBD in only the left colon for at least fifteen years, should have a colonoscopy every one to two years to check for dysplasia. Recent studies show that colonoscopy is the most effective way of finding colon cancer in its earliest, most curable stage.

How Ulcerative Colitis Can Affect You Over Your Lifetime

As with Crohn's disease, ulcerative colitis can affect women during their reproductive years.

Reproduction

Fertility among women with ulcerative colitis seems to be unaffected by the disease itself. However, women who undergo removal of their colon may have trouble conceiving after the surgery, according to a study in the January 2002 issue of the journal *Gastroenterology*. The study, from Denmark, compared fertility rates of women with UC to women without the condition. Those women who had not undergone colectomy had an equal or higher fertility rate as women without ulcerative colitis. Those women who underwent colectomy had a significantly lower fertility rate and an increased use of in-vitro fertilization.

Around a third of women with active ulcerative colitis who become pregnant will improve, and a third will worsen, notes Dr. Sunanda Kane. UC can also occur during pregnancy and the postpartum period. However, sulfasalazine is safe to use during pregnancy, and the 5-ASA agents also appear safe.

Midlife and Beyond

Osteoporosis is a major concern for women taking corticosteroids, especially later in life. Corticosteroids tend to complicate and worsen diabetes, high blood pressure, and other age-related diseases. Women with UC may need antiresorptive agents called *bisphosphonates*, such as alendronate (Fosamax) or risedronate (Actonel) to stem bone loss.

One form of colon inflammation, called *ischemic colitis*, can occur in later life and is caused by poor circulation and can mimic the symptoms of IBD. One study found that 75 percent of people with colitis after the age of fifty actually had ischemic colitis, and neither form of IBD. Older women may also develop an antibiotic-associated colitis.

> *I was diagnosed with celiac disease as a child. Apparently it runs in my family. My grandmother later told me one of her sisters died of diarrhea and dehydration as a baby; they thought it was colic. But I thought it was something you outgrew . . . I found out by accident that you don't really outgrow it. I never had a digestive system that worked properly, from what I can tell. Once every few weeks, I'd have what they called a "stomach virus." I thought I was just susceptible to that. No matter how much I ate, I felt full. If I didn't eat, I'd drop five pounds. If I looked at my stool, I'd see whole pieces of undigested food, and globs of fat. I'd think, "I'm not digesting my food."*

I didn't know anything about celiac. Except they made you live on nothing when you were a kid, then they thought you outgrew it and you were fine. I made an appointment with an internist and told him I don't know that much about celiac disease, but maybe there's a relationship between that and what's going on with my digestive system. I said, "I think you need to do a stool analysis because I'm not digesting my food." And he said no. Celiac disease has nothing to do with it. This was in 1975 when this happened. I was eighteen or nineteen. I thought I was being completely logical. But he dismissed it. He gave me a blood test of some kind, which showed nothing. So I figured celiac had nothing to do with it, and I gave up. I didn't pursue it until much later on.

RONNIE, FORTY-FIVE

Celiac Disease

Celiac disease is an autoimmune disease that damages the small intestine and interferes with absorption of nutrients. In celiac disease, the immune system mounts an inflammatory reaction against *gluten*, a protein found in wheat (similar proteins are found in rye, barley, possibly oats), in the process destroying the numerous tiny villi in the lining of the small intestine.

You'll recall that villi absorb nutrients from food; without villi you become malnourished, no matter how much you eat. Celiac disease (or *celiac sprue*) affects the parts of the small intestine where iron and calcium are absorbed, so most people with celiac have *iron deficiency anemia* and bone loss. The disease also destroys cells in the intestinal lining containing the receptors for vitamins A, D, E, K, and B_{12}. Vitamin B_{12} deficiency results in another form of anemia, *macrocytic anemia* (in which abnormally enlarged red blood cells crowd out normal cells).

Celiac disease runs in families, and genes are thought to play a role. It was once thought to be relatively rare in this country (it's commonplace in Ireland and Italy), but a recent study by the University of Maryland found that as many as 1 in every 200 Americans may have celiac sprue. Women are affected three times more often than men and, because symptoms are similar to irritable bowel syndrome, some may be mistakenly diagnosed with IBS.

Warning Signs of Celiac Disease

- Recurrent abdominal bloating and pain
- Chronic diarrhea
- Weight loss
- Pale, foul-smelling stool
- Anemia
- Gas
- Bone loss
- Muscle cramps
- Fatigue and depression
- Joint pain
- Tingling and numbness in the legs (*neuropathy*)
- Pale mouth sores
- Painful skin rash (*dermatitis herpetiformis*)
- Discolored teeth; loss of enamel
- Missed menstrual periods

Celiac typically arises during early childhood, but it can also be triggered (or become active for the first time) after surgery, pregnancy, childbirth, viral infections, or even severe emotional stress. People were once thought to "outgrow" celiac disease. But we now know that's not true. And untreated celiac disease can have serious complications, including an increased risk of certain types of cancers.

What Causes Celiac Disease?

Unlike other autoimmune diseases, in celiac the immune system doesn't attack self-antigens. The attack is actually directed against water-insoluble proteins, or *prolamins*, in grains as they pass through the digestive system. These proteins—*gliadin* (found in wheat), *secalin* (from rye), and *hordein* (contained in barley)—trigger an inflammatory reaction in the small intestines of genetically susceptible individuals.

When the immune system senses a prolamin, it sends white blood cells to attack them. These lymphocytes infiltrate the lining of the small intestine, and the resulting inflammation causes overgrowth of the valleys (*crypts*) between the villi, and eventually the destruction of the villi themselves.

"It's not a case of mistaken identity or molecular mimicry. The villi are not the targets; they are innocent bystanders," remarks Peter H. R. Green, MD, clinical professor and director of the Celiac Disease Research Center at Columbia University. "Celiac disease is an unusual autoimmune disease because we know what the environmental antigen is." What *isn't* known is when or how the initial sensitization to gluten occurs. In people who are genetically susceptible to celiac disease, "tolerance" to gluten may not occur.

Technically, all the foods we eat are "foreign" antigens. But as we gradually start eating solid foods as babies, the immune system becomes programmed to tolerate them. The immune system has to reach a certain maturity before it can do this, however. That's one reason breastfeeding is beneficial. It not only contains a perfect balance of proteins, carbohydrates, and fat to nourish an infant, but because these nutrient antigens come from the mother, they are less likely to set off an immune reaction. Breast milk also contains many important antibodies that help an infant fight off infections, and creates a protective environment in the intestines. Baby formulas contain cow's milk that's been altered to closely resemble human milk (but it lacks the key antibodies). In families where food allergies or lactose intolerance is common, soy baby formula is used. In the case of milk allergies, babies are fed *protein hydrolysate* formulas, which contain cow's milk proteins broken down in a way that mimics digestion and is less likely to provoke allergic reactions. (Allergic reactions also involve the immune system and often occur in people with autoimmune disease.) The first solid food babies eat is rice cereal, which does not contain gluten.

One factor thought to play a role in when and how celiac appears is whether (and how long) you were breastfed. Some experts believe that the longer you were breastfed, the later symptoms of celiac disease may appear (and the more atypical those symptoms). Other risk factors may include the age at which you began eating foods containing gluten, and how much gluten you ate. (Celiac most often arises between four and twenty-four months.) But, again, when the initial sensitization to gluten takes place is not known.

A majority of people with celiac disease produce antibodies against gliadin, setting off a process that leads to production of autoantibodies. These include *antireticulin antibodies* (*ARAs*), which react to a component of connective tissue in the gastrointestinal tract called *reticulin*, and *antiendomysium antibodies* (*EMAs*), which react against components of smooth muscle tissue in the esophagus and the upper part of the small intestine (jejunum). "It's thought that all the autoantibodies in celiac are somehow related to the fact that you have an intestinal disorder that allows your immune system to 'see' a lot of foreign proteins," explains Dr. Green. "The intestines become so permeable that many proteins go through and are presented as foreign to the immune system where that would not normally occur, which may result in a 'saturation' of the immune system, in an overreactive immune system, that eventually reacts against self."

In fact, celiac disease is closely associated with other autoimmune diseases, including type 1 diabetes, thyroid disease, and Sjögren's syndrome, which are often the initial diagnosis in adults with celiac sprue. "It's thought that you get the celiac disease first, then you get these autoantibodies to other organs, and then you get the other organ disease, and much later the celiac gets diagnosed," explains Dr. Green. "If you take a bunch of kids with celiac disease, they will often have autoantibodies to the pancreas or to the thyroid. If you put them on a gluten-free diet, those autoantibodies go away. So maybe if you can diagnose celiac early enough, you may prevent these other autoimmune diseases."

Genes play a major role in celiac disease. Among identical twins (who share identical genes), if one twin has celiac there's a 70 percent chance the other twin will have it too. Among nonidentical twins, this *concordance* rate is 40 percent. But sharing the same human leukocyte antigens (HLAs) may not be the only factor that predisposes people to celiac disease.

"We don't know the genes that are responsible. Celiac is associated with certain HLA genes, but they are also common in the general population. So there are probably multiple genes involved," observes Dr. Green.

It's not clear whether female (or male) hormones play a role in celiac disease. "We have looked at male-female differences in celiac disease, and men seem to have more severe manifestations than women. Men have lower bone density and lower total cholesterol, suggesting more malabsorption. But more women get it than men," remarks Dr. Green. "Hormones have not been looked at closely in women with celiac disease, but in men you have low testosterone levels. There's a circulation of estrogen within the liver that gets secreted in bile and then reabsorbed. So potentially, you don't get reabsorption of secreted estrogen. Women may well have lowered testosterone, too. But it hasn't been studied."

> Ronnie's story continues:
> *I actually learned about celiac disease from a free magazine I got in a health food store . . . the article talked about all the symptoms I had been having for years. It mentioned a book, and I ordered it. It told you what to eat and not to eat. So I tried eliminating all the gluten in my diet. I went to a bookstore that had a medical text section and found two books that had something on celiac and took notes. That's how I learned everything . . . the tests that diagnose it, which does include a stool analysis to look for evidence of undigested fat . . . and they described all the damage to the villi. I did go to see another doctor who didn't want to hear about anything I had learned. She just wanted to run tests. She got very huffy and said, "You think you know so much . . . I'm the doctor." I have other problems along with the celiac. I've had chronic fatigue . . . I had fibromyalgia . . . on both sides of my family there's diabetes, and I am very prone to hypoglycemia. But aside from avoiding gluten and fat, I figured there was nothing the medical profession could really do for me.*

Symptoms of Celiac Disease

Celiac disease affects each person differently. You may have more diarrhea and abdominal pain, while another woman may have anemia or bone loss as signs of malabsorption. Some women may have no symptoms at all; the undamaged parts of their small intestine are able to absorb enough nutrients to prevent GI problems or malabsorption. This hidden (*occult*) disease may contribute to the notion that celiac disease is rare in this country, says Dr. Green.

But even people with no symptoms are at risk for complications, including certain cancers (see page 224).

The classic symptoms of celiac include diarrhea, flatulence, weight loss, and fatigue. Your stool may appear grayish or tan in color, smell rancid, and float. If celiac is severe and involves most of the small intestine, fat absorption will also be impaired, and fat goblets may appear in stool (*steatorrhea*) and there may be oil floating in the toilet. Some women may experience constipation with celiac.

Symptoms can also depend on specific areas of the intestine affected by celiac disease. When the duodenum and nearby parts of the small intestine are involved, iron is poorly absorbed, leading to iron deficiency anemia. This is also the area where fat-soluble vitamins—A, D, E, and K—are taken in, and celiac disease may cause them to be poorly absorbed as well. Vitamin B_{12} is absorbed in the furthest part of the small intestine (the *ileum*), which is less frequently involved in celiac disease. But if the disease causes a deficiency of vitamin B_{12}, it can lead to *macrocytic anemia*. Poor absorption of calcium and vitamin D leads to bone loss. In serious, untreated celiac disease, women can develop severe malnutrition, osteoporosis, and even malignant tumors of the small intestine (see page 237).

"The classical presentation is probably uncommon in this country, and many women might be misdiagnosed with irritable bowel syndrome. One study from London found that one in twenty people diagnosed with IBS might actually have celiac disease. Iron deficiency anemia may be blamed on menstrual blood loss when some women might have celiac disease," remarks Dr. Green. "With women there may be a delay in diagnosis because they are seen as a complaining patient, they're told 'It's all in your head,' or 'It's irritable bowel syndrome.' Gastroenterologists are taught that IBS is the most common diagnosis, and if they see a woman with altered bowel habits and all the other manifestations, they may not think of celiac disease."

Celiac disease can manifest at any time in life. "Kids can get diagnosed and they go on a gluten-free diet, and many years ago people were told they 'grew out of it.' But that was because during adolescence they tolerated going back to gluten. Then later on in life they get rediagnosed and may present with osteoporosis or a malignancy. So making this diagnosis is important," says Dr. Green.

You may develop a rash as a consequence of gluten intolerance. The itchy, blistering rash—dermatitis herpetiformis—affects the arms, legs, trunk, and scalp. Less commonly, there may be leg ulcerations.

Diagnosing Celiac Disease

Diagnosing celiac disease can be difficult because some symptoms are similar to irritable bowel syndrome, Crohn's disease, ulcerative colitis, diverticular disease, intestinal infections, chronic fatigue syndrome, and depression. Some of those diseases may also occur in women with celiac.

The longer you continue undiagnosed and untreated, the greater the chance of developing malnutrition and other complications. In Italy, where celiac disease is common, all children are screened by age six, says Dr. Green. In fact, Italians are tested for the disease as soon as they show any symptoms. As a result, the time between when a person first experiences symptoms and a diagnosis is usually only two to three weeks. In the United States, where celiac has been considered rare, the time between the first symptoms and a diagnosis averages about ten years.

"It's actually an easy diagnosis to make. Most people with celiac test positive for antibodies to gliadin, which is the part of wheat that people mount the immunological reaction to. Then you test for tissue autoantigens. Those tests are widely available. If they are positive, the next step is a small intestinal biopsy done with endoscopy," explains Dr. Green. Because celiac disease is hereditary, first-degree family members—your parents, siblings, and children—should also be tested, he adds. Additional tests are done to detect complications of celiac, such as anemia and osteoporosis.

Tests You May Need and What They Mean

Antigliadin antibodies are present in up to 40 percent of people with celiac disease, but they are not specific to celiac; they can also be found in people with small-bowel Crohn's disease and, in low amounts, in the general population. The level of antigliadin antibodies will fall if you stick to a gluten-free diet.

Antiendomysium (**EMA**) and **antireticulin** (**ARA**) antibodies are antibodies against components of connective tissue in the gastrointestinal tract. ARAs react against a protein called reticulin; EMAs recognize parts of smooth muscle tissue in the esophagus and the upper part of the small intestine. EMAs are considered specific for celiac disease (they will decline if you're on a gluten-free diet.) ARAs are also found in people with rheumatoid arthritis and Sjögren's.

Small-intestine biopsy is considered the gold standard for diagnosing celiac disease. Under sedation (to make you more comfortable and quiet your gag reflex) a long, thin hollow tube called an *endoscope* is passed through the mouth, esophagus, and stomach into the small intestine. A small sample of tissue from the upper area of the small intestine is taken with instruments passed through the endoscope. In celiac disease the biopsy will reveal atrophy of the villi. The test takes about ten minutes and no special preparation is needed. Small-intestine biopsy is also done to test the effectiveness of a gluten-free diet; damage to the small intestine is often healed if the diet is followed carefully.

A **complete blood count** (**CBC**) includes a count of the iron-carrying red blood cells (RBCs) and *hemoglobin*, the component in red blood cells that transports iron. A low red blood cell count and low hemoglobin diagnose iron deficiency anemia, caused by malabsorption of iron from the small intestine. Women normally have lower levels of hemoglobin than men, between 12 to 16 grams of hemoglobin per deciliter of blood (g/dl). In macrocytic anemia, caused by malabsorption of vitamin B_{12}, red blood cells will become enlarged and crowd out normal RBCs. Borderline deficiency of vitamin B_{12} is considered to be 258 picomoles per liter of blood (pmol/l); clinical deficiency is a B_{12} level of 148 pmol/l or below.

Dual-energy x-ray absorptiometry (**DEXA**) measures bone density and can detect osteoporosis, a frequent complication of celiac disease. The DEXA is a painless test that uses very low doses of radiation. You lie on a table with your legs elevated while a special x-ray device slowly moves up and down above you, taking pictures of your hips and spine to measure bone density at key areas, including the vertebrae in the lower spine, and the upper part of the thigh (femur) inside the hip joint. The test takes around ten minutes.

You get DEXA results in two numbers: the *T-score* and the *Z-score*. The Z-score compares your bone mineral density (BMD) to that of women in your age and ethnic group, and a T-score compares your BMD to the average for Caucasian women between the age of twenty-five and thirty-five, when bone density is at its peak. These scores are reported as standard deviations (ST) from the norm in each group, which is set at zero. You can be above or below, plus or minus, the mean. The more important reading is the T-score. You're considered to have osteoporosis if your BMD is 2.5 standard deviations below the mean for young adult women; a T-score between −1 and −2.5 standard deviations below the peak bone mass is considered to be *osteopenia*, or mild bone loss.

Treating Celiac Disease

The only treatment for celiac disease is a gluten-free diet. That means avoiding foods that contain wheat (including kamut, a form of wheat; spelt, an older form of wheat; and triticale, a blend of rye and wheat), rye, barley, and possibly oats—that includes most grains, pastas, cereals, and breads, as well as foods containing fillers made from grain. You need to follow this diet even if you don't have GI symptoms, since damage may be occurring silently.

Within days of starting a gluten-free diet, your symptoms start to ease and the condition of the small intestine begins to improve. Within three to six months, the small intestine is usually completely healed—meaning the villi are intact and working (in older adults, this may take up to two years). An endoscopic small-intestine biopsy can determine whether you're responding to the diet.

Many gluten-free products are made with corn, rice, soy, sorghum, or chestnut flower. Some products are labeled gluten free; with others you may have to read the list of ingredients carefully. Ingredients derived from grain may not be obvious. For example, malt is a common ingredient used to give foods flavor; you may not know it's made from barley. Another common ingredient, hydrolyzed vegetable protein, is actually made from grain. On the other hand, buckwheat may have wheat in its name, but it's a grain that doesn't contain gluten.

"Gluten can even be found in medications. The bulk of a pill or capsule is filler, or binder, usually cornstarch or wheat starch. So people with celiac are advised to check all their drugs once a year, because drug companies can change their suppliers," advises Dr. Green. "A surprising source of gluten is communion wafers."

Eating even the tiniest amount of gluten can provoke damage to the small intestine. So if you have celiac disease, you'll need to educate yourself about safe food ingredients. The Celiac Foundation website has lists of gluten-free foods, products, and manufacturers (see Appendix A).

In addition to a gluten-free diet, you may also need pancreatic enzymes to aid digestion. "When you eat, the gut secretes hormones that stimulate the pancreas to produce enzymes needed for digestion. If you have celiac disease you don't secrete these hormones, and therefore the pancreas doesn't respond well when you eat. So if people are feeling unwell at diagnosis, we give them pancreatic enzymes," explains Dr. Green.

A small percentage of people with celiac don't respond to a gluten-free diet; their small intestines may be so damaged that they can't heal. Some people with celiac develop an associated autoimmune disease, *lymphocytic colitis.* "The intestine looks normal endoscopically, but on biopsy is found to have lymphocytic infiltration. And that's a cause of failure to respond to a gluten-free

---

Celiac Disease Clusters

Celiac disease is associated with a number of autoimmune diseases, especially type 1 diabetes. Take a look at the chapters on the diseases that cluster with celiac, since early diagnosis of celiac could well prevent or aid in diagnosing other diseases.

- Type 1 diabetes
- Thyroid disease
- Sjögren's syndrome
- Primary biliary cirrhosis
- Myasthenia gravis
- Pernicious anemia

diet," says Dr. Green. Other people may have such severe intestinal damage that they can't absorb enough nutrients to maintain health and may need intravenous supplementation. "Some patients have refractory, nonresponsive celiac disease and they may require steroids or immunosuppressants. These include prednisone or azathioprine," he adds.

Related disorders include *collagenous sprue*, which resembles celiac disease but a thick layer of collagen is deposited beneath the inner lining of the intestines. This condition may not respond to a gluten-free diet and may require immunosuppressants.

A small number of people with celiac disease develop mucosal ulcerations. If this occurs in the duodenum, it can be mistaken for peptic ulcers; if it occurs farther down in the small intestine, it may be mistaken for Crohn's disease. The condition, called *ulcerative jejunitis*, is more common in the elderly.

Celiac disease is associated with an increased risk of certain kinds of cancers, including non-Hodgkins lymphoma, intestinal T-cell lymphoma, small bowel and esophageal cancer, and melanoma. "However, it's been shown in Europe that once you put people on a gluten-free diet, the risk of developing these cancers eventually goes back to that of the general population. So this makes it especially urgent for people to be diagnosed as early as possible," says Dr. Green.

How Celiac Disease Can Affect You Over Your Lifetime

Celiac disease can cause special complications for women, including delayed puberty and menarche, menstrual irregularities, miscarriages, infertility, and premature menopause. In childhood, the complications are due to delayed development, but it's not clear how celiac can cause reproductive problems, says Dr. Green.

While celiac can show itself at any time, diagnosis in adults seems to peak around age fifty. And the irritability and depression of celiac may even be mistaken for symptoms of menopause.

Celiac poses the threat of osteoporosis for women of all ages. But if a woman is diagnosed with low bone density during her forties or fifties, the underlying cause is often assumed to be estrogen loss, and the standard treatment of bisphosphonates (Fosamax, Actonel) to prevent bone resorption may create problems. "Potentially, if the osteoporosis is due to malabsorption of calcium, and a woman is actually maintaining a normal serum calcium, the calcium is being leached out of bones because it is not being absorbed from the gut," he explains. "If people have osteoporosis due to celiac disease and are just put on Fosamax, the body would not be able to remove calcium from the bones, and serum calcium could potentially drop to dangerous levels. So we don't recommend that people with osteoporosis and celiac disease be put straight on Fosamax, because we have to increase their calcium absorption first. And that must be done through a gluten-free diet."

Malabsorption of calcium can also lead to *hyperparathyroidism*; about 20 percent of women with osteoporosis and celiac disease will develop this problem. The four tiny parathyroid glands are buried in the thyroid and produce parathyroid hormone (PTH), needed along with calcitonin (produced by the thyroid gland) and vitamin D to regulate the balance of calcium in the body. If there's too little calcium in the blood, the parathyroid glands secrete more PTH, taking calcium from the bones to correct the imbalance. In celiac disease, calcium isn't properly absorbed and passes out of the body. Vitamin D isn't being absorbed, either. So the parathyroid produces more PTH. Chronic low levels of calcium can cause the gland to become overactive, causing even more calcium to be removed from the bones.

Hyperparathyroidism is diagnosed by measuring levels of PTH, urinary calcium, and vitamin D. In hyperparathyroidism, PTH is elevated, as is one form of vitamin D (*1,25-dihydroxy vitamin D*), and urinary calcium is high (signaling malabsorption). Hyperparathyroidism is treated by surgically removing abnormal parathyroid tissue, and giving oral calcium and 1,25-dihydroxy vitamin D supplements (Calcitriol) to normalize calcium.

Pernicious Anemia

An autoimmune disease common in women over age sixty is *pernicious anemia*. It results from an autoimmune attack on the *parietal* cells lining the stomach, which secrete a chemical called *intrinsic factor* (*IF*) that binds to vitamin B_{12} and helps it absorb in the small intestine. The destruction of the parietal cells impairs production of intrinsic factor, and autoantibodies against IF prevent it from binding to vitamin B$_{12}$ so it can't be absorbed.

The resulting vitamin deficiency can cause atrophy of the surface of the tongue (*atrophic glossitis*), producing a red, smooth appearance; diarrhea; and nerve damage (*peripheral neuropathy*) that leads to tingling and numbness. Nerve damage is a result of lesions caused by autoantibodies, and in severe cases lesions can develop in the brain, leading to memory loss and even psychosis (in some cases, it may be mistaken for Alzheimer's disease). It can also occur in women with celiac disease and other autoimmune diseases.

Pernicious anemia is diagnosed with blood tests to measure vitamin B$_{12}$ and levels of folate, another B vitamin. Red blood cells become enlarged in pernicious anemia (they're called *megaloblasts*). More than 90 percent of women will have autoantibodies to parietal cells; nearly half of patients have autoantibodies to intrinsic factor.

The treatment is simple: monthly injections of 100 micrograms (mcg) of vitamin B$_{12}$. This remedies the anemia and, in many cases, corrects the nerve-related complications.

In some elderly people, the lining of the stomach may atrophy, and a daily supplement of 25 micrograms of vitamin B$_{12}$ is recommended to prevent deficiency.

9

An Attack of Nerves—
Multiple Sclerosis

*When I was told I had multiple sclerosis it knocked me for a loop . . . it
was like being blown across the room. I couldn't quite believe it. It was
so unexpected. I tried to be very calm when I got the results of the tests,
but one night I just sat down and decided that I would let it all out,
and cried hysterically. But my dog got so upset, I had to calm myself
down. I still haven't quite gotten used to it. Every time I get a cold, it
seems to flare. It seems like it's there all the time. My greatest fear is
ending up in a wheelchair. Even though my doctor reassures me that
won't happen, I still worry about it. I guess the worry will never leave.*

ANA, FIFTY-TWO

If you can imagine an electrical cord with insulation that's frayed and worn
away in places, causing a short in the wire and then shorting out the electrical system, then you can visualize multiple sclerosis (MS).

In MS, autoantibodies, immune cells, and inflammation damage the "insulation" (called *myelin*) wrapped around nerve cell fibers in the brain and spinal
cord that carry messages to the rest of the body, causing a variety of symptoms, from vision problems to limb weakness. Two-thirds of the 500,000
Americans with MS are women, and the number of new cases among women
is rising. The reasons why are unclear; it may be due to better diagnosis or a
real increase.

Warning Signs of MS

- Fatigue
- Vision problems—blurred or double vision
- Tingling, numbness, burning sensations in the arms or legs
- Muscle weakness, especially in the legs
- Muscle stiffness or spasticity
- Problems with balance or coordination
- Problems with short-term memory
- Dizziness or vertigo
- Slowed or slurred speech
- Change in bladder or bowel function

More people are now being diagnosed at an earlier stage and started on drug treatments that can slow the progression of the disease. Where once MS could mean disability and confinement to a wheelchair, today most women with the disease lead normal, fully functional lives.

What Causes MS?

Myelin is usually compared to the insulation around electrical wires that helps electrical transmission and protects the wires from being damaged and shorting out. But it's not really like the single, smooth layer of rubber found on electrical wires. It's a fatty substance manufactured by specialized cells called *oligodendrocytes* that coils around nerve fibers (*axons*), more like multiple layers of electrical tape.

Both myelin and oligodendrocytes find themselves under attack in MS. Autoantibodies reacting to proteins in myelin (including *myelin basic protein*) and other toxic products of immune cells eat away one or more layers of the myelin sheath and the cells producing it. Since a single oligodendrocyte may spin out myelin for fifty to one hundred axons, an attack on one of these cells can result in problems for multiple axons, notes Anthony J. Reder, MD, asso-

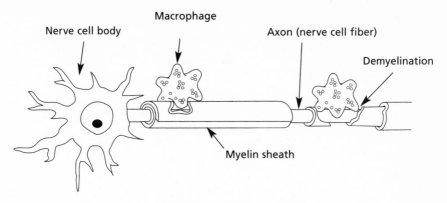

Macrophage

Nerve cell body

Axon (nerve cell fiber)

Demyelination

Myelin sheath

How MS Affects Nerve Cells

ciate professor of neurology at the University of Chicago. However, because there are so many layers of myelin, it may take a while for the damage to produce symptoms. And myelin may regenerate over a period of months in the beginning (the brain may even reorganize some of its circuits to compensate for minor damage). But the new myelin is not as stable, and eventually spots along the sheath are totally eaten away (*demyelination*). Inflammation of the sheath at areas of demyelination, which may come in cycles or bursts of activity, is believed to be responsible for MS flares. Immune attacks and inflammation can occur in any area of the central nervous system—the brain, the spinal cord, or the optic nerve—but early on, most of this damage occurs silently.

As myelin is eaten away, messages between nerve cells are increasingly disrupted. When the axon is exposed, it can become damaged or even severed. Accumulated damage to axons can be widespread, eventually leading to irreversible loss of function and permanent disability.

As myelin is stripped away, it's replaced by scar (*sclerotic*) tissue, which forms *plaques* that build up at numerous spots around the central nervous system—hence the name *multiple sclerosis*. Plaques and inflammation show up as white spots on magnetic resonance imaging (MRI). MRI is an important diagnostic tool because it reveals plaques even when there are no symptoms. The number of myelin-producing cells are reduced (or they're absent altogether) within plaques.

For all of this newfound knowledge about the underlying process of MS damage, it's still unclear what triggers it in the first place. Faulty genes may predispose people to the most common form of MS. Up to 20 percent of MS patients have at least one relative with the disease. While there's no evidence that MS itself can be inherited, having certain genes may also make people vulnerable to environmental toxins or viruses. Some MS experts believe female hormones may protect nerve cells to some extent.

The agents of destruction in MS are thought to be cell-killing (*cytotoxic*) T-cells, activated as if to rout a foreign invader, along with hordes of scavenger macrophages attracted by chemicals released by the activated T-cells. In fact, there may *be* an invader hidden in nerves. Some viruses can infect the body and then remain dormant in nerve trunks. To T-cells, those viruses may look similar to proteins in myelin (molecular mimicry). There are dozens of suspects—including *Epstein-Barr virus* (*EBV*, which causes *infectious mononucleosis*), the respiratory virus *Hemophilus influenzae*, the mumps and measles viruses, and a herpes virus that causes the childhood illness *roseola*. We've all been exposed to them, and it's unclear whether they actually trigger the initial MS attack.

Antibodies to these viruses (evidence the body has reacted to an infection) are elevated in people with MS; antibodies have also been found in cerebral spinal fluid (CSF). Evidence of viral infections in the central nervous system and in MS plaques have also been detected. EBV antibodies are increased during MS exacerbations, notes Dr. Reder. "One out of every three upper respiratory viruses triggers an MS attack, probably caused by the activation of the immune system," he says. Respiratory infections are known to prompt MS relapses (probably through a reaction in "memory cells" programmed by a previous encounter with a virus). But so far there's no direct evidence that viruses actually *cause* MS.

One recent study suggests that EBV infection increases the *risk* of developing MS. Researchers from Harvard analyzed blood samples from 144 women with definite or probable MS and 288 healthy women taking part in the ongoing Nurses' Health Study. Eighteen of the women developed MS over a ten-year period; 126 had MS or MS symptoms at the start of the study. The researchers found elevations of anti-EBV antibodies in blood collected from the 18 women before they were diagnosed with MS, and antibodies in blood from the other 126 women collected after their diagnosis; levels were all higher than in their age-matched healthy counterparts. A fourfold elevation in antibodies to one fragment of the virus was associated with a fourfold increase in the risk of MS, according to the study reported in the *Journal of the American Medical Association* (*JAMA*) in December 2001.

Since 90 percent of people have been exposed to EBV at some point, other factors must be involved in MS, such as genetic predisposition, the age at which a woman is infected, or even infection with other microbes, the researchers speculate.

But how would the destructive T-cells get through the blood-brain barrier that protects the brain from toxins? New research indicates that cells in the brain membrane (*endothelial cells*) somehow become activated and secrete chemicals that attract T-cells, then literally pull them through the cells, crossing the normally impervious blood-brain barrier, says Dr. Reder. These chemicals are called *adhesion molecules*, because they act like glue. Once inside the brain, myelin-reactive T-cells multiply and likely release chemicals that bring more inflammatory cells into the area to cause damage.

Some scientists believe MS may actually be several different disorders, some of which may be autoimmune and others more like damage from toxins or viruses. Recent research has identified four possible categories of disease based on the appearance of brain lesions; studies are under way to correlate those findings with actual brain tissue samples and MRI images.

The first symptom I had was actually vision loss in one eye. I went to an ophthalmologist who suspected that I had MS and wrote in my file that he suspected nerve damage, but he told me it was "only optic neuritis" and that it would go away. I immediately went and looked up optic neuritis in the encyclopedia, and it scared me because it said it was inflammation of nerves. And that led me to believe it wasn't going to stop. And I became very frightened and thought I was going to be completely blind, but I decided to ignore it. I went on for about six years with various symptoms that were not really conclusive enough to make a diagnosis, which I know now . . . I didn't realize that fatigue was a part of MS, and I had other symptoms as well . . . like problems with my bladder, and dizziness if I sat down and stood up too fast. But the symptoms of MS are things everyone has at one time or another, but they're just more magnified and chronic. Everyone has the tingling hand or the limb that falls asleep, everyone's been tired and fatigued. So I could easily chalk up all of my symptoms to other problems. I didn't even think about pulling all this together. I was in my early twenties, I was going to college, I had a lot going on, and I chose to ignore it. I saw various doctors, but no one wanted to make a definitive diagnosis.

Mariana, thirty-nine

Symptoms of MS

MS can be sneaky—the first symptoms can come and go, and you might not pay much attention to them. A mild tingling in one leg, a little trouble with your eyes. Perhaps some fatigue, joint pain, or trouble remembering things. Sometimes these symptoms last a few days and may include balance problems, slurred speech, and stiffness. Symptoms can resemble other conditions, including Lyme disease, which may delay a diagnosis.

The most common symptom is actually fatigue, reported by up to 85 percent of MS patients. "MS fatigue is very distinctive. It's not a function of physical disability, or of not sleeping, but if you don't sleep well that can aggravate it. These women sleep eight hours and wake up feeling like they are just drained. It's generally made worse with heat, and generally gets worse later in the day," says Barbara S. Giesser, MD, an associate clinical professor of neurology at the University of California, Los Angeles. Unlike other autoimmune diseases, chronic fatigue syndrome (CFS) and fibromyalgia are not usually fellow travelers with MS. "However, I certainly have had patients who were initially diagnosed with fibromyalgia or CFS and turned out to have MS," she adds.

Depression is actually the second most common symptom of MS, reported by up to 70 percent of patients at some point during the course of their illness. Some women may experience wide mood swings, unprovoked and uncontrollable euphoria followed by extreme depression. In fact, Dr. Reder speculates that sometimes the mood swings attributed to *bipolar depression* (also called *manic depression*) could be an early symptom of MS. No brain lesions are found in manic depression, but may be seen in early MS.

Depression in MS may be due to brain lesions or immune dysregulation; depression may also induce abnormalities of immune function that may contribute to MS. A recent study found that treating depression is accompanied by a reduction in interferon-gamma production, one of the inflammatory proteins in MS.

Vision problems are very common, especially *optic neuritis*. This can take the form of blurred or hazy vision, usually in the central area, or even a complete loss of vision. Problems can come on gradually or suddenly, and resolve quickly. Pain around the eyes may precede loss of vision, sometimes by a few hours, sometimes by a few days. An eye exam may reveal paleness at the back of the eye, indicating optic nerve damage.

Motor symptoms can include a vague feeling of weakness or heaviness in the legs (one leg may tend to drag), as well as a tendency to trip or fall. Five percent of MS patients present with a tremor, while 2 percent may suffer from nerve pain that affects the jaw called *trigeminal neuralgia*, notes Dr. Reder. Some women may have trouble swallowing or experience facial twitches.

The most common cognitive changes are slowed thinking and memory retrieval, especially visual memory. Corresponding brain changes may even be seen, such as thinning of the corpus callosum, which connects the two hemispheres of the brain, and a degeneration of nerve fibers.

Some of the sensory changes experienced in MS include tingling, numbness, or feelings similar to small electrical shocks in the limbs or other areas of the body. Some women may experience vertigo or clumsiness. Five percent of women may initially experience bladder problems, a sense of urinary urgency along with more frequent urination, or incontinence. In some women, the bladder may not empty completely and they may have frequent urinary tract infections. Bladder or urinary problems may be the only initial symptoms of MS. Heat can cause a worsening of symptoms, making it even harder for damaged neurons to communicate.

Four types of multiple sclerosis can be diagnosed, based on general patterns of symptoms:

1. **Relapsing-remitting**: This is the most common type of MS, in which symptoms flare and then go into remission. This respite may be due to bursts of inflammation that subside or to the regeneration of myelin. That inflam-

mation can be seen on MRI using a special contrast agent. Up to 75 percent of people with MS display the relapsing-remitting type.

2. **Primary progressive**: In this type of MS there are continual attacks on nerves and inflammation, with no remissions, causing increasing disability; about 10 percent of patients have primary progressive MS. (This is actually more common in men.)

3. **Secondary progressive**: About two-thirds of people with the milder relapsing-remitting MS evolve into a secondary progressive form. This can occur with or without occasional flares, minor remissions, and even long plateaus of stability in the disease. But eventually the disease keeps worsening, with a progressive loss of axons.

4. **Progressive relapsing**: This is a relatively rare type of MS, occurring in about 5 percent of patients. In this type of MS, there's a steady worsening of disease from the start, but with distinct flare-ups, that may or may not get better. But there's continued disease progression in between flare-ups.

Ana's story continues:
I had a bad cold and sinus infection the winter before I was diagnosed. It seemed like it would never go away. And I had started to feel dizzy. I felt dizzy all the time. I figured it was from the sinus infection, so I went to see an ear, nose, and throat doctor. I was tested for Lyme disease, which came back negative. I had all kinds of other tests, but nothing showed up. The doctor was concerned about the dizziness, and sent me to a balance function center. I went through a whole set of tests. But they couldn't determine what was wrong. I was eventually sent for a brain scan, and that's when they saw small lesions. I also had a spinal tap. I was told I probably had had MS for some time. I was lucky to be diagnosed so quickly.

Diagnosing MS

In the spring of 2001, an expert panel convened by the National Multiple Sclerosis Society issued new criteria for diagnosing MS, reflecting the latest research. There are now three diagnostic categories: *MS*, *possible MS*, and *not MS*.

The new guidelines keep the threshold of two separate attacks as a requirement for a formal diagnosis of MS. An attack is defined as a neurological disturbance typical of those seen in MS, either reported by the patient or observed by the physician, lasting at least 24 hours. A single episode of muscle weakness would not qualify, but multiple episodes would. The onset of the two attacks must be at least 30 days apart. A clinical evaluation and sometimes three tests—MRI, analysis of cerebrospinal fluid (CSF), and analysis of Visual Evoked Potentials (VEPs)—are used to confirm a second attack. The clinical guidelines also allow for the diagnosis of people who've had only one attack, so they can be started on medication if needed. Evidence of a second attack must be seen on MRI.

There are also people who've had no obvious MS attacks, but have had steady progression of disability. For those people, the diagnostic criteria require a positive CSF test, plus multiple lesions in the brain or spinal cord seen on MRI, or an abnormal VEP with fewer brain and spinal cord lesions.

Depending on the symptoms, the neurologist must also exclude other conditions that mimic MS. Blood tests may be needed to rule out other autoimmune diseases or Lyme disease; those tests usually turn out normal in MS patients.

Tests You May Need and What They Mean

Magnetic resonance imaging (MRI) of the brain is the most frequently used test for multiple sclerosis, clearly showing the white plaques characteristic of MS. The addition of a contrast agent (*gadolinium*) can "light up" areas where inflammatory cells have crossed into the brain, causing demyelination.

Plaque that is seen in certain areas of the brain, such as the optic nerve, can be correlated with symptoms. The amount and location of plaques are taken into account in assessing the stage, severity, and progression of the disease. *White matter* makes up most of the brain, and gets its name from the color of the myelin insulation. *Gray matter* makes up the cerebral cortex, the multifold outer layer of the brain where most information processing occurs. To be diagnosed with MS with an MRI, separate scans must find at least one gadolinium-enhanced lesion (or a new lesion suggesting inflammation), plus plaques in characteristic areas of the brain or in the spinal cord.

A 2002 study in the *New England Journal of Medicine* says MRI scans can pick up the earliest signs of the disease in people who have only mild, inter-mittent symptoms, allowing them to be put on medication as soon as possible. The study followed 71 patients given periodic MRI scans, and among those whose initial test showed plaques in the brain, 88 percent developed MS.

Evoked potentials (EPs) are noninvasive tests that can reveal problems in myelin conduction. During a VEP test, you look at a checkerboard pattern or series of flashing lights while being monitored by a device that measures the conduction of visual images from the eyes to the brain. A delay or pro-longation of conduction signals (or weaker conduction) is seen when there's demyelination. EPs are especially useful in confirming a diagnosis of MS, because they can often detect lesions not seen on MRI.

Lumbar puncture or spinal tap tests a sample of *cerebrospinal fluid* for antibodies and proteins that result from the breakdown of myelin. Under local anesthesia, a hollow needle is inserted into the spine to withdraw a small sam-ple of the fluid bathing the spinal cord and brain. The fluid is then examined for the presence of abnormal levels of *immunoglobulins* (which are occasion-ally autoantibodies), fragments of myelin basic protein produced by inflam-mation, and for immune cells. This helps to distinguish MS from other nervous system diseases.

Looking for traces of myelin basic protein in urine, along with MRI scans, may help identify women whose disease is transforming from relapsing-remitting MS to secondary progressive MS (a sign of more damage to come). A study of 662 MS patients reported in 2001 by researchers at the Univer-sity of Alabama, Birmingham, and other centers found that such a test could be helpful in predicting the course of the disease.

The severity of MS is scored using a numerical scale. The *Extended Dis-ability Status Score (EDSS)* measures vision, sensation, coordination, strength, and walking ability. For example, a score of 0 indicates a normal neurologi-cal exam. A score of 1.0 to 1.5 indicates an abnormal neurological exam, but no disability. A score of 2.0 to 2.5 shows mild disability, while a score of 3.0 to 3.5 shows mild to moderate disability. By the time a patient has a score of 6.0, they need a cane to help them walk.

Some clinical signs of MS can provide helpful clues along with the EDSS. For example, women who present with optic neuritis show paleness in the back of the eye after symptoms resolve; the paleness indicates a lesion on the

---

MS Clusters

The problems that often cluster with MS are not all autoimmune. But the fatigue and depression of an underactive thyroid may not be apparent if you're having similar symptoms from your MS. So it's important to be aware of anything that occurs in addition to MS symptoms.

- Hypothyroidism
- Fibromyalgia and arthritis pain
- Epilepsy (may occur in 5 percent of patients)
- Ulcerative colitis
- Interstitial cystitis

---

optic nerve that caused demyelination, says Dr. Reder. Some women may show an impaired response to a pinprick, heat, or light touch in areas that correlate to areas of nerve damage. Clumsiness and an impaired ability to sense vibrations can be signs of demyelination that can sometimes be correlated with an MRI (however, often MRIs do not correlate with symptoms).

Ana's story continues:

I recall that when I was trying to get pregnant in 1988, and was losing each pregnancy after a few weeks, I was told I had some kind of "autoimmune" problem. I didn't pay much attention to it at the time. I was seeing a fertility specialist and she took some blood tests. I was told I had IgG antibodies, and that my body was rejecting the pregnancy. I was put on heparin, this blood thinner, and they wanted to put me on prednisone and put me in some kind of clinical trial. But I wouldn't take it. Eventually I decided to adopt. But I think now there must have been some kind of autoimmune thing going on even then.

The Female Factor

Over the years, there have been hints that female hormones may play a role in MS. For one thing, there are fewer MS relapses during pregnancy, when estrogen levels are increased. This may be partly due to pregnancy-associated elevations of a weaker form of estrogen called *estriol*, normally produced in small amounts in fatty tissues. Lower levels of estrogen that are usually present in the body may not be enough to protect against MS. Animal studies also show that testosterone may be protective, and this may be one reason men get MS less frequently (and later in life).

"There are all sorts of immunosuppressant substances produced during pregnancy. When you look at women with relapsing-remitting MS who become pregnant, the relapse rate during the nine months of pregnancy goes dramatically down, especially in the third trimester, compared to prepregnancy levels," says Dr. Giesser. "There's an increase in the relapse rate immediately postpartum, in the three to six months after delivery, and then the relapse rate returns to prepregnancy levels." She cites one study that included MRIs of pregnant women with MS. "Two women who were in a study protocol happened to get pregnant, and they elected to stay in the study. They were given MRIs during pregnancy, and lesion activity went down during pregnancy and rebounded after they delivered. But we just don't know why."

Studies that have followed women with MS for long periods of time after pregnancy have found that they do not have increased long-term disability compared to women who have not been pregnant. "And there are a couple of studies to suggest that pregnancy may even have kind of a protective effect, that people who became pregnant may have a little longer time before increased disability, or the onset of things may be delayed," she adds. Again, it's not clear if that's due to hormones.

"A lot of the sex differences in MS may be due to the protective effects of testosterone, and pregnancy-associated levels of estriol. But that's probably not the whole story. Sex chromosomes may also have a role in making the disease better or worse," says Rhonda Voskuhl, MD, associate professor of neurology at the University of California, Los Angeles. Dr. Voskuhl is studying the effects of estriol on MS.

Relapsing-remitting MS is largely inflammatory, and estrogen may act as an anti-inflammatory agent, observes Dr. Voskuhl. When female mice, engineered to develop an MS-like disease, *experimental autoimmune encephalomyelitis (EAE)*, are given estrogen, they produce higher levels of an anti-inflammatory cytokine. And the effects of estrogen during pregnancy also dampen inflammation in the immune system, she notes.

Dr. Voskuhl initially studied the effects of estriol in mice with EAE and found that they had fewer exacerbations, less disability, and improved health compared to mice not treated with the hormone. Based on these results, she conducted a small pilot study of estriol among twelve women, six of whom had relapsing-remitting MS and the other six with secondary progressive disease. "We saw a beneficial effect on the immune system, we saw lesser reactions to skin testing. On MRI we saw about a 50 percent reduction in gadolinium-enhanced lesion volume in relapsing-remitting patients, and the number of lesions was reduced by around 20 percent. The secondary progressive patients did not show any benefit." During the treatment period, there seemed to be some stabilization of lesions caused by T-cells, as well. "What we are doing now is a larger study among relapsing-remitting patients to see if we can have statistically significant results."

Dr. Voskuhl also hopes to see clinical trials of estriol in combination with the so-called ABC drugs (Avonex, Betaseron, and Copaxone) to see whether it will enhance their effects. Estriol, made from soybeans, is widely used in Europe to treat hot flashes, but is not yet approved for use in the United States.

Another sex difference may be due to inflammatory cytokines. During pregnancy, levels of *interferon gamma* (a damaging inflammatory cytokine associated with MS) are lower. A small study at the Cleveland Clinic Foundation revealed that when T-cells from women with MS were stimulated with a myelin protein, they produced higher levels of interferon gamma compared to men. At the same time, women with MS produced *none* of a regulatory cytokine that may dampen the disease process. It's not clear what role, if any, sex hormones may play in this response.

However, the inflammatory immune response does switch to a regulatory response during pregnancy (so the body doesn't reject the fetus), and MS typically improves during pregnancy, when estrogen and estriol levels are high. Researchers at the Cleveland Clinic Foundation say a possible new direction in MS therapy would be stimulating that regulatory response.

Another recent study found that a combination of estrogen and a T-cell receptor vaccine completely prevented EAE in female mice, and those mice getting either estrogen or the vaccine developed fewer symptoms than mice getting no treatment. The researchers, at the Neuroimmunology Research Program at the Portland Veterans Administration Medical Center in Oregon, developed a vaccine that blocked certain T-cell receptors, preventing them from interacting with myelin. The vaccine also increased the number of regulatory immune cells that keep autoreactive T-cells in check, the researchers reported in 2001. They plan to design a pilot study for humans.

Another new avenue of therapy may come from studying estrogen's effects on specific brain cells. One of the ways estrogen suppresses EAE in mice is by changing the action of T-cells and the activity of brain cells called *microglia*, which can produce toxic molecules that attack myelin-producing cells. Studies are under way to see whether female hormones can suppress these attacks. Dr. Voskuhl is also looking into adding progesterone to estriol, which she believes may enhance its effects.

But all of this doesn't mean estrogen can be prescribed as a treatment for MS yet. "We've only done a pilot study. The results are interesting, but must be confirmed in a placebo-controlled trial. Also, the doses we used are pregnancy doses, which are high levels of estriol. So I don't know what effect the estrogens and doses found in birth control pills or hormone replacement will have on symptoms," remarks Dr. Voskuhl. "Conjugated equine estrogens are made from the urine of pregnant mares, so they contain estriol. So Premarin may help—or it may do nothing. We simply don't know."

However, Dr. Voskuhl and Dr. Giesser believe estrogen—either in birth control pills or in hormone replacement therapy—can be safely used by women with MS, as long as they're being followed by a gynecologist.

Ana's story continues:
I had a hard time getting used to the Avonex. They had to put me on half-doses, and then took me off it. I was then put on Copaxone for a while, and felt great. But then they noticed that I had an allergic reaction at the injection site, and I had to go back on Avonex. And that was rough. So I started with tiny doses and gradually increased the dose until I could get acclimated to the drug. You learn to live with a lot. I had to learn to give myself injections. That was difficult. What is wonderful is that these drugs are shipped right to your home, and there are nurses you can call with questions. And that makes it easier. For example, the nurses told me to drink a lot of water the day I get the injection and the day after, to keep me hydrated. You use every piece of information they give you, and it all makes you feel that much better.

I was also fortunate to have a gynecologist who works with my neurologist, and when I started to have hot flashes she said I should absolutely be on estrogen. Since heat can make MS feel worse, I thought it was a good thing to do. Menopausal symptoms are just one more thing I don't want to worry about.

Treating Multiple Sclerosis

Under the new diagnostic criteria, a woman who experiences a single MS attack can be started on medications that have been shown to slow the progression of the disease—in many cases preventing permanent disability.

This change in treatment was largely brought about by a major study reported in the September 28, 2000, *New England Journal of Medicine*. The trial, known as the CHAMPS study, was conducted among 838 men and women at 50 clinical centers in the U.S. and Canada judged to have a high probability of developing MS based on symptoms and findings on MRI. The group was randomly assigned to weekly injections of *interferon beta-1a* (*Avonex*) or placebo. The trial was supposed to last three years, but after a planned pause to survey interim results, the trial was stopped early because the effects were so positive. The upshot: weekly injections of Avonex were found to delay the onset of clinically definite MS by 44 percent and produced a lower rate of brain lesions. New research also found that Avonex slows the brain atrophy associated with MS.

Since CHAMPS, many women can begin treatment after the earliest symptoms of MS appear. The medical advisory board of the MS Society recommends that treatment be started as soon as possible (except in pregnant women) with one of the new MS drugs: Avonex, *interferon beta-1b* (*Betaseron*), or *copolymer-1* (*Copaxone*), known as the "ABC drugs." A new interferon drug, *interferon beta-1a* (*Rebif*), is now available.

Interferon beta-1a (Avonex) works like natural human interferon to dampen immune system activity. Avonex was approved by the FDA in 1996 to reduce the frequency and severity of exacerbations in people with relapsing-remitting MS, but is now being used to treat people who have experienced a single MS attack, to slow down the disease. The drug is given by self-administered injection once a week into the large muscles of the thigh (or hip or upper arm muscle). Avonex reduces relapses by about 18 percent, slows MS progression, and studies show it may help cognitive impairment in relapsing MS.

Side effects include flulike symptoms (chills, fever, aches) after the injection, which lessen as time goes on. In rare cases, Avonex can cause mild anemia and elevated liver enzymes (suggestive of liver inflammation), so patients must be monitored.

Interferon beta-1b (Betaseron) was the first of the ABC drugs, approved in 1993. It also works like natural human interferon to inhibit immune system activity and reduces MS relapses by about 30 percent. It's injected under the skin every other day.

Betaseron also causes flulike symptoms after an injection (which also lessen after a while). Women can also experience reactions at the site of the injection (which can be serious and require medical attention in about 5 percent of cases). It can also cause elevated liver enzymes and low white blood cell counts, increasing the risk of infection.

A study comparing Betaseron to Avonex found it was more effective in reducing relapses, but further studies are needed. Avonex and Betaseron both can cause menstrual irregularities in about 15 to 25 percent of women.

Glatiramer acetate (Copaxone) is a synthetic protein that looks like myelin to the immune system. Its neuroprotective effects haven't been proven in MS, but it seems to block attacks on myelin by T-cells, apparently acting as a decoy for myelin. Copaxone is approved for relapsing-remitting MS. A long-term clinical trial among more than 250 patients with relapsing-remitting MS found that most of those who stayed on Copaxone had an improvement in their neurological status or remained unchanged after eight years. Interim results of the twelve-year trial, led by the Maryland Center for MS at the University of Maryland in Baltimore, were reported at the 2002 annual meeting of the American Academy of Neurology. Another study found that Copaxone stopped new brain lesions caused by MS flares and reduced the amount of damaged brain tissue over time, with the protective effects appearing three to four months after treatment began.

Copaxone is available in prefilled syringes and given by injection once a day. It can cause reactions at the injection site. In rare cases, there may be anxiety, chest tightness, shortness of breath, and flushing right after an injection, but there do not seem to be any long-term consequences.

"I like to think that these drugs give the brain a 'breather,' allowing more of the normal remyelination to occur," says Dr. Reder. The ABC drugs all cost around $10,000 a year, but are available at a reduced rate through the manufacturers.

Interferon beta-1a (Rebif) was approved by the FDA in March 2002 for relapsing-remitting MS. It also works like natural human interferon. Studies showed Rebif reduced the frequency of MS exacerbations, reduced disease activity seen on MRI, and slowed the progression of disability. A 2001 study comparing Rebif to Avonex showed it produced a 32 percent reduction in relapses compared to Avonex. Another trial showed Rebif could delay MS development as the ABC drugs did in the CHAMPS study.

Rebif is prescribed in prefilled syringes and given by self-injection three days a week at the same time of day, with each injection forty-eight hours apart. There can be reactions at the injection site (soreness, redness, pain, bruising), so you're advised to pick a different spot each time to lessen the chance of an infection or other problem. Side effects include flulike symptoms (fever, chills, muscle aches, and tiredness), depression and anxiety, liver problems, a drop in red and white blood cell counts, changes in thyroid function, and allergic reactions. Periodic blood testing is needed to monitor liver or blood changes. Like the ABC drugs, Rebif cannot be used during pregnancy.

Mitoxantrone (Novantrone) is an anticancer drug that suppresses T-cell, B-cell, and macrophage activity, and seems to lessen attacks on myelin. It is usually given intravenously every three months for up to two years (or up to a specific cumulative lifetime dose). A 2002 study from France, where it has been used for more than a decade, found that an initial "induction" course of more intense mitoxantrone therapy for six months significantly reduced relapse rates, and kept 43 percent of patients relapse free for a five-year period. Recent studies also suggest that combining Novantrone with Betaseron is safe and may reduce disease progression without significant toxicity in people with aggressive relapsing-remitting disease, or secondary progressive disease, whose MS wasn't controlled by Betaseron.

Novantrone can affect the heart, raising the risk of congestive heart failure. So you must have normal heart function to take the drug, and tests of cardiac function are necessary before and during treatment.

Targeting Common Symptoms

Other treatments for MS target symptoms, such as pain, tremor, bladder or bowel dysfunction, and fatigue.

"Up to 85 percent of MS patients have fatigue, and it may be the single most disabling symptom," remarks Dr. Giesser. An antiviral medication called *amantadine* is widely used to treat MS-related fatigue. Some patients benefit from a stimulant used for hyperactivity, *methylphenidate hydrochloride* (*Ritalin*). A newer stimulant, *modafinil* (*Provigil*) has been very effective in clinical trials against MS-related fatigue. Antidepressants such as *fluoxetine* (*Prozac*) may also help fatigue.

Physical, occupational, and/or cognitive therapy may sometimes be recommended. A landmark 1996 study at the University of Utah found that aerobic exercise produced many physical and emotional benefits for MS patients, including improved bowel and bladder control and reduced fatigue.

Most MS patients are sensitive to increases in body heat, so exercising in an air-conditioned room is highly recommended. Dehydration can exacerbate fatigue, but many women with MS don't drink enough water because of bladder incontinence. But getting enough water during exercise is extremely important.

Anti-seizure medications like *carbamazepine* (*Tegretol*) and *gabapentin* (*Neurontin*) help nerve pain. Other drugs used for MS-related pain include the tricyclic antidepressants *amitriptyline* (*Elavil*) and *imipramine* (*Tofranil*), which interfere with pain signals from nerves. Antispasmodic drugs, such as *baclofen* (*Lioresal*) or *tizanidine* (*Zanaflex*), can help leg or back spasms. Prednisone may be given for *optic neuritis*.

MS patients have specific bladder problems. "In MS, the bladder often doesn't store urine properly. So instead of holding a normal volume of urine, around two or three cups, before you have the urge to go or before you empty reflexively, a patient's bladder may hold only a cup or so. The result is urgency, a spastic, nervous bladder that wants to go all the time," says Dr. Giesser. "Or, MS patients may have a bladder that doesn't empty itself completely, so when you void there's still urine in the bladder, which leads to urinary tract infections, urine reflux (it can theoretically back up into the kidneys), and kidney disease. And there are women who have a 'mixed' bladder, a bladder that wants to empty all the time, but doesn't empty well."

For a purely spastic bladder that doesn't store urine well, patients are prescribed *anticholinergic* agents, drugs that relax the bladder and allow it to hold more urine. In some cases, women are taught how to use urinary catheters. "For 'mixed' bladders we may use medication along with self-catheterization. It's very individual." A new procedure, *sacral nerve stimulation*, a kind of "pacemaker" that helps eliminate abnormal nerve signals to the bladder, may work for some women with MS, she adds.

Another common problem is constipation. "Women who are less mobile are more prone to constipation. Some of the drugs we give cause constipation. A lot of women with bladder problems self-treat by restricting liquids and become dehydrated, which contributes to constipation. And MS probably has some effect on gut motility, as well," says Dr. Giesser. In general, women with MS are advised to increase fiber intake, take bulking agents, keep well hydrated, and eliminate on a schedule to help keep regular.

Studies conducted by the NMSS show that two out of three people with MS will remain ambulatory twenty years after diagnosis, and those numbers should improve as more people are treated earlier for the disease. Again, just because you're not experiencing a relapse doesn't mean there's no disease progression. So medication is needed.

What's Next?

New drugs in the pipeline include *natalizumab* (*Antegren*), now in Phase III clinical trials. The drug, a new class of therapeutics called *alpha 4 integrin inhibitors*, is designed to prevent the migration of inflammatory cells from the blood to other sites in the body. (In MS, it would block adhesion molecules that attach T-cells to cells lining the blood vessels in the brain and draw them across the blood-brain barrier.) Preliminary results reported in 2001 showed that Antegren slowed the relapse rate by 50 percent and lesions seen on MRI by 80 percent, notes Dr. Reder. It's also being tested in Crohn's disease.

Avonex and Betaseron are being tested against secondary progressive MS, and Copaxone and Avonex are being tested in primary progressive MS.

Scientists are also investigating the possibility of stimulating immature (or *progenitor*) myelin-making cells or transplanting those cells into patients with MS. Other experimental treatments being tested in animals include exposing autoreactive T-cells to large amounts of myelin basic protein in an effort to induce programmed cell death. Monoclonal antibodies and immunoglobulins are also being tested in animal experiments to regrow myelin.

Ritonavir, a drug used to treat human immunodeficiency virus (HIV), has shown potential benefits in preliminary animal studies. Ritonavir is a protease inhibitor, which affects an enzyme (called a *proteasome* enzyme) thought to play a role in the activation of lymphocytes that attack the myelin sheath in MS. Daily doses of ritonavir prevented clinical symptoms in the animal model of MS in such a way that researchers feel it may have a protective effect when given early in the disease. MS also seems to respond to other antiviral therapies.

Drugs used to treat Alzheimer's disease are also being tested to see whether they can slow cognitive decline in MS. Preliminary indications are that *donepezil* (*Aricept*), slightly improved cognitive function in the small group of patients who have tried it, Dr. Reder reports, but definitive data will have to come from clinical trials. Newer drugs such as *galantamine* (*Reminyl*) may be even more effective.

A small, preliminary study reported at the American Academy of Neurology annual meeting in 2002, suggested stem cell transplants might be effective in severe MS.

Mariana's story continues:

I was formally diagnosed when I was thirty, when I started to have my first problems with walking. Then it was completely undeniable that I had MS, there was no way I could ignore it. I found myself a good neurologist . . . and my husband dragged me to my first support group, which scared me to death. Because there were a lot of people there who were worse off than I was. And that frightened me. I'd been told for years it could be MS. But I hadn't accepted it in my mind until that point. I finally came to grips with it . . . I didn't go back to the support group until later and I ended up being the program coordinator because I didn't like the way it was being run; everyone would just sit around and complain. So we started getting people to come in to talk to us about MS and things to do to take charge of your life. And we also talked about touchy subjects like sexual dysfunction. For me, it was the emotional issues that were hardest. For example, it was hard to get my groceries in and out of the house and it was good to find out how to make that easier. But how does it make me feel as a person that I can't do that anymore, that I have to ask neighbors to help me? That was the hardest part for me. To me, it's a sign of weakness. You make yourself vulnerable and indebted to them. Some people like to do for others, do community service. But I had no way to "pay them back." I felt very inadequate. That was an emotional stumbling block I had to get over.

How MS Can Affect You Over Your Lifetime

While MS flares and relapses seem to be affected by hormones in younger women, there's little research on the subject, and menopause is largely uncharted territory.

Premenstrual Flares

Women with MS often report that symptoms get worse in the days before their periods, but there have been only a few studies. "We published the first abstract in 1990 on premenstrual fluctuations. We surveyed 149 women, who completed a questionnaire that asked, 'Do you ever notice an increase in your symptoms during your menstrual cycle? If so, when?' Seventy percent said they had changes in their symptoms every month, most of them saying this occurred during the week prior to menses," said Dr. Giesser. "About 40 percent noticed exacerbations—different than symptom fluctuation—came at a particular time during their cycle. Since 1990, there have been several other reports, self-report questionnaire samples, that have also reported this. There have also been three small studies that reported some changes in MRIs correlated with different phases of the menstrual cycle. So we have uncontrolled, preliminary data in very small samples of women that yes, there seems to be an association with neurological symptoms and the premenstrual period. But we don't know what is causing it."

It's not clear whether this is related to a temporary worsening of preexisting symptoms or disease exacerbation, comments Dr. Voskuhl. "These are very different. If you are getting a relapse, this could be an indication of inflammation and new demyelination. In contrast, when a woman is exposed to heat, her symptoms get worse, but it doesn't mean her disease is *worsening*," she points out. Most likely it is a temporary worsening of symptoms, not a relapse of MS.

According to Dr. Giesser, the most common symptoms that worsen premenstrually are fatigue, imbalance, difficulty walking, and spasticity. Specific symptoms can be individually treated (see page 256). It's not known whether there are menstrual cycle changes in the metabolism of various medications.

Pregnancy/Postpartum

The good news is that MS doesn't seem to hamper a woman's ability to get pregnant and carry to term, and MS symptoms get better during pregnancy. This is thought to be partly due to high estrogen levels (especially estriol), which appear to reduce immune system activity and reduce the frequency of MS attacks. The relapse rate seems to be lowest in the third trimester, and spikes in the three to six months after delivery as hormones return to normal levels (depending on whether a woman breastfeeds).

The ABC drugs cannot be taken during pregnancy and, Dr. Giesser says, for the most part they are not needed because of pregnancy's favorable effects. "Women should be off any one of these drugs for at least two menstrual cycles before they try to get pregnant," advises Dr. Giesser. "There are a lot of reports about women who happened to become pregnant while they were on these drugs, stopped the drugs, and had perfectly healthy babies. But we prefer to be cautious."

During pregnancy, standard urine and blood tests are done to monitor for preeclampsia and other problems. A neurological exam would be given once or twice over the course of the pregnancy. Women with MS do not have a higher rate of birth defects or miscarriages.

Medications must be resumed as soon as possible after delivery, unless a woman is planning to breastfeed. Because of a lack of safety data, the ABC drugs and Rebif can't be used during breastfeeding.

Aside from a spike in the relapse rate after delivery (as estrogen levels return to normal), women who breastfeed do not seem to have more relapses than women who don't. "It's not clear why there is a relapse rebound after delivery. It could be the effects of all the hormones returning to normal levels. All the immunosuppressant chemicals do, too. There's an increase in prolactin during lactation, but I don't think you can hang it on any one hormone."

The biggest problem for many women who decide to become pregnant is fatigue and caring for their children in the event of a relapse. Strong support is needed from family members to share the load.

Menopause and Beyond

It's not known whether the wide shifts in hormones during perimenopause or the decline in estrogen after menopause affect the course of MS.

"There are no data on menopause and MS. A woman in her late forties or early fifties probably has had MS for twenty to thirty years, and she may stop having defined relapses as her disease becomes secondary progressive. So there are fewer relapses in menopause, but it may be for reasons that have nothing to do with hormones and more to do with the natural history of the disease," remarks Dr. Giesser.

Menopause may have some effects on the symptoms of MS. For example, hot flashes raise body heat, which can worsen fatigue and other symptoms. Menopause itself may not have any effect on the inflammatory process that underlies MS. However, there's simply not enough information on the effect of hormone replacement on MS. "Right now, we have no data to suggest that it's good for them, although it may be, we certainly don't have any data to suggest that it's bad. So if a woman's gynecologist or internist thinks she should be on hormone replacement for any kind of medical or gynecological reason, I tell them go ahead," says Dr. Giesser.

Dr. Voskuhl concurs. "I think if a woman wants to take hormone replacement, there's no reason not to. However, I don't think very-low-dose estrogens will be very helpful." Cooling vests can help dampen symptoms in hot weather and they may also be helpful to women experiencing hot flashes.

Some women may want to investigate herbal remedies like *black cohosh* (the branded product is *Remifemin*) or *red clover* (*Promensil*) for menopausal symptoms.

Corticosteroids cause bone loss, but the ABC drugs do not. So bone-building drugs are needed if a woman is taking steroids for MS attacks.

Throughout life, women are twice as likely as men to suffer from depression—and it's also a more common symptom in people with MS. A small study from the University of California at San Francisco, reported in the *Archives of Neurology* in 2001, found that the antidepressants known as *selective serotonin reuptake inhibitors* (*SSRIs*) not only help relieve depression, but also significantly reduce levels of gamma interferon. The researchers suggest that treating depression could also be an important factor in down-regulating autoreactive T-cells.

Ana's story continues:

In a sense, MS has actually freed me . . . giving me a chance to do more things that I love. I decided to apply for disability since the fatigue had started to interfere with my work. At first, the idea depressed me, but then I realized that I would now have more time to paint and to write, two things that I'd had to put on the back burner because of the demands of my job. So MS has provided me the great luxury of time for myself, which many women never get, trying to keep up with their careers and their family life. I found hidden blessings and opportunities in a disease that initially seemed like it would limit me.

10

Weak in the Knees— Myasthenia Gravis

There were signs that there was something wrong for a while. My husband and some of my friends had thought I was taking prescription tranquilizers, because my voice would start slurring. And my secretary said it had gotten to the point that I would dictate a letter to Mr. Smith and say Mr. Jones. I would forget phone numbers. I was clumsy, I would step wrong and fall . . . I couldn't put the backs on earrings. Or use a little calculator. Little things like that. But because I'm such a Type-A person, I masked the symptoms. Then I collapsed in church on July 4, 1999 . . . after the service, I walked over to hug a friend, and suddenly I didn't know where I was. And my legs were like real rubbery. My husband got me out of there, got me in the car, and drove to the emergency room. The neurologist thought maybe it was a TIA or an aneurysm and was going to send me to a larger hospital, but the doctor on call said it was stress: "Stress does funny things to you," he said. They did a bunch of tests but couldn't find anything, so they sent me home. The following morning, after my husband left for work, I went to brush my teeth and choked. And I panicked. I crawled upstairs to the phone and paged him, and then we went back to the hospital. They did the blood test and they did the Tensilon test. It was unreal. When they gave me the Tensilon, all of my symptoms disappeared. And we cried because we knew what was facing me. I started on medication that day.

JACKIE, FORTY-NINE

Warning Signs of Myasthenia Gravis

- Weakness or drooping of eyelids in one or both lids
- Double vision
- Eye closing can be weak
- Difficulty chewing, swallowing, or speaking
- Regurgitating fluid up the nose
- Difficulty with facial muscles, smiling
- Weakness in upper limbs
- Difficulty breathing

Myasthenia gravis (MG) involves communication between nerves and muscles. It results from an autoantibody attack on the receptors for a chemical that carries signals between the nervous system and voluntary muscles—the muscles we have direct control over. MG affects three to four times more women than men up until the age of forty. In older age, more men than women are affected.

Once considered a fatal disease, MG can now be controlled successfully, and a majority of people with MG live productive lives.

What Causes MG?

When we pick up a pencil or take a walk, we may not be conscious of directing specific muscles, but our brain has to tell those muscles to move. That message is sent by a chemical called *acetylcholine (ACh)*, released at the *neuromuscular junction*, the spot where the motor nerve terminal meets a folded muscle membrane called the *end plate*. When the brain stimulates the motor nerve, acetylcholine is sent out in little packets (*vesicles*) that cross the space between the muscle and nerve (called the *synapse*) and binds to receptors concentrated on the peaks of each end-plate fold. When the vesicles bind to *acetylcholine receptors (AChR)*, it stimulates the muscle to contract. We couldn't pick up that pencil without ACh.

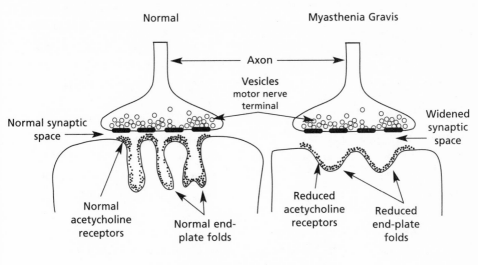

Normal   Myasthenia Gravis

The Neuromuscular Junction

In myasthenia gravis, autoantibodies to proteins on ACh receptors (*anti-AChR autoantibodies*) cause the loss of those receptors, so that fewer remain. The muscle end plate also loses its folded shape, further reducing the number of ACh receptors and widening the space between muscle and nerve. While there's plenty of ACh, there are fewer receptors to pick it up, and the membrane becomes less sensitive. The effects of ACh are reduced, so there's less chance that a nerve impulse will provoke a muscle contraction, leading to muscle weakness, explains Arnold I. Levinson, MD, chief of allergy and immunology at the University of Pennsylvania School of Medicine, who is researching the origins of MG.

"The hallmark of the disease is a marked reduction in the number of receptors but a normal amount of acetylcholine. There is also actual destruction of the muscle end plate by the autoantibodies and complement," says Dr. Levinson. The fewer the ACh receptors, the worse the symptoms of MG.

Abnormal cell growth in the thymus may lead to production of autoantibodies. Ten percent of people with MG have small, benign tumors in the thymus (called *thymomas*); 60 to 70 percent have abnormal development of B-cell–enriched areas (germinal center hyperplasia) in the thymus, says Dr. Levinson. Thymic abnormalities may result in sensitization of cells to produce anti-AChR autoantibodies. "Years ago, before we even knew about immune cells, it was clear the thymus was involved in myasthenia, so the thymus was routinely removed in patients with myasthenia. And patients got better. We still don't know why they get better, but to this day thymectomy is still a first-line therapy for patients before the age of sixty," remarks Dr. Levinson. "Levels of autoantibodies drop after thymectomy, but the improvement is not necessarily due to lower antibody titers. The amount of circulating autoantibodies does not correlate to the severity of myasthenia."

"We think the thymus plays a primary role in myasthenia, and we think that self-tolerance is actually broken in the thymus. There are AChR-reactive cells that are not eliminated in the thymus and are exported into the circulation. We're testing the hypothesis in animals that some inflammatory event allows these T-cells, which react with acetylcholine receptors, to travel *back* to the thymus, where they're activated by locally-expressed AChR in people with myasthenia," says Dr. Levinson.

Some research suggests that *molecular mimicry* may play a role in myasthenia, with immune cells mistaking ACh receptors for a virus (possibly a herpes simplex virus) or bacteria.

MG may also have a genetic component, since a variety of autoimmune diseases are associated with myasthenia (in both patients and their family members—see MG Clusters, page 271). It's possible that an inherited defect in immune regulation may predispose people to myasthenia gravis.

Jackie's story continues:
I was lucky I was diagnosed quickly. And I think it was because I had a female doctor . . . I knew, and my husband Joe knew, that I wasn't crazy. But you feel that way when doctors dismiss you and say, "Oh, it's just stress." Even one of my best friends said to me "Maybe you just need to chill out and take some time off." And really, the symptoms were deceptive. Now we look back and we know what was going on. But I was extremely fortunate. I've heard horror stories from other women with this disease going two and three years and even more before they're diagnosed. Going from doctor to doctor, and all of them saying it's all in their heads. After I was diagnosed with MG, the doctor who told me it was stress came into my room and I told him, "I'm going to make you a better doctor. You blew off my symptoms as stress, and embarrassed me in front of my family and friends. You

have to start to think about your attitude." He needed to know that. And he did change the way he treats his patients. But he wasn't unusual. Many doctors tell a woman who has complaints he can't pin down, "Oh, it's in your head," when he would start doing every kind of test if it was a man. And it shouldn't be that way.

Symptoms of MG

The first symptom of MG is usually droopy eyelids (*ptosis*). Muscle weakness around the eyes (*ocular muscles*) and/or the development of double vision (*diplopia*) are usually what bring women to see their doctor. The eyes may not close completely, and eye movements may be difficult or tiring. For example, looking upward and trying to hold the eyes open may result in eyelid drooping that gets progressively worse.

There can be problems with the *bulbar muscles* around the mouth and throat, causing problems speaking, chewing, swallowing, and even smiling. Women can also experience weakness in the arms or legs. Usually, muscle weakness is less severe in the morning and worsens as the day goes on, especially if the affected muscles are used for long periods of time.

While MG is a progressive disease, it doesn't always cause rapid deterioration. In 10 to 15 percent of cases, weakness is restricted to the eye muscles. Many women will have some progressive weakness during the first year or two involving the mouth and throat (*oropharyngeal*) muscles and/or the limb muscles. But the disease can stabilize over time. "If myasthenia doesn't become severe early on, it may stay on a plateau. For example, if muscle weakness is restricted to the eyes for the first three years, it's likely to remain there in 90 percent of cases. It's unusual for the disease to be mild for ten years and then start progressing," remarks Janice M. Massey, MD, professor of neurology and director of the Myasthenia Gravis Clinic at Duke University Medical Center.

Often a woman may have mild weakness and not attach much importance to it, and up to 25 percent of people may see some remission of initial symptoms. So it can be a while before she sees a doctor, especially if she doesn't have classical symptoms such as drooping eyes or double vision. Mild symptoms also may not be constant; ptosis may get worse toward the end of the day, or with exercise, and improve after rest. "In fact, it's not unusual for patients not to realize the degree of weakness they had until it's improved by treatment," adds Dr. Massey, who serves on the medical advisory board of the Myasthenia Gravis Foundation.

Conversely, if MG worsens rapidly over days to weeks, especially in the muscles involving speaking, chewing, or swallowing, that can indicate a case that needs swift and aggressive treatment, says Dr. Massey. "In rare cases we see a patient whose symptoms have been stable for over ten years get the flu or another illness, something that sets the immune system off, and their disease can start to progress to a more serious level."

In mild cases, a diagnosis may be delayed until symptoms start to worsen, sometimes by coexisting thyroid disease. An overactive thyroid (hyperthyroidism) or an underactive thyroid (hypothyroidism) can cause muscle weakness, and Graves' disease may mimic the eye muscle weakness of MG. In women with myasthenia, mild symptoms that had not caused concern previously may worsen with the onset of thyroid disease to the point where a woman may finally seek medical attention. "Changes in thyroid function, either hypo- or hyperthyroidism, can produce true worsening of disease activity," comments Dr. Massey.

Myasthenic symptoms can be worsened by medications. The most common drugs that affect myasthenia are antibiotics, particularly mycin drugs (like streptomycin), beta-blockers, and other cardiac drugs, which have a direct effect on neuromuscular transmission. Even nonprescription drugs can exacerbate symptoms of MG—for example, milk of magnesia, because magnesium affects the neuromuscular junction. A partial list of medications that exacerbate myasthenia appears on page 277.

Myasthenic symptoms can also be worsened temporarily by illness (particularly respiratory viral infections), increases in body temperature in hot weather (especially in high humidity), stress, emotional upsets, and pregnancy. "Women can become profoundly weak after walking in the heat or working in the garden. After they cool off and rest, within a day or so they completely recuperate. That exacerbation doesn't indicate a worsening of disease," Dr. Massey emphasizes. "If a patient comes in whose symptoms have gotten worse out of the blue, I will ask her if she's had a recent viral infection, if she has been put on any new medications, of if she is pregnant. I will also check her thyroid function. Sorting out the causes of symptoms and what may be causing them can be complicated, since there are many factors that could contribute."

Fifteen percent of myasthenia patients will present with thymoma, although this is more common in men. In this case, removal of the tumor and the residual thymus tissue (thymoma/thymectomy) can cure the disease.

Diagnosing MG

While muscle weakness is a primary symptom of MG, it's not specific to myasthenia gravis. Again, muscle problems, especially around the eyes, can be caused by Hashimoto's thyroiditis or Graves' disease, and medications may produce or exacerbate muscle weakness. So other causes must be definitively ruled out.

"A good clinical evaluation with a thorough history is really at the heart of making a diagnosis of myasthenia. Lab tests can be useful, but are not as useful as a good clinical evaluation," stresses Dr. Massey.

Among the tests that can help confirm a diagnosis is a test for antibodies to the acetylcholine receptor and tests that involve electrically stimulating muscle fibers, either a single muscle fiber or repetitively stimulating specific groups of muscle fibers. "We may have to do other routine electrophysiological studies to verify key abnormalities we see on these tests, or to make sure there's no other underlying problem causing the muscle weakness," explains Dr. Massey.

Tests You May Need and What They Mean

Anti-acetylcholine receptor (AChR) antibody test: A majority of people with myasthenia gravis have anti-AChR antibodies, but unlike some markers of inflammation, the serum concentration of anti-AChR antibodies is not associated with the severity of disease (antibody levels can be low at the onset of the disease and increase later on). AChR antibodies are also increased in women with lupus, inflammatory neuropathy, *amyotrophic lateral sclerosis*

(*ALS*), thymoma, in women with rheumatoid arthritis taking D-penicillamine, and even in healthy relatives of MG patients. You can even have a false-positive test if blood is drawn within forty-eight hours of a surgical procedure involving general anesthesia and muscle relaxants. But generally, elevated AChR antibodies—together with key clinical symptoms—confirms the diagnosis of myasthenia gravis, says Dr. Massey.

Electromyography repetitive nerve stimulation (RNS) uses a harmless, low-frequency electrical signal to stimulate nerves, and the reaction in muscle is measured. In people with myasthenia, the muscle response becomes progressively weaker with each separate stimulation. Multiple muscle groups may be tested. This decreasing response is seen more often in facial muscles, arm muscles (biceps, deltoids), and shoulder muscles (trapezius). A significant decrease in response to repetitive stimulation in either a hand or shoulder muscle is found in about 60 percent of patients with myasthenia gravis. The response is not specific to MG, but an abnormal finding is a good predictor of the disease.

Single-fiber EMG (SFEMG) involves recordings that can be made from pairs of muscle fibers supplied by branches of a single nerve fiber. It's time consuming and difficult, and requires special equipment, but is the most sensitive clinical test of neuromuscular transmission abnormalities. However, it's not specific for MG. What's seen is a "jitter" in some muscles in almost all patients with myasthenia gravis. Patients with mild or purely ocular muscle weakness may have increased "jitter" only in facial muscles. The test is sensitive for MG in greater than 90 percent of cases.

The **edrophonium chloride test** is done if electrophysiological studies prove inconclusive or a patient has coexisting problems that may complicate her case. The test uses an intravenous infusion of a chemical called *edrophonium chloride* (*Tensilon*) to temporarily slow the breakdown of acetylcholine. Tensilon takes effect rapidly, in a minute or less, improving muscle weakness (such as ptosis) *if* it's caused by the abnormal neuromuscular transmission that occurs in MG. Tensilon's effects last only five to ten minutes. If you have ptosis, and after the injection the ptosis goes away, that's a fairly good indication that you may have MG.

A small test dose is usually given to make sure there's no unusual sensitivity or side effects, such as a slowed heartbeat (a dose of atropine is kept on hand to counteract its effects). The test cannot be given to people with heart

MG Clusters

A variety of autoimmune diseases have been associated with myasthenia gravis (in both MG patients and their family members), ranging from endocrine to blood disorders, and symptoms may overlap. Thyroid disease occurs in up to 15 percent of people with MG.

- Graves' disease, Hashimoto's thyroiditis
- Type 1 diabetes
- Systemic lupus erythematosus
- Rheumatoid arthritis
- Sjögren's syndrome
- Pernicious anemia
- Alopecia areata
- Autoimmune thrombocytopenia purpura

problems or the elderly. The edrophonium test is not completely specific for MG; patients with other conditions may also show a response.

A similar drug, *neostigmine*, can be given as an intramuscular injection. Neostigmine takes effect more slowly and lasts longer, but has less potential for side effects. In some people, a trial of the drug *pyridostigmine* (*Mestinon*) may produce improvement in muscle weakness that can't be seen after only one dose of edrophonium chloride or neostigmine.

Because thyroid disease occurs so often with MG, **thyroid function tests** are needed to rule out Graves' disease, hyperthyroidism, or hypothyroidism as a cause of muscle weakness. These tests may include *thyroid stimulating hormone* (*TSH*) and thyroid antibody tests.

A **CT scan** of the chest is also needed to examine the thymus, since many women may have thymomas or thymus abnormalities.

Jackie's story continues:

I was diagnosed with pernicious anemia two years before I found out I had MG; I was told I had rheumatoid arthritis around the same time I was diagnosed with MG, in December. And over the years I had several falls and injured myself, and now we look back and almost all of it was clumsy behav-

ior. So I probably had myasthenia for a long time, and probably these other illnesses, too. Now every six months I get tested with bloodwork for thyroid.

The Female Factor

Myasthenia gravis appears to affect more women than men in their twenties and thirties, and more men than women during the sixties and seventies. But things may not be that clear-cut.

"Presumably there's some hormonal relationship, but what that relationship may be is unknown. Some of the more recent statistics, especially with the aging of the population, give a more equal ratio between men and women after age fifty," remarks Dr. Massey. As the over-fifty population has increased, so has the prevalence of MG and the average age at diagnosis. As far as it's known, there are no sex differences in what occurs in the thymus or in the presentation of the disease, she adds. However, gender does play a role in the way MG is treated, mostly in the choice of medications for women of child-bearing age.

Treating Myasthenia Gravis

Because myasthenia gravis can be so varied and differs in each person, treatment is highly individualized according to the severity of disease, age, sex, and the degree of functional impairment. The major difficulty in treating MG is that a response may be difficult to measure; symptoms can improve spontaneously, or the disease can go into remission, especially early on.

For the majority of women with MG, treatment begins with drugs that slow the breakdown of acetylcholine and relieve symptoms. The second-line treatment is removal of the thymus (*thymectomy*) or immunosuppression. Sometimes they are all combined.

Cholinesterase inhibitors are the mainstay of treatment for symptoms of myasthenia gravis. *Anticholinesterase drugs* neutralize an enzyme that breaks down acetylcholine at the neuromuscular junction, increasing the amount of acetylcholine and giving it a better chance to be taken up by receptors, which have been reduced in number by the disease process. *Pyridostigmine* *bromide* (*Mestinon, Regonol*) and *neostigmine bromide* (*Prostigmin*) are the most commonly used oral medications, and may be given in combination. Prostigmin can be given by injection. *Ambenonium* (*Mytelase*) may be used in moderate to severe cases. Edrophonium chloride (Tensilon) may also be given intravenously.

"Cholinesterase inhibitors reduce muscle weakness, but do not affect the underlying disease that causes it," stresses Dr. Massey. "These drugs are usually given in conjunction with other treatments, particularly thymectomy in younger patients."

Some women can show substantial improvement with cholinesterase inhibitors, while there may be little to no effect in others. The need for medication can vary from day to day (even during the same day) in response to menstruation, emotional stress, infections, and hot weather. Various muscles may even respond differently; some may get stronger, some become weaker, and others show no change at all. Muscle strength rarely returns to normal with cholinesterase inhibitors, but people can be quite functional.

The side effects are due to the drugs' effects on receptors in smooth muscle, skeletal muscle, and certain glands. These can include: narrowing of the muscle of the iris in the eye, causing the pupil to become smaller; increased nasal and bronchial secretions; and increased salivation and urination. Gastrointestinal effects can include loose stools and diarrhea, queasiness or nausea, vomiting, and abdominal cramps. Cholinesterase inhibitors may also worsen urinary tract infections.

If you have problems with swallowing or breathing, the increased bronchial secretions and saliva can be a serious problem. If too much ACh accumulates at receptors in other muscle tissue (such as in smooth muscle), it can cause weakness and, in rare cases, respiratory failure.

Thymectomy, removal of the thymus, increases the frequency of remissions in MG, and is recommended for most patients, especially if they have thymomas.

Thymectomy seems to be most effective in people younger than fifty years, particularly those with early disease, and those with moderate to severe disease who have not responded to other treatments. Improvement in symptoms may not be seen immediately; it may take place gradually over several years. Some studies suggest that African-Americans may have somewhat less improvement after thymectomy, but not enough to advise avoiding the surgery. "Women, particularly those who have germinal center hyperplasia in the thymus or who were diagnosed in the previous two years, tend to do better after thymectomy," remarks Dr. Levinson.

Corticosteroid drugs, usually *prednisone*, decrease the buildup of antibodies to acetylcholine receptors and speed up the normal death (*apoptosis*) of the cells that produce the antibodies. Corticosteroids are used to prepare patients for thymectomy, and sometimes after the surgery, in people who fail to respond completely. More than 75 percent of patients show a marked improvement, or complete relief of symptoms, with prednisone (usually in the first six to eight weeks), often followed by a total remission. Afterward, some people may be able to take prednisone every other day.

Around one-third of patients become temporarily weaker in the first week to ten days after starting prednisone. While treatment can be started at a low dose to minimize the problem and slowly increased until there's improvement in muscle strength, it's hard to predict when the worsening from prednisone may take place and it may be confusing. People with early MG usually respond best, but the severity of disease does not predict the ultimate improvement. Patients with thymoma have an excellent response to prednisone before or after removal of the tumor. The major disadvantages of corticosteroid therapy are the side effects (see pages 34 to 35).

For women, the major concern is the development of osteoporosis, and estrogen or bone-building drugs may be needed. "The fact that prednisone accelerates bone loss is something that, on occasion, would lead me to choose another medication over prednisone," comments Dr. Massey. "We do use bone-building drugs, such as alendronate, if there is significant osteoporosis as a complication of steroid therapy. This is something we would closely follow."

Immunosuppressant drugs dampen the activity of the immune system, and may be needed when a woman fails corticosteroid treatment, can't tolerate prednisone, or is unable to take steroids.

Azathioprine (*Imuran*) reverses symptoms in most women, but the effects may not be seen for four to eight months, and a woman may not achieve a full remission for one to two years. Once there's improvement in muscle strength, it will be maintained as long as the drug is taken; if azathioprine is discontinued, symptoms recur within two to three months. Some women may respond better to treatment with both prednisone and azathioprine than to either drug by itself. Both medications can be started simultaneously, and the dose of prednisone can be tapered once azathioprine becomes fully effective. Approximately one-third of patients have mild side effects (depending on the dose) that may require lowering their doses.

Cyclosporine A is sometimes helpful. It mostly inhibits the T-cell–dependent immune responses. Most patients will see an improvement in muscle strength within one to two months after starting cyclosporine, but maximum benefits take six months. After achieving a maximum response, the dose of cyclosporine is gradually reduced to the lowest level that will maintain symptom improvement. Adverse effects include kidney damage and high blood pressure.

Cyclophosphamide (Cytoxan) is occasionally used to treat MG. It is used to treat some cancers and interferes with rapidly proliferating cells (including T-cells and B-cells), and reduces the production of autoantibodies. Cytoxan can be given intravenously or orally. More than half of patients become asymptomatic after one year on cyclophosphamide. Side effects include nausea, vomiting, hair loss, appetite loss, anemia, thrombocytopenia, leukopenia, and infertility. Antinausea drugs (like *ondansetron*) given to chemotherapy patients can help relieve the nausea and vomiting. Cyclophosphamide also causes birth defects and is contraindicated in pregnancy. Infections are always a risk with any immunosuppressant drug.

Plasma exchange (plasmapheresis) is an exchange of the clear fluid component of the blood (plasma, in which blood cells float) with plasma from healthy individuals. The effect is to reduce the amount of damaging antibodies and immune complexes. Plasma exchange involves several treatments to exchange three to four liters of plasma over a two-week period. It produces rapid improvement, and is a short-term treatment for patients who experience a sudden worsening of symptoms (myasthenic "crisis") or in those rare cases where there's a rapid onset of disease involving the muscles of the mouth and throat (posing the threat of serious airway problems). It's also used to quickly improve muscle strength before surgery, and as an intermittent therapy for patients who don't respond to other treatments.

Some women may improve right after the first treatment, or it may take as many as five to seven treatments to see an increase in muscle strength. Improvement can last for weeks or months, making it an effective short-term or stopgap therapy, says Dr. Massey. However, the temporary effect will be lost unless immunosuppressant drugs are given or the thymus is removed.

While most women who benefit from the initial plasma exchange will respond to subsequent exchanges, repeated treatments do not have a cumulative benefit. Plasma exchange is usually followed by thymectomy and/or immunosuppressant drugs.

Intravenous immunoglobulin (IVIG) can be used as an alternative to plasma exchange in cases of severe myasthenic exacerbation. IVIG is usually given over a period of two to five days. It's not clear how IVIG works; it may suppress the production of antibodies against acetylcholine receptors. Between 50 to 100 percent of patients show improvement, usually within a week, and the effects of IVIG can last for weeks or months. However, recent studies suggest IVIG is not as effective as plasma exchange.

Jackie's story continues:
Before I was diagnosed, I had planned to go skydiving with a group of people the next Saturday. They didn't think I would do it. But I did. I knew I was fixing to have major surgery . . . they had scheduled a thymectomy for the next Friday, and that's like open-heart surgery. So I said I'm going to do it. And I did. It was awesome.

At first, I was on high doses of Mestinon, but after the thymectomy they tapered it down. Now I'm on normal doses. And I can pretty much do what I want as long as I take my medicine and get plenty of sleep. And I have to take something to sleep, which I don't like. Before all this, give me four hours of sleep and I was ready to go. I went to law school when I was married with two kids . . . now, unfortunately, I'm in bed early. But I'm not complaining; I still get plenty of work done.

I have my ups and downs. When you have myasthenia, your muscles and ligaments are more susceptible to injury, and I've had a couple of knee injuries. I now have an electric muscle stimulator; it's a pad that you put on your legs or arms. You program it, and when it's on you tighten muscles, and when it's off you relax. It's a minute on and a minute off. And that helps to build muscle tone. I try to walk a little, even if it's only ten minutes a day, three times a day. Recently I started to have hot flashes . . . that's not external heat, but it's heat and it affects you as much as external heat does. So my doctor put me on estrogen, Cenestin, and it keeps them pretty much under control. With the myasthenia, the more Mestinon you take, the more you sweat, especially at night. I woke up some nights just drenched in

Drugs That Can Worsen MG

A number of drugs can exacerbate symptoms of myasthenia because they block transmission at the neuromuscular junction. These include:

- Tetracycline
- Streptomycin
- Neomycin (and other aminoglycoside antibiotics)
- Clindamycin
- Ampicillin
- Lithium
- Chloroquine (and other quinine derivatives)
- Cipro
- D-penicillamine

Because they affect muscles, these drugs can induce respiratory depression after surgery. Penicillin and cephalosporins can safely be used to treat infections in immunosuppressed women with myasthenia.

---

sweat. My doctor thought it was a combination of the Mestinon and the hot flashes. But if I have night sweats now, I think it's mostly from the Mestinon, and I hardly ever have them. That's one of the best things about my doctor; I could tell her anything. And she took my concerns seriously.

How Myasthenia Can Affect You Over Your Lifetime

As with other autoimmune diseases, there's a lack of research into how MG affects women at different times of their lives. Most of the information we have is anecdotal, gleaned from the experience of neurologists who treat women with myasthenia.

Premenstrual Fluctuations

Many women with MG report that their symptoms get worse during the premenstrual period. According to the Myasthenia Gravis Foundation of America, it's believed that progesterone is responsible for the worsening of muscle weakness during this period (especially since symptoms improve once a period begins and progesterone drops off). However, it may be difficult to distinguish between possible hormonal effects, the effects of premenstrual syndrome, and a true exacerbation of symptoms.

"A small percentage of women report a worsening of myasthenia premenstrually. It's something that the literature has repeated over the years, but it's never been studied, to my knowledge," remarks Dr. Massey. "It really is unclear whether there's a worsening of symptoms or that women with premenstrual syndrome generally feel worse during that time, especially in terms of fatigue or stress, and that affects their myasthenia."

For example, fatigue is usually a product of muscle weakness rather than a symptom of the disease itself (as it is in RA or lupus), she notes. If PMS brings increased irritability and stress, that may worsen muscle weakness and fatigue. Women with myasthenia have to pace themselves and need to make extra accommodations during the premenstrual period, says Dr. Massey. Discomfort from symptoms that are clearly PMS related, such as bloating, breast tenderness, irritability, and mood swings, needs to be dealt with separately and in consultation with a gynecologist.

Pregnancy

Myasthenia itself doesn't affect your ability to become pregnant, and generally doesn't affect the normal growth and development of a fetus. (In rare cases, *arthrogryposis*, a congenital abnormality causing limb contractures, is seen in infants of MG mothers.) There is a risk of the disease worsening and of the baby developing a temporary neonatal myasthenia (see page 280). MG can even be triggered by pregnancy.

"Some women initially present during the first trimester or immediately after delivery. The progression of symptoms can be fairly dramatic over a period of days or weeks. The immune system is markedly altered in pregnancy to allow a woman to carry a fetus, and that is partly hormonally driven," observes Dr. Massey.

For women with myasthenia, prepregnancy counseling is extremely important. "We have no way of predicting how a particular woman will do during pregnancy. If we need to continue treatment, there are safety factors to consider. Women also need to know that they'll need more rest than usual to avoid symptom exacerbations," says Dr. Massey. "The course of myasthenia can be unpredictable during pregnancy. In general, it may worsen early in the pregnancy or right after delivery. However, after that exacerbation, the disease may stabilize again, as it does in MS." There's no way to predict which women will worsen after pregnancy, she adds.

Cholinesterase inhibitors like Mestinon have not been shown to cause birth defects, but some muscle weakness has been reported in newborns whose mothers took the drugs. They cannot be given intravenously, since it can lead to premature labor. Prednisone carries minimal risks to the fetus and is used during pregnancy. If you experience an exacerbation of MG during pregnancy, you can be admitted to the hospital, where you can undergo plasmapheresis and the baby can be monitored.

Late in pregnancy, the growing fetus can restrict the movement of the diaphragm, causing some shortness of breath. The drug *magnesium sulfate*, given to control eclampsia (high blood pressure in pregnancy), exacerbates MG, so other medications must be used to control blood pressure. In rare instances, a ventilator for respiratory support may be needed, says Dr. Massey.

While labor can be extra exhausting when you have MG, the disease doesn't affect the onset and duration of labor, since the uterus is smooth muscle. However, the voluntary and skeletal muscles can become weakened if labor is prolonged, and you can become extremely exhausted. Pain relief medication is given on an individualized basis. Muscle relaxants used during labor anesthesia may temporarily exacerbate muscle weakness. As in women without MG, cesareans are done when indicated.

"Women with myasthenia need to be followed in a high-risk obstetrical facility, in conjunction with a neurologist, and there has to be close communication by the care team," stresses Dr. Massey. "We usually admit women for the last week or two prior to delivery, so they and their baby can be closely followed."

Breastfeeding

There's no reason to avoid breastfeeding, but you may find it extremely fatiguing. While antimyasthenics have not been reported to cause problems in nursing babies, Mytelase has not been rated for safety during lactation. The

Physicians' Desk Reference (*PDR*) advises caution with Prostigmin, since risk cannot be ruled out. Mestinon is excreted in breast milk, but since no effects have been reported in infants it can be used (however, newborns should be monitored). Steroids are excreted in low levels, and the risk to the baby is considered low, adds Dr. Massey. Azathioprine, cyclosporine, and cyclophosphamide pass into breast milk and are not used in breastfeeding women.

AChR antibodies not only cross the placenta but can be found in low levels in breast milk, discouraging many women from breastfeeding. "Getting up during the night to breastfeed may completely wear a woman out. It's difficult to deal with caring for a newborn and a chronic disease. Most of my patients opt not to breastfeed so that someone else can feed the baby at night, and because they are worried about medications and the antibody issue," says Dr. Massey.

Neonatal Myasthenia Gravis

Between 10 and 20 percent of children born to women with MG develop a temporary *neonatal myasthenia gravis*. However, having one child with neonatal MG does not necessarily mean subsequent children will have it.

As in neonatal lupus, neonatal MG is thought to be caused by autoantibodies from the mother's circulation that cross the placenta. Neonatal MG may occur from birth to ten days after delivery (usually within the first twenty-four to forty-eight hours), with the baby showing poor sucking and generalized muscle weakness. Babies may also show eyelid drooping and have difficulty swallowing, and may not display facial expressions because of muscle weakness. In rare cases, some infants may have trouble breathing. Symptoms can be mild to severe, and usually continue for three to five weeks, until the baby has cleared the mother's antibodies.

Treatment usually involves giving low doses of oral Mestinon every few hours, along with intensive monitoring and, in some cases, use of a respirator if breathing difficulties arise. Blood transfusions rather than plasma exchange may be done, but severe cases may require plasma exchange. Most babies recover completely from neonatal MG. "Usually we are able to support and watch the child without aggressive treatment," adds Dr. Massey.

Children can also develop *juvenile myasthenia gravis*. The peak onset of the disease is between the ages of one and four, and between ages eleven and sixteen. As with adults, other autoimmune diseases can cluster with juvenile MG, especially Graves' disease. The treatment is the same as for adult MG, with thymectomy usually performed after puberty. About 20 percent of all cases of myasthenia gravis develop during childhood; one-quarter of those children have complete remission with treatment.

Midlife and Beyond

While heat can exacerbate MG, hot flashes don't seem to make symptoms worse. "I've actually never had a patient tell me that her myasthenia got worse with hot flashes. No one likes hot flashes, but the heat is brief and may not be enough to truly exacerbate the myasthenia. The core temperature of the body may not really change with hot flashes, so it's more of a perception of heat," Dr. Massey remarks.

The decision to take estrogen for menopausal symptoms is usually not based on having myasthenia. If a woman is taking prednisone, estrogen replacement would help prevent bone loss. "I would defer to a woman's gynecologist in this decision," Dr. Massey adds. In the case of corticosteroid use, other bone-building drugs may be used. "A family history or personal history of breast cancer would outweigh any other factor, for me, in the decision whether to take estrogen."

In later life, there's an increased risk of pernicious anemia, a condition in which the stomach does not absorb vitamin B_{12}, which can be treated with supplements. So older women with MG need to be periodically checked for the condition.

Menopause can also affect the quality of sleep. "Sleep can be a big issue. If you haven't had a good night's sleep, it's hard to deal with your disease. If this becomes an issue, ERT would be advised if hot flashes were interfering with sleep," remarks Dr. Massey. Newer sleep medications like *zaleplon* (*Sonata*) and *zolpidem* (*Ambien*) can be used for short periods, without daytime drowsiness.

Myositis

Myositis describes a group of inflammatory muscle diseases, thought to be autoimmune, that cause degeneration of skeletal muscle tissues, resulting in muscle weakness. They are *polymyositis* (*PM*) (*myo* means "muscle," *itis* means "inflammation," and *poly* means multiple muscles are involved), *dermato-myositis* (*DM*) (which has a distinctive red facial rash), and *inclusion-body myositis* (*IBM*). Polymyositis affects the *proximal* muscles (those nearest to the trunk), including the arms, legs, and neck, and in rare cases the *distal* muscles (those farthest from the trunk, like the fingers); inclusion-body myositis involves both groups of muscles. As with myasthenia, muscle weakness comes on gradually in PM and IBM, sometimes over a period of years. Polymyositis affects more women than men; inclusion-body myositis occurs more frequently in men. Dermatomyositis is more common in women.

Symptoms of polymyositis can include difficulty swallowing or breathing; about a third of patients have muscle pain. In IBM, about half of patients have swallowing difficulties, and there can be weakness of the wrist and finger flexor muscles, and atrophy (or shrinkage) of the forearm and quadriceps muscles. In contrast to the other myopathies, IBM often begins after age fifty.

The rash of dermatomyositis is distinctive from the classic butterfly rash of lupus; it erupts over the eyelids, cheeks, and bridge of the nose and on the chest, knuckles, elbows, and knees. It's a reddish purple or dusky lilac in color, rather than bright red. People with DM may also develop hardened, calcified bumps under the skin. In contrast to the other myopathies, dermatomyositis can also come on suddenly over days or a period of months. The muscles of the trunk, hips, shoulders, and neck are usually involved. Polymyositis can be associated with malignancy.

These diseases are diagnosed through muscle biopsies, electromyography (see page 270), and blood tests. The treatment for PM and DM is high-dose prednisone and, sometimes, immunosuppressants like azathioprine (Imuran, see page 274), and *methotrexate* (*Rheumatrex*, see page 130). Unfortunately, there's no effective treatment for IBM, although preliminary studies show some benefits for *intravenous immunoglobulin* (*IVIG*, see page 276). IVG also helps patients who don't respond to corticosteroids.

Jackie's story continues:
You just have to keep on going. Everything's good when I'm feeling good and my medicine is level; I can do pretty much what I want. But then I get up some mornings and it's all I can do to drag myself upstairs. In the last year,

I have tried to put a self-imposed twenty-four-hour limit on a pity party. I can go twenty-four hours, in my pajamas, lying around and whining "poor pitiful me" and I can cry, and then I make myself get up. There are some days I would rather stay in bed with the covers up. But you can't do that . . . self-pity is worse than any illness. And I'm lucky. Some people with this illness are in wheelchairs. I figure there are two things I can control: my faith and my attitude. The rest of it, you just have to play the hand you're dealt.

11

A Fury in the Blood— Antiphospholipid Syndrome, Immune Thrombocytopenic Purpura, and Vasculitis

It took me almost ten years to get a diagnosis. I had a history of head-aches and started having blood clots in my legs in 1986. The vascular surgeon I was seeing found that my platelets were sky high, and I was told I had essential thrombocytosis. He put me on Coumadin to thin my blood. Almost immediately, my headaches went away, and after a while I stopped having the leg clots. My platelet count went back to normal, so they took me off the Coumadin, and right away I started having headaches again, and I had a ministroke. But when I told my primary care physician about it, he said that a stroke was unlikely for a woman my age who had good blood pressure and cholesterol. He said it was probably an episode of low blood sugar, and didn't do any tests.

I was in my daughter's room when I had another stroke. I felt this stabbing pain in my head, like an ice pick. I thought I was speaking normally, my words sounded normal to me. But my daughter said, "Mom, your words are slurry and one side of your mouth is droopy. You're having a stroke," and she called 911. When we got to the ER the doctor on duty didn't think I had had a stroke (he also said I was too young, my blood pressure was too good, and so on) and sent me home. But the next day I couldn't get out of bed, and we went to another hospital closer by. They did an MRI and it showed that I had actually had five small strokes. They ordered a bunch of blood tests; one of them was a cardiolipin antibody test. The odd thing was that years before, my ophthalmologist had asked if I had had a cardiolipin workup. He said that anybody with unusual clotting under age forty should have the test, and he even wrote down the name . . . But my doctor said I didn't need it, that it was expensive and difficult to do. Which wasn't true, it turns out. And in the hospital, after my stroke, the neurologist I saw suspected I had antiphospholipid syndrome, but my doctor dismissed the idea, too. It took me months to get the results of the blood test they did after that stroke. The hospital claimed they faxed it to my doctor, but he said he never got it. By that time I had gone to a bigger hospital in the city to see a specialist, and he was the one who made the diagnosis of antiphospholipid syndrome. When we finally saw the results of that first blood test, it was positive for antiphospholipid antibodies. Maybe some of my strokes could have been avoided if my doctor had taken my symptoms seriously.

MARGARET, FORTY-SIX

Antiphospholipid Syndrome

Antiphospholipid syndrome (APS) is a disorder in which autoantibodies promote blood clots that can affect virtually any area of the body—causing seemingly unrelated problems like miscarriages and stroke.

First identified in the mid-1980s, antiphospholipid syndrome is an insidious disease that may not be diagnosed until after a woman has suffered several strokes, as in Margaret's case. In fact, APS is now thought to account for one-third of all strokes in people under age fifty, as well as 20 percent of clots in the veins of the legs (*deep vein thrombosis, DVT*), and up to 15 percent of recurrent miscarriages. APS may actually have more widespread effects in the body than systemic lupus, since blood clots can block just about any blood vessel, from the tiniest capillaries in the eyes to the large vessels supplying the heart and brain.

The formation of blood clots involves *platelets*, which are blood cells that originate in the bone marrow along with white and red blood cells, and proteins called *coagulation* or *clotting factors*. When you have a cut, platelets rush to the area to start plugging up the wound. First, each platelet adheres to the damaged blood vessel and becomes activated so they attach to each other (*aggregate*). Platelets are activated partly by chemicals secreted when a blood vessel is injured and by *thrombin*, a protein released during the clotting process itself (activated platelets also secrete chemicals needed for clotting). These chemicals stimulate coagulation factors in the blood and form a stringy protein called *fibrin*, creating long filaments that enmesh the platelets and other blood cells to form a semisolid plug in the wound that stops bleeding. Abnormal clot formation occurs when a blood vessel has not been punctured or cut.

This "coagulation cascade" is a complex process; anything that interferes with one step can cause either a tendency to abnormal bleeding or formation of blood clots (*thromboses*). In APS, it's thought that autoantibodies react with proteins involved in the coagulation cascade, and yet-unknown mechanisms can disturb this process and lead to abnormal clot formation in veins or arteries. APS can cause clots in leg veins called (DVTs) or clots in major arteries leading to strokes or "ministrokes" called *transient ischemic attacks* (*TIAs*). In pregnant women, these autoantibodies can lead to clots in the placenta that block blood flow to the fetus, causing recurrent miscarriages.

Antiphospholipid syndrome is five times more common in women than in men, and sometimes runs in families. APS can occur with other autoimmune diseases, but it can also affect otherwise healthy women whose only outward sign may be repeated pregnancy loss.

Warning Signs of APS

- Repeated miscarriages (generally second trimester)
- Blood clots (including *deep vein thromboses*)
- Transient ischemic attacks (TIAs), or ministrokes
- Migraine headaches
- Thrombocytopenia
- Red, mottled rash on the legs (*livedo reticularis*)
- Heart valve disease

---

288 THE AUTOIMMUNE CONNECTION

What Causes APS?

The name *antiphospholipid syndrome* is actually a misnomer. Newer research suggests that autoantibodies involved in APS, *antiphospholipid antibodies (APLs)*, probably don't react against *phospholipids*, fatty molecules that make up most of the membranes of all cells. Instead, APLs act against key *proteins* involved in clotting.

There are two main antiphospholipid antibodies: *anticardiolipin antibodies (aCLs)* and the *lupus anticoagulant (LA)*. Recent research has changed our understanding of the targets and actions of these antibodies, so the names originally given to them aren't really descriptive. The lupus anticoagulant (LA) doesn't have anticoagulant properties, but produces an increased risk of blood clotting. And it turns out aCLs don't actually bind to cardiolipin (a phospholipid found in high concentrations in heart and muscle tissue but present in all tissue). The main target of these antibodies is *beta$_2$ glycoprotein 1 ($\beta_2 GP1$)*, a protein that binds to cell membranes and has natural anticoagulant properties, and *prothrombin*, a normal blood protein that also binds to cell membranes and is essential for clotting.

Antiphospholipid antibodies (APLs) are present in higher amounts in up to a third of women with lupus, and in women with rheumatoid arthritis, Sjögren's syndrome, and other autoimmune diseases, but they don't always cause clotting problems. Other types of APLs can be produced after infections (especially in older people) and do not seem to clot. Infections linked to antiphospholipid antibodies include *parvovirus* (the respiratory virus that causes *fifth disease*), rubella, mumps, Lyme disease, and hepatitis A, B, and C. APLs are also found in women with *immune thrombocytopenia purpura* (a condition in which there are low platelet counts, see pages 299 to 315).

There are a number of theories as to how these antibodies may come about. "Perhaps you get an infection, and there's inflammation and the cell phospholipids turn over and are exposed on the cell surface. But after the infection and inflammation go away, the normal antibody response doesn't die down, the antibodies start mutating, and sooner or later they start binding to an important blood clotting protein," suggests Joan T. Merrill, MD, an expert on APS and head of the department of clinical pharmacology at the Oklahoma Medical Research Foundation in Oklahoma City.

Or, an infection may set off another process that leaves clotting-related proteins exposed to an immune system attack. "When there is inflammation, these proteins bind to the surface of the cells of the bloodstream, and may fold in such a way that exposes little pieces of the protein that aren't normally seen by the immune system. Antiphospholipid antibodies may be binding to parts of these proteins that normally stay hidden until they are needed to stop blood clotting. So when the protein unfolds and exposes certain areas, instead of stopping blood clotting, the protein is attacked by antibodies," says Dr. Merrill who also heads up the Registry for the Anit-phospholipid Syndrome.

There may be something about the placenta itself that attracts anticardiolipin antibodies, which cause cell death and other adverse effects that can lead to fetal loss.

Perhaps molecular mimicry might be involved, where invading microbes have a similar structure to clotting proteins, so the immune system attacks both. While the bacteria are eventually eliminated, in vulnerable women immune cells may continue to target the normal proteins. In fact, a recent study by the Center for Autoimmune Diseases at the Sheba Medical Center at Tel-Aviv University in Israel suggests that *Hemophilus influenzae* and other common bacteria may trigger production of certain antiphospholipid antibodies. "Most probably antiphospholipid syndrome, like other autoimmune diseases, is induced by common infectious agents. And when this infection occurs in someone with the right genetic background they will develop full-blown antiphospholipid syndrome," explains Yehuda Shoenfeld, MD, lead author of the study.

Several genes are probably involved in APS, and it can run in families. One recent study found that as many as one in three relatives of APS patients had antiphospholipid antibodies in their blood. Some of the genes associated with rheumatoid arthritis, and other autoimmune diseases (like the DR4 gene) are also found in women with APS, which may explain its coexistence with those diseases. Your genes may also determine the amount of APLs you make. For example, women with higher levels of aCLs have more clotting events.

I can tell you exactly when this all started. It was in February of 1989. I woke up in the middle of the night with a severe headache and joint pain. I had had a little fever all week, I developed a kind of rash on my arm, and I was extremely tired. I went to bed that Friday night, and must have awakened around two in the morning in such pain that I couldn't bear to have the sheets on me. It was that bad and that fast. It was like I went to bed and woke up someone else. And the fatigue the next day was just crushing. Not like when you've cleaned your whole house and you're very tired. More like you've been turned inside out. But we thought it was the flu, because that's how flu hits. I had also had periods of confusion before that; I'd be at the grocery store and just stop and wonder what I was doing there with these coupons and this list. I went to my family doctor and he tested me for lupus, for Lyme disease, for mono, everything. But the tests all came up negative . . . and if you're a woman, they say, "Are you premenstrual, are you pre-menopausal, are you depressed?" Well, I wasn't depressed. I was very happy. I had just met a wonderful man. We don't live far from Yale (where it turns out they were studying this disease). I went there, and tested positive for antiphospholipid antibodies. They also did an MRI and saw evidence that I had had multiple small strokes. They counted a dozen lesions in the mid-brain; they looked like little grains of rice on the MRI. This explained the confusion. And that was a relief, because after they run all those tests and find nothing, you begin to feel as if you really are going crazy.

ELAINE, FIFTY-EIGHT

Symptoms of APS

Elaine's and Margaret's stories are not that unusual. Women with APS tend to have dramatic case histories, remarks Robert A. S. Roubey, MD, an associate professor of medicine at the University of North Carolina at Chapel Hill, and director of the Antiphospholipid Syndrome Collaborative Registry (one of several APS registries). "A woman comes into the office and says 'I have been pregnant five times and lost all the babies, and I have never been able to carry a pregnancy to term.' Or a young woman has a stroke out of the blue. Or a young woman has recurrent DVTs. Those are the three key symptoms of APS, and they are striking," says Dr. Roubey.

Recurrent miscarriages occur at specific points in a pregnancy in APS. "The most typical fetal loss associated with antiphospholipid antibodies occurs late in the first trimester or in the second trimester, which is a very unusual time to have a loss. Perhaps 10 to 15 percent of these losses are associated with antiphospholipid antibodies," says Dr. Roubey. "Very early loss, before ten weeks, is very common and there can be many causes, so it's difficult to make an association with these antibodies."

Repeated episodes of blood clots in leg veins (especially in the deep veins) and strokes (major and mini) are the other major symptoms of APS. Deep vein thrombosis is dangerous because a piece of the clot can break off and travel to the heart or lungs.

Some women with APS also have reduced platelet counts (*thrombocytopenia*), often detected during routine bloodwork. Although these women have longer than usual clotting times, they typically don't have bleeding episodes, Dr. Roubey points out.

Other complications of APS include heart attacks (often before age forty-five, possibly because of accelerated atherosclerosis), epileptic-type seizures, headaches (often migraines), vision problems caused by blockages (*infarcts*) in the blood vessels of the eye, memory problems or dementia caused by ministrokes (*multi-infarct dementia*), blood clots in the lungs (*pulmonary embolism*), and heart valve disease.

"With heart valve disease in APS, you have fibrin deposits on the valves, most often the mitral valve, which thickens the valve so it doesn't close properly—this allows some blood to flow backward, which we call regurgitation," explains Dr. Roubey. "These fibrin deposits can break off and cause occlusions, and clots can also form on the valve. This also occurs in lupus, and is associated with anticardiolipin antibodies."

APS can cause skin problems, including a red or bluish rash on the legs (*livedo reticularis*), which looks like a "mesh network of veins underneath the skin," says Dr. Roubey.

These problems can appear sporadically, separated by months or years, and seem unrelated. In some women, a series of clotting-related events affecting multiple organs (especially the kidneys and the heart) suddenly occurs over a period of days or weeks, sometimes after infections, surgery, or giving birth. This is called *catastrophic APS*, and it can be life threatening.

When APS occurs by itself it is called *primary antiphospholipid syndrome* (*PAPS*), and is more common in younger women with recurrent, unexplained miscarriages. *Secondary APS* can be associated with underlying autoimmune diseases (such as lupus) and can even be drug induced. Patients are generally categorized by age, sex, and the complications they have, since symptoms may be caused by an underlying problem rather than by APS itself. Finding out whether other family members have APS can help women to recognize symptoms and be treated earlier. One study found that 20 percent of women with APLs who suffer recurrent miscarriages go on to develop leg clots.

Diagnosing APS

Any kind of abnormal blood clotting, whether in an artery or vein, and pregnancy losses that occur between the end of the first trimester to the middle of the second trimester, should make a physician think of testing for antiphospholipid syndrome.

The presence of both the lupus anticoagulant (LA) and anticardiolipin (aCL) antibodies, together with clinical signs and symptoms, are the gold standard for diagnosing APS, says E. Nigel Harris, MD, a pioneer in APS research and dean of the Morehouse School of Medicine in Atlanta. "Sixty percent of APS patients will have both of these antibodies, while only 16 percent will be positive for the lupus anticoagulant alone. Since one test may be positive without the other, both are needed. The anticardiolipin antibody test will also be positive in women with lupus, and in other autoimmune diseases, including rheumatoid arthritis, and infectious diseases," explains Dr. Harris.

Under the most widely accepted diagnostic criteria, you need a history of a clot and the presence of an antiphospholipid antibody to be diagnosed with APS. However, if you have antibodies but have never had a clot, your risk seems to increase along with the *level* of the antibody. So specific testing for these two antibodies (one of which is a test to measure clotting times) are needed for a definitive diagnosis. Positive tests may help to predict which women are at risk for problems as well as for management of their treatment.

Antibodies are also called *immunoglobulins*. There are several categories of immunoglobulins—including *immunoglobulin G (IgG)*, *immunoglobulin M (IgM)*, and *immunoglobulin A (IgA)*. It's important to know the subcategory (or *isotype*) that the antiphospholipid antibody belongs to if you're suspected of having APS, since the IgG isotype is associated with a greater risk of blood clotting. So your blood tests will not only report the level of antibodies, but also their isotype. In the future, even more specific antibody testing may be able to help doctors tell which women are most at risk for fetal loss, says Dr. Harris.

According to the accepted diagnostic criteria for APS, you need to have one or more of the following clinical signs, along with antiphospholipid antibodies of the IgG (or IgM) subtype:

- Recurrent early pregnancy loss
- Unexplained fetal loss after ten weeks
- One or more premature births due to severe preeclampsia or placental insufficiency
- Venous blood clots
- Arterial blood clots

In addition, these clinical signs may factor into a diagnosis:

- Leg ulcers
- Thrombocytopenia
- Hemolytic anemia

Tests You May Need and What They Mean

There are four ways to test for antiphospholipid antibodies:

Anticardiolipin antibodies (aCLs) are measured using a test called an *ELISA* (*enzyme-linked immunoabsorbent assay*), in which the clear part of the blood (plasma) is analyzed for the presence of antibodies. An ELISA test is very sensitive and can detect even low levels (*titers*) of aCLs and other antibodies. The tests are reported as high titers (over 80 units), medium titers (20 to 80 units), or low titers (10 to 20 units); they also indicate whether aCLs belong to the IgG subgroup (and their titers).

Anticardiolipin antibodies need to react with certain proteins (called *cofactors*) in order to promote blood clots. A conventional ELISA test can detect whether aCLs react to beta$_2$ glycoprotein 1. Why have this additional test? For one thing, it's more specific for APS than measuring the amount (titer) of aCLs. Studies have also shown that aCLs produced by infections don't react with beta$_2$ glycoprotein 1 and are less likely to cause clotting. Finding aCLs that react with this cofactor is considered to be a good predictor of thrombotic events.

Beta$_2$ glycoprotein 1 antibodies (ß$_2$GP1) can also be detected using an ELISA test. Finding specific antibodies to this cofactor is also considered to be a good predictor of a woman's risk for clotting problems. The test for ß$_2$GP1 is relatively new, but further studies may show it to be one of the most important and sensitive tests for APS, comments Dr. Merrill.

Lupus anticoagulant antibodies (LACs) this test is an important marker for a high risk of blood clots and fetal loss. Tests to measure the presence of a so-called lupus anticoagulant include an *activated partial thromboplastin time (aPTT)* test, in which clot-promoting factors are added to a sample of blood plasma from a patient with suspected APS and to normal plasma, and the time both samples take to coagulate is compared.

A **venereal disease research laboratory (VDRL)** test may sometimes be done. Part of this antigen is similar in structure to the bacteria that cause syphilis, and a false-positive test for syphilis may actually be the first clue to the presence of antiphospholipid antibodies (and was one of the first assays used to detect APS). A false-positive VDRL test is usually not considered to have as strong a correlation with clotting.

Laboratory tests may also include assays for other, less common antiphospholipid antibodies (such as phosphatidyl serine); tests for deficiencies in antithrombin and in the clotting cofactors *protein C* and *protein S* (that protect against excessive clotting), and for *homocysteine* (a naturally occurring amino acid in the body that is harmful to blood vessels in high amounts and is a risk factor for clots); and genetic tests for clotting disorders. A complete blood count (CBC) measures white and red blood cells, as well as platelets. The normal range for platelets is 150,000 to 450,000 per cubic microliter of blood. A platelet count of less than 150,000 of blood is considered to be thrombocytopenia (see pages 304 to 305).

Magnetic resonance imaging (MRI) may be done if it's suspected that a woman has had strokes or ministrokes. The damage from TIAs is seen as small white spots scattered around the brain.

The Female Factor

Can female hormones play a role in APS? The answer is unclear. "It probably has something to do with hormones, but it's not as simple as 'female hormones are bad, and male hormones are good.' There's a very complicated system of checks and balances in which hormones play an important role, and it looks as if people who get autoimmune diseases have a slightly different balance of hormones. But we don't really understand these issues very well," says Dr. Merrill.

Naturally occurring estrogens in the body keep blood vessels supple, and seem to prevent clogging and hardening of the arteries. On the other hand, it's important to know that estrogen increases production of clotting factors by the liver; therefore, adding estrogen (whether in oral contraceptives or hormone replacement therapy) can increase the risk of blood clots. Estrogen can also lower levels of a clotting cofactor called *protein S*, an anticoagulant protein, that may be abnormally low in APS.

"So it's a question of balance, what other hormones are present or not present. We do not know that women with antiphospholipid antibodies should not take estrogen. The relationship of hormones to APS requires further study," adds Dr. Merrill.

Elaine's story continues:
You really need to take a careful family history. You can't just ask about one disease—you throw out a name and people may not know what it is. Or someone would say, "What's my thyroid got to do with anything? You have arthritis." People don't make the connections. I know I didn't. And until I

APS Clusters

Antiphospholipid antibodies are found in women with a number of autoimmune diseases (including lupus, scleroderma, polymyositis, and vasculitis), but they're not always associated with clotting problems. The autoimmune diseases that can cluster with APS include the following:

- Lupus
- Immune thrombocytopenia purpura
- Raynaud's phenomenon
- Inflammatory bowel disease

was diagnosed and had my daughter tested, because she kept having mis-carriages, I never would have connected the dots. But it turns out that my mother had arthritis, colitis, thyroid disease, and terrible migraines and died of a stroke when she was forty-eight. Her father and two of my uncles died of strokes. My eldest daughter has had several miscarriages, she has headaches, and she has Crohn's disease. My other daughter has tested posi-tive for APLs. So autoimmunity runs in my family, but it never had a name.

Treating APS

Treatment for antiphospholipid syndrome usually involves measures to pre-vent blood clotting. This can include aspirin (which prevents platelets from clumping together) or anticoagulants like heparin or warfarin. The dose and length of treatment depends on whether you've had recurrent miscarriages and/or clots.

Corticosteroids and other drugs that dampen inflammation and immune system activity are not generally used in women with APS, since it's not con-sidered an inflammatory disease. Immune thrombocytopenia can occur in APS, and although it responds to steroids, the coexisting tendency for bleed-ing due to low platelet counts and the tendency for abnormal clotting poses a major problem for women receiving anticoagulants. So treatment for women with both disorders can be a delicate balancing act.

Anticoagulant therapy with **warfarin** (**Coumadin**) is prescribed if you have APLs and have had any kind of clotting episode (including deep vein thromboses and transient ischemic attacks). Treatment is usually prolonged, often lifelong, because the risk of recurrent vascular thromboses is so high. However, your level of anticoagulation will need to be monitored carefully with regular blood tests to make sure that you're not at risk for bleeding because your blood has been overtreated and does not clot at all.

Regulating the level of anticoagulation is based on a numerical system called the *international normalized ratio* (*INR*). In the past, coagulation stan-dards were set at each lab; the INR is a means of standardizing the coagula-tion assay. The INR measures the balance of bleeding to coagulation by measuring your actual clotting time against an expected or control time. Your

INR will be measured with daily blood tests when you're first prescribed warfarin, until your doctor is sure clotting time is within a safe range. Blood tests will then be gradually reduced in frequency if your clotting time is stable.

The goal for APS patients with vascular thromboses is an INR of 3.0 or greater. At this range there's a higher risk of bleeding complications, so careful monitoring is needed. (A slightly lower level of anticoagulation may be needed in women with both APS and thrombocytopenia.) In addition, other risk factors for thromboembolic events—including high blood pressure and high cholesterol—must be aggressively controlled.

Aspirin and heparin are usually prescribed together or separately to prevent miscarriages in women with APS who have had recurrent pregnancy losses.

Women who have had recurrent early miscarriages regardless of whether they have had a history of clotting episodes when not pregnant are usually given injections of low-molecular weight heparin twice a day, along with low-dose aspirin (81 milligrams). Low-molecular weight heparin is fractionated to include only smaller heparin molecules. Low-molecular weight heparin (*Lovenox, Fragmin*) is generally longer acting and carries less risk of bleeding than regular (or unfractionated heparin). It's given in injections, usually twice a day.

Prophylactic therapy may be needed even if you have antiphospholipid antibodies but no other clinical signs, or if you have APS and have experienced miscarriages but not thromboses, since there's a risk for developing clots later on in life. The first step may be low-dose (81 mg) aspirin.

APS patients at high risk of clots may need a single injection of heparin before air travel, since sitting for long periods on lengthy flights increases the risk of deep vein thromboses (dubbed "economy-class syndrome").

Women with APS should avoid certain drugs that may increase their risk of clotting, including oral contraceptives and estrogen replacement therapy (which increase production of clotting factors by the liver). COX-2 inhibitors prescribed for pain relief do not have the anticlotting effects of aspirin and there is the possibility that they can increase the risk of clots.

Future treatments may include an experimental drug aimed at turning off the B-cells that make antibodies to beta$_2$ glycoprotein 1. Early clinical trials of the drug are under way.

How APS Can Affect You Over Your Lifetime

The effects of APS vary throughout the stages of a woman's life.

Fertility and Pregnancy

If you have APS, you will probably not have a problem getting pregnant, but you can lose the pregnancy—most commonly during the second trimester, but even in the first trimester.

The negative effects of APS on pregnancy may be due to abnormal function of the placenta. In normal pregnancies, the end portions of the spiral-shaped arteries that supply the placenta are open, and there's no smooth muscle layer, so blood flows freely to the fetus. In women with APS, some researchers have found narrowing of these small arteries, with a thickened inner lining and deposits not unlike those in cardiovascular disease, so blood flow to the fetus can be impeded (*placental insufficiency*). In addition, there are blood clots and even placental tissue death. Investigators are looking into the possible role of complement in damage to the placenta. Right now, the exact mechanism that causes nonthrombotic problems in the placenta in APS is not understood, so therapy to prevent pregnancy loss remains aimed at avoiding blood clots.

"In women with clearly established APS, if the last pregnancy resulted in early loss, the chances of the next pregnancy also resulting in a loss are something around 70 to 80 percent, if you don't treat with anticoagulants," says Dr. Roubey. The treatment is generally a low dose of heparin and baby aspirin (see page 297). "There's some evidence that if you just take the baby aspirin, you can get the success rate up to 40 percent or so. But with low-molecular weight heparin, you usually can maintain the pregnancy 70 or 80 percent of the time."

If pregnancy loss occurs despite treatment with heparin, infusions of intravenous gamma globulin (IVIG) over a four- or five-day period may be a safe (but costly) alternative.

Menopause and Beyond

If you have APS you should not use estrogen replacement to treat menopausal symptoms because of the risk of blood clots. "Antiphospholipid antibodies give you one risk factor for clotting, and you don't want to add another," remarks Dr. Roubey.

Nonhormonal menopausal remedies might be helpful as long as they don't promote clotting (as does *evening primrose oil*) or interfere with blood thinners and aspirin (as *red clover/Promensil* does). Potential remedies include vitamin E (which may help relieve hot flashes) and B vitamins (especially vitamin B_6) for mood swings. The B vitamin folic acid has the added advantage of lowering homocysteine, which can damage blood vessels and lead to atherosclerosis. *Wild yams*, which contain *diosgenin*, a precursor to natural progesterone (used by some drug companies to make prescription progestins), may also relieve hot flashes and other menopausal symptoms without promoting clotting. You should discuss *any* herbal or vitamin regimens with your doctor. (For details on nonhormonal menopause remedies, see pages 46 to 47.)

It's important to note that the risk of recurrent thromboses may increase with age, so anticoagulant therapy must be continued with careful monitoring.

Around ten years ago I noticed I was getting these fried-egg-sized bruises on my forearm. If I bit my tongue it would bleed for a long time . . . I would also have very heavy periods. At the time, I was a systems analyst for a pharmaceutical company. My tongue kept bleeding, and I didn't feel well. I went to a doctor, who eventually ran blood tests. My platelets were around 6,000—there were virtually none in my blood. He told me I had a platelet disorder. He wrote down the name of the disease. At the time, I didn't even know what platelets were.

JOAN YOUNG, FIFTY-SIX, FOUNDER AND PRESIDENT,
PLATELET DISORDERS SUPPORT ASSOCIATION

Immune Thrombocytopenic Purpura (ITP)

Immune thrombocytopenic purpura (ITP) is a disorder in which the immune system attacks and destroys platelets in the blood, interfering with normal blood clotting.

You'll recall that when you get a cut, platelets gather in the area and almost immediately start to form a clot to seal off the area and limit bleeding. It's kind of like plugging up a leaky pipe. But if you don't have the materials to make that plug, the pipe keeps leaking. In ITP (sometimes called *autoimmune thrombocytopenic purpura*), there's a shortage of platelets to form the plug because the immune system has targeted them for destruction in the spleen. As a result, blood clots don't form properly, allowing bleeding to continue for longer periods.

The spleen is a kidney bean–shaped organ located in the upper left abdomen, just behind your ribs, that produces some of the antibodies and immune cells that help fight off infections, removes worn-out red blood cells, and antibody-coated particles like bacteria. Normally, platelets circulate in the blood for eight to ten days before being cleared by the spleen and replaced by others produced in the bone marrow. In women with ITP, this process of platelet clearance is sped up by autoantibodies. These antibodies bind to platelets and cause the spleen and other organs to remove them from the blood prematurely. So platelets remain in the blood for only a few days or even a few hours, depending on how severe the disease is. The platelets are destroyed faster than they can be replaced. A *thrombocyte* is a clotting cell, *penia* means low blood levels; *thrombocytopenia* means low platelets.

Since platelets are essential for stopping leakage of blood from damaged blood vessels, severe thrombocytopenia can cause bleeding, especially from smaller blood vessels in the skin and other parts of the body.

Low platelets can lead to prolonged and heavy menstrual periods, and bleeding from tiny blood vessels in mucosal surfaces such as the nose or gums. Bleeding can occur even with a minor injury that doesn't break the surface of the skin, so you bruise easily. Small bleeds can arise from blood vessels beneath the surface of the skin or mucosa, producing small red spots called *petechiae* inside of the mouth and on the legs. When the platelet count gets too low, bleeding can occur without provocation in the intestines or even the brain.

Normally you have 150,000 to 450,000 platelets per cubic microliter of blood (cu/μl). In severe cases of ITP, platelets are so depleted that the count can be close to zero; in milder cases, your platelet count may hover around 100,000 cu/μl. However, bleeding usually does not occur until platelet counts fall below 30–50,000 or even 10,000.

Platelets have another function that has nothing to do with clotting. They store the mood-elevating brain chemical *serotonin*, which has effects not only in the brain but also in the body. Platelets store about 2 percent of the body's serotonin (and 99 percent of its parent or *precursor* chemical *L-tryptophan*,

---

Warning Signs of Immune Thrombocytopenic Purpura

- Tiny spots of bleeding inside the mouth
- Easy or spontaneous bruising
- Petechiae on the lower legs and ankles
- Bleeding gums
- Nosebleeds
- Fatigue
- Depression
- Muscle aches

---

which is converted to serotonin once it gets into the brain). Serotonin is involved in mood regulation, appetite, biological rhythms, and our sleep-wake cycle. So another consequence of having too few platelets can be a low level of serotonin, which may cause depression and fatigue.

ITP can occur at any age, but in adults it most often occurs between ages twenty and forty, affecting three times as many women as men. It can also occur in the elderly. In some cases, ITP occurs along with other autoimmune diseases such as lupus, rheumatoid arthritis, inflammatory bowel disease, and thyroid disease (see page 311). When it occurs by itself, the disorder is called *primary thrombocytopenic purpura.*

While ITP can develop slowly in adults, in children it can come on suddenly (usually between ages two and four)—sometimes a couple of weeks after a viral illness—then resolve on its own after a few weeks or months.

What Causes ITP?

The destruction of platelets is caused by autoantibodies called *antiplatelet antibodies.* But this autoantibody doesn't directly attack the platelet cell; it binds to the cell membrane and makes the cell a *target* for destruction by macrophages in the spleen.

You'll recall that macrophages (the "big eaters") are programmed to recognize foreign antigens like bacteria, ingest them, and take them out of circulation. While some macrophages patrol the bloodstream, some are produced by the spleen to help fight infectious agents there. When a receptor called *Fc* on those macrophages targets the antiplatelet antibody on the surface of a platelet, the macrophage thinks it's a foreign cell and gobbles up the platelet, explains hematologist S. Gerald Sandler, MD, professor of medicine and pathology at Georgetown University Medical Center in Washington, D.C.

Antiplatelet antibodies are first produced by B-cells contained in the spongelike outer layer (or *capsule*) of the spleen, lymph nodes, and even the bone marrow. Even after the spleen is removed, people with ITP have elevated antiplatelet antibodies. So those B-cells must also be present in the circulation. The number of antibody-producing B-cells may be increased in women with ITP, says Dr. Sandler. Numbers are also increased of "helper" T-cells, which signal B-cells to produce autoantibodies, perhaps telling other B-cells to secrete antiplatelet antibodies. Platelet destruction can also occur in the liver (another organ that helps cleanse the blood).

What prompts the formation of these autoantibodies is not clear. When the body is invaded by viruses or bacteria, production of antibodies called *immunoglobulins* may be stimulated. These antibodies act against proteins on platelets. Most of the platelets destroyed in the spleen become coated with a normally occurring immunoglobulin—immunoglobulin G (IgG), and the amount of platelet surface IgG correlates with the degree of thrombocytopenia.

The structure of the platelet is thought to be totally normal; it's the coating that's not. "What the macrophage is really looking for are bacteria that are coated with the immunoglobulin, the body's normal defense. And it will take bacteria and eat it up, get it out of the circulation, if it's got the antibody on it as part of the defense. In this case, abnormally, we've got a platelet that's cruising through with an abnormal antibody on it, so that's what's going to get picked up by the Fc receptor on the macrophage," says Dr. Sandler. "So what you have is a disorder where normal-looking platelets get taken out of the circulation by a cell in the spleen because they are coated with an antibody that shouldn't be on their surface."

At the same time, animal studies suggest ITP may in part be due to a problem with the development of platelets from stem cells, the cells in bone marrow that also develop into red and white blood cells. A growth factor produced in the liver called *thrombopoietin* (*TPO*) acts on stem cells to transform (or *differentiate*) them into cells called *megakaryocytes*, which mature into platelets and are released into the bloodstream. TPO levels are not increased to compensate for low platelets. This compounds the situation, and may be one reason platelets are destroyed faster than new ones are made.

Infections and medications can also cause formation of antibodies. The fact that some cases of ITP are caused by drugs, occur after a virus, or worsen after a viral infection may mean that there are environmental triggers. ITP has been associated with Lyme disease, *cytomegalovirus*, *Epstein-Barr virus* (*EBV*, infectious mononucleosis), *mycoplasmal pneumonia*, hepatitis C, and the ulcer-causing bacteria *Helicobacter pylori*.

"There are infections that you don't completely clear that are associated with ITP. When you suppress them, it makes the thrombocytopenia better. For example, antiviral therapy boosts platelet counts in people with ITP with HIV-related thrombocytopenia or in hepatitis C," says hematologist James B. Bussel, MD, professor of pediatrics and director of the Platelet Disorders Center at the Weill Medical College of Cornell University. "H. pylori is another example. In a recent study in Italy of 30 patients with chronic ITP, among those found to have H. pylori infections who were treated, some showed sustained platelet increases. We can diagnose H. pylori with a breath test or an antibody test, and this may turn out to be a strategy for treating certain patients. It has not worked yet in the U.S. and more investigation is needed."

There may be genes involved that increase the risk of developing ITP, but they have not been isolated yet. Potential genetic variations could include a gene that affects the Fc receptor, TPO, or other components of the immune system. "If we could find such genes it would then allow us to do tests in people and determine the optimal treatment for that individual," comments Dr. Bussel.

Joan's story continues:

If I had four hours a day when I could actually do something, that was a good day. I was incredibly fatigued; I couldn't walk out to get my mail . . . I was obsessed with the marks on my body. I had red spots on my legs, and I would get enormous bruises. I had blood blisters in my mouth that looked like grapes. I went to my doctor to get a platelet count twice a week. Once it was zero; it was very frightening. I tried to keep my brain active with crosswords. I changed my diet, I adopted a macrobiotic diet, and that seemed to help a little bit. Then I got the flu, and my platelets fell to 10 . . . I had a number of treatments, but nothing seemed to work for me. Finally, I agreed to have a splenectomy . . . but two weeks after that, my platelets were as low as they were before. I tried herbs, I went on a macrobiotic diet, I did many other things to improve my health and tried a new regimen of drugs . . . and finally my platelets came back to a normal level.

Symptoms of ITP

ITP typically develops over months or years in adults, and there's typically no spontaneous bleeding until platelets fall below a certain level, usually around 50,000.

Your first symptoms may be heavy periods that last longer than usual. You may have nosebleeds (*epistaxis*), and your gums may bleed during routine dental work. Bleeding can occur even with a minor injury that doesn't break the surface of the skin, so you bruise easily (*purpura* means "bleeding under the skin"). Sometimes this bruising (*thrombocytopenic purpura*) can occur on the arms or legs with no provocation at all, as it did with Joan.

Skin lesions develop as the tiny blood vessels beneath the surface of the skin or mucous membranes bleed, forming small purple spots (petechiae) inside the mouth and on the ankles and legs. The petechiae don't itch and they're not raised (in contrast to those in vasculitis). Petechiae can merge together and form large bruiselike areas called purpura, which may occasionally develop into hemorrhagic blisters (*bullae*).

As your platelet count falls, there may be blood in the urine (*hematuria*), gastrointestinal bleeding, and, in rare cases, bleeding in the brain (*cerebral hemorrhage*).

Some women may become alarmed at the frequency of bruises, and seek medical care. But in 50 percent of cases, ITP is diagnosed during routine blood tests, says Dr. Bussel.

Diagnosing Immune Thrombocytopenic Purpura

The diagnosis of thrombocytopenia is straightforward: a platelet count that falls below 150,000. What isn't so simple is determining the *cause*.

A number of diseases can cause low platelet counts, including lupus, antiphospholipid syndrome, Crohn's disease, Graves' disease, and primary biliary cirrhosis. Other diseases that can cause low platelet counts include chronic lymphocytic leukemia, B-cell lymphoma, and Hodgkin's disease. In some cases, a low platelet count occurs without apparent cause or other diseases (*idiopathic* or *nonimmune thrombocytopenic purpura*).

Secondary immune thrombocytopenia occurs in a number of multisystemic autoimmune diseases. At least 30 percent of women with systemic lupus also have ITP and, in certain cases, it may be the first symptom that presents itself, says Dr. Bussel. ITP may also occur in rheumatoid arthritis and scleroderma.

However, unlike diseases where antibody testing can help make a diagnosis, testing for antiplatelet antibodies isn't useful in diagnosing ITP. "The diagnosis is based on a platelet count of under 150,000, large platelets seen on a blood smear, and an otherwise normal blood count and physical exam, except for signs of bleeding, such as petechiae," explains Dr. Bussel.

Tests You May Need and What They Mean

Complete blood count (CBC) is the most important test for diagnosing thrombocytopenia. But you need the CBC, not just a platelet count, stresses Dr. Bussel. "You need to know the white cell count, the level of hemoglobin, the size of the red blood cells, the mean cell volume, all the red cell indices, to see if there are abnormal cells circulating," he explains.

In some people with thrombocytopenia, red blood cells may either be cleared faster by the spleen because of antibodies directed against them or they have bleeding from heavy menses, so a red blood cell count may be lower than normal. *Hematocrit* (percent of red cells per volume of blood) and level of *hemoglobin* (the oxygen-carrying component of red cells) also indicate the amount of red blood cells.

A **peripheral blood smear** can reveal enlarged platelets (*megathrombocytes*), which are frequently seen with ITP and may be a sign that platelets are being destroyed and new large ones rushed out of the blood marrow to compensate. In the test, a blood sample is smeared onto a slide, stained, and viewed under a microscope.

A **direct Coombs test** may be done to see whether red cells have an antibody or complement on their surface (which is important in treatment with a drug called WinRho, pages 308 to 309). "You can have the same problem with red blood cells as you do with platelets, where there's an antibody that causes them to be broken down faster by the spleen," explains Dr. Bussel. "We might do this test to determine which patients could receive a treatment that places an immunoglobulin antibody on the red cells to make them a target instead of platelets. But if the red cells already have antibody on their surface, the drug would cause more red cell breakdown, or *aggravated hemolysis*."

Bone marrow aspiration may be needed in some cases to determine whether the number of megakaryocytes, the precursor cells to platelets, is normal. If megakaryocytes are increased, it can indicate that platelets are being destroyed by the spleen. *Myelodysplasia* (abnormal growth of bone marrow), a preleukemic syndrome found more often in people over age sixty, can lead to abnormal megakaryocytes and low platelet counts and can be picked up with a bone marrow test. Bone marrow aspiration can also detect leukemia or marrow failure.

Lupus autoantibody testing may be advisable if symptoms of arthritis exist with thrombocytopenia and other autoantibodies are present (such as antiphospholipid antibodies). "If other organ systems appear to be involved, it may be appropriate to see whether a woman has lupus. In this case, the thrombocytopenia would be the tip of the iceberg," says Dr. Bussel. Key autoantibodies in lupus include *antinuclear antibodies, anti-DNA antibodies*, and *antiphospholipid antibodies* (see pages 59 to 61.)

Thyroid stimulating hormone (TSH) tests may also be done, since there's as much as a 10 percent overlap with hypothyroidism in ITP, Dr. Bussel adds (see page 91).

Treating Immune Thrombocytopenic Purpura

ITP is an unpredictable disease. Some women simply have lowered platelet counts, but never progress to bleeding or other symptoms, and no treatment is needed. Other women may have platelet counts so perilously low that they are in danger of cerebral hemorrhage or other life-threatening bleeds, and immediate intervention is needed.

"There are really no hard and fast numbers. But in general, if your platelets are greater than 30,000, we don't start treatment unless you have symptoms or bleeding or need to undergo surgery," says Dr. Bussel. "For newly diagnosed women whose platelets are under 10,000 or with bleeding symptoms, we would give IVIG in combination with prednisone. In some cases the platelet count will return to normal levels and retreatment may not be needed. Unfortunately, there's no way to predict which women will respond and which will need more therapy."

The most effective treatment to rapidly increase platelet counts—intravenous immunoglobulin (IVIG), *intravenous Rh (D) immune globulin (IV RhIG, WinRho)*, and steroids—interfere with the destruction of platelets. Removing the spleen (*splenectomy*), the only curative treatment for ITP, gets rid of the main site of platelet destruction. However, after the surgery, the destruction of platelets can resume in other sites, like the liver. Oral corticosteroids are the most commonly used nonsurgical treatment to maintain the platelet count. Because of the serious side effects, women cannot continually take high doses and, in some patients, a short course of steroids followed by IVIG or WinRho will bring about a long-term remission.

Corticosteroids, most often prednisone, suppress overall immune function, decreasing the destruction of platelets and possibly increasing platelet production. The usual dose is 1 milligram of prednisone per kilogram of body weight (2.20 pounds) a day for approximately two weeks until platelet counts come up to a "safe" level (over 30,000). The drug is then tapered off.

"No medication that can be taken orally has been shown to get the count up higher and quicker than prednisone. For this reason, it is usually part of all initial treatments for ITP," remarks Dr. Sandler. "Steroids are more useful for acute treatment, which we call *induction*, than they are for keeping platelet counts up over the long term, which we call *maintenance*."

Because of the side effects of high-dose steroids, they are not optimally continued for more than four weeks at a time. However, some women may need repeated cycles or prolonged use of steroids, increasing the risk of hypertension, diabetes, cataracts, and bone loss.

Intravenous immunoglobulin (IVIG) is prepared from human plasma and contains immunoglobulins for IgG, or gamma globulin. IVIG may work by blocking the receptors on macrophages that look for platelets coated with the IgG antiplatelet antibody. "On these receptors there's a lock-and-key mechanism. If we flood the circulation with these other IgG molecules, then they're going to fit into the lock on that receptor and let the platelets go free," explains Dr. Sandler. "We call it a *medical splenectomy*. The spleen can't do two things at once, and if you occupy it with some other molecule, it won't eat platelets. You're really taking the spleen out of action." Recent research suggests that IVIG actually turns on inhibitory receptors and in that way prevents platelets from getting destroyed.

Although IVIG can raise platelet counts within a day or so, large doses are required, which take three or more hours to be infused into the body. IVIG is also expensive—around $3,000 or more per infusion. Adverse side effects can include sudden headaches, backaches, flushing, chills, and (rarely) irritation of the membranes around the brain (*aseptic meningitis*), kidney dysfunction and failure. The platelet count starts going down within days of an infusion as receptors become cleared of the IgG, so by the end of two to four weeks another infusion may be needed. However, the side effects are not as toxic as those of high-dose steroids (and IVIG doesn't cause bone loss).

Intravenous Rh (D) immune globulin (IV RhIG, WinRho) is also prepared from human immunoglobulins in plasma, but contains a specific antibody to a marker on red blood cells called "D," making them a target instead of platelets.

Rh is a substance (actually an antigen) on the blood cells of 85 percent of people; if you don't have it, you're called *Rh-negative*. Rh is used in blood typing, along with blood grouping (whether or not there are specific protein markers on blood cells that make your blood A, B, O, or AB, positive or negative), to match blood from donor to recipient.

When given to Rh (D)-positive women with ITP who haven't had a splenectomy, the drug (dubbed "anti-D") causes macrophages to target the D protein marker on red blood cells. "Anti-D goes onto normal red blood cells much as the IgG antibody attaches to platelets. Red cells are larger than platelets, and since these people have normal red count, there are more coated red cells than platelets. So the red cells go in and literally stuff the mouth of the macrophage and the platelets are spared," explains Dr. Sandler.

The normal life of a red cell is around 120 days; WinRho accelerates the process of removal and keeps the macrophages in the spleen busy gobbling red cells. Platelet counts begin to rise within one to two days after an infusion of WinRho, and peak within a week or two. The response can last up to thirty days before another infusion is needed.

Studies of anti-D have shown a response rate of over 70 percent, bringing platelet counts to over 100,000 in many people, depending on the dose. It also contains special "detergents" and solvents that destroy viruses (such as hepatitis B and C) and remove other viruses, ensuring the drug's safety (since it's made from human plasma). WinRho takes around five minutes to infuse (a quick infusion is called a "push"), has fewer side effects, and is less costly than IVIG. But again, it works only in Rh (D)-positive women and those who have not had a splenectomy. In rare cases, WinRho may also cause excessive red cell breakdown. When red cells are broken up too quickly, hemoglobin is released in the bloodstream and excreted in urine, turning it pink. The direct Coombs test may be able to weed out patients at risk for excess hemolysis. A dose of prednisone before an infusion will help prevent fever and chills.

Anti-D may be used in adults as maintenance therapy. "In a pilot study we conducted, over 40 percent of patients discontinue all treatment over a two-year period. Some maintained platelets of over 100,000 six months after receiving anti-D. The median time to get off treatment is twelve months," adds Dr. Bussel. "So it may be appropriate to wait six to twelve months to see whether people get better before we consider splenectomy."

WinRho is as effective as IVIG for maintaining remissions and is less toxic. However, only 85 percent of patients are Rh (D)-positive. For the remaining 15 percent of women who are Rh (D)-negative, infusions of IVIG may be used as maintenance therapy.

If IVIG or WinRho infusions every three or four weeks maintain a safe platelet count, there's no reason to consider immediate splenectomy in most cases, remarks Dr. Sandler.

Splenectomy is 80 percent effective in bringing up platelet counts within days, and 60 to 70 percent of patients will have a lasting and substantial increase in platelets. Despite its function as a blood filter and fighter of infections, the spleen is actually not an essential organ. Once it's removed, many of its jobs are taken over by other parts of the lymphatic system; the liver filters the blood, and antibodies can be produced elsewhere. And the destruction of platelets will also take place elsewhere in the body, notably in the liver. You may also have small "accessory" spleens, which must be removed with the primary spleen. Splenectomy also carries a very small risk of serious infections.

The surgery can now be done laparoscopically, using small incisions, rather than as major abdominal surgery; you remain in the hospital for one to three days and can resume most normal routines in a week. Splenectomy may be riskier in older people, and is done less frequently after age sixty-five.

Other treatments: Some women's platelet counts fail to go back up after treatment with prednisone, IVIG or WinRho, and splenectomy. "These are the most difficult people to treat, so we use a combination of drugs, which is more effective than single agents, but can be more toxic," says Dr. Bussel. These can include a male hormone, *danazol* (*Danocrine, Cyclamen*); immune-suppressing agents such as *azathioprine* (*Imuran*), *mycophenolate mofetil* (*CellCept*); the chemotherapy drugs *vincristine* (*Oncovin*) or *vinblastine* (*Velban*), and *cyclophosphamide* (*Cytoxan*). Other drugs that can raise platelet counts in severe unresponsive ITP include *colchicine* and *cyclosporine* (which is more toxic).

Danazol is a weak version of testosterone, and causes a temporary menopause as well as androgenic side effects like acne, growth of facial hair, and a rise in LDL cholesterol. It may cause liver problems; so liver function tests must be normal before danazol is used. If you have any neurological problems, vincristine can't be given, since it causes nerve damage. If you've been in remission and platelets start to fall again, corticosteroids and, in some cases, a combination of vincristine, IVIG, solumedrol, danazol, and/or aza-thioprine are given.

Studies suggest that a drug called *rituximab* (*Rituxan*), approved for treating lymphoma, may help half of the patients with unresponsive ITP. "It has been used in a quarter of a million people worldwide, and is relatively non-toxic, which makes it more attractive to use," says Dr. Bussel.

Bone marrow transplants (where after the marrow is destroyed with high-dose chemotherapy, stem cells are infused back into the patient) are being tried in severe, refractory ITP. In one preliminary study of fourteen ITP patients sponsored by the National Heart, Lung, and Blood Institute, four patients achieved complete responses, with platelet counts staying over 100,000 for more than two years, and two other patients obtained partial responses, with higher platelet counts and a reduced need for other medications, Dr. Bussel reports.

ITP Clusters

ITP is seen in as many as 30 percent of women with lupus and in other autoimmune diseases that affect multiple organ systems. In some cases, your doctor will monitor platelet counts as part of your regular bloodwork. However, you should be alert for symptoms of ITP if you have any of the following autoimmune diseases:

- Antiphospholipid syndrome
- Rheumatoid arthritis
- Scleroderma
- Graves' disease, Hashimoto's thyroiditis
- Inflammatory bowel disease (Crohn's disease, ulcerative colitis)
- Primary biliary cirrhosis

I was diagnosed when I was twenty-two. I was in my senior year in college in California, and I was feeling extremely fatigued. At first I chalked it up to staying up half the night to study; I wanted to graduate with highest honors. But after I had the flu that winter, I never really recovered. And I started to notice these little blood blister things in my mouth and had a couple of bad nosebleeds. I went to the university's medical center—we had a major medical school there—and the blood tests came back showing that my platelets were extremely low, around 1,900 . . . a hematologist explained that I had thrombocytopenia, that my platelets were disappearing from my body, and that the flu virus had probably made it worse. I figured they would be giving me a blood transfusion or something (that's how little I knew then), but they put me on steroids, 60 milligrams of prednisone, which they said would bring my platelet count up. It did, but the side effects were awful. My face ballooned, I gained thirty pounds, and I had mood swings. They finally tapered me off it when my counts went up to 230,000. I was thrilled to be off that drug!

I went to our medical library and started reading all I could about this disease, and what I read really scared me to death. I had always had very heavy periods, which seemed to go on forever; I figured that was just me. But I must have had ITP since my teens. The disease changed a lot of my habits; I stopped shaving my legs and used a cream hair remover. I bought an electric toothbrush so I wouldn't brush my teeth too hard (once I ended up with a mouthful of blood after I accidentally bit my tongue). I stopped playing handball (which I used to love), because I was afraid of the bruising. After I got off the prednisone, I worked hard at losing the weight and my face started to look normal. My fiancé and I had planned to be married at Christmastime and I wanted to look nice. I made it through the wedding, and then my platelets dropped again and I was right back on prednisone. I went through three cycles of the stuff and my platelets finally seemed to stabilize, and I thought I was out of the woods.

When I was twenty-seven I became pregnant. Fortunately, my hematologist referred me to an OB who had handled a number of ITP pregnancies. My platelets stayed in the 90s during my first and second trimester, but when they started falling again, I was back on prednisone. My OB assured me that prednisone would not harm my baby, but there was an outside chance that my baby would be born with ITP. When Callie was born they found she had a platelet count of 28,000, so they took her to the neonatal intensive care unit, and she stayed there for a few days. She was put on a liquid form of prednisone for four weeks, and her platelet count went up to 250,000 and has stayed normal ever since, thank God. After that, I decided to have a splenectomy—I was tired of the way this disease seemed to dominate my life. My platelets have been normal ever since the surgery, and we hope to have a second child. The only catch is that my ITP could come back during pregnancy. But it's a chance I guess I'll take.

AUDREY, THIRTY-TWO

How ITP Can Affect You Over Your Lifetime

Having low platelets can affect menstrual periods and can complicate pregnancy; some cases of ITP may even be caused by pregnancy.

Menstruation and Fertility

Low platelet counts that delay clotting can cause extremely heavy menstrual periods that last longer than a week. For some women who have had ITP for years with no other symptoms, heavy periods may simply seem "normal." Iron replacement may be important.

Some women who experience heavy menstrual bleeding take oral contraceptives to regulate their cycles and lessen bleeding, and this is generally safe for women with ITP, says Dr. Bussel. Women taking the antidepressant *fluoxetine* (*Sarafem*) for premenstrual dysphoric disorder may lower their platelet counts, since the drug interferes with the reuptake of serotonin.

Pregnancy and Postpartum

Many cases of ITP are first diagnosed during pregnancy and, in fact, the disease can be triggered by pregnancy. (There is a separate, non-autoimmune problem called *gestational thrombocytopenia* that often occurs during the third trimester, where platelet counts may drop slightly, to around 80,000 or 90,000, but return to normal after delivery.)

It was previously thought that pregnant women with ITP might experience some worsening of their disease. But this may not always be the case, says Daniel W. Skupski, MD, an associate professor of OB/GYN at the Weill Medical College of Cornell University. Dr. Skupski and colleagues studied ninety-six pregnancies in fifty-three women over a sixteen-year period to look at the severity of ITP in pregnancy, recording how often women had bleeding episodes (especially around the time of delivery), and kept track of whether the disease worsened or improved over time. "Major bleeding complications were limited to one case of early placental separation and four cases of postpartum hemorrhage, which is no different from the rate of these types of problems in women without ITP," says Dr. Skupski. "It appeared that, as a general rule, ITP improved in the early part of pregnancy, returned to baseline later in pregnancy, was not different in severity during pregnancy as opposed to when not pregnant, and did not appear to worsen in subsequent pregnancies."

During pregnancy your platelet counts will be monitored, and, if need be, you'll be put on oral corticosteroids if they drop too low. IVIG is used only when clearly indicated. "Our experience with IVIG is that it doesn't produce problems for the pregnancy or for the fetus," says Dr. Skupski. When platelet counts were below 50,000 around the thirty-eighth week of pregnancy, treatment with IVIG produced an increased count such that labor could be induced and epidural anesthesia could safely be used. Premature births do not seem to be associated with ITP.

Neonatal thrombocytopenia can occur in up to 15 percent of infants born to women with ITP, because of maternal antibodies crossing the placenta. Having a previous baby born with thrombocytopenia increases the chance another child will be affected. Your platelet count does not have any bearing on your baby's.

In neonatal thrombocytopenia, a baby may be born with a low platelet count or platelets may begin to drop in the first week after delivery. Oral corticosteroids and intravenous immunoglobulin can help bring platelet counts up. However, the baby's platelet count usually stabilizes and starts to rise within three to four weeks, as maternal antibodies gradually decrease (interestingly maternal antibodies may not fully clear until about six months).

While ITP itself doesn't appear to worsen because of pregnancy, in some women platelet counts may settle at a lower level after giving birth and dip further with each subsequent pregnancy, says Dr. Skupski. This may be because the disease tends to worsen over time, rather than any effect of pregnancy. And it does not necessarily cause bleeding or other symptoms.

Menopause and Beyond

Estrogen replacement therapy (ERT) for menopausal symptoms may lower platelet counts in some women with ITP, says Dr. Bussel. Preliminary studies suggest that taking a higher dose of progestin for ten days every month with estrogen may counter those effects. Progestin also prevents overgrowth of cells in the uterus that can lead to cancer, and women who have not had a hysterectomy are generally advised to take combined hormone replacement therapy.

"However, because it can lower platelet counts, I generally do not advise women to take estrogen for osteoporosis prevention. There are other drugs that are more effective for this purpose," he adds. "If a woman feels that she needs estrogen for menopausal symptoms, I would advise her to do so in conjunction with measuring platelet counts regularly, to make sure it is not having any adverse effects on her ITP."

Nonhormonal menopausal remedies like vitamins or herbs may be helpful for some women. However, *red clover* (sold under the brand name of *Promen-*

sil) can promote bleeding and should not be used by women with bleeding disorders like thrombocytopenia.

If you've ever taken prednisone or other corticosteroids, you have an increased risk of osteoporosis, so you should have regular bone mineral density testing, especially after menopause. You also need to take supplemental calcium and vitamin D, and possibly drugs, to prevent or treat osteoporosis.

As you get older, you're more likely to be taking one or more medications for other health problems, such as high blood pressure or high cholesterol. There are prescription drugs (as well as over-the-counter drugs and supplements) that can lower platelet counts. For example, the cholesterol-lowering drug *atorvastatin* (*Lipitor*) binds to plasma proteins and may infrequently cause severe thrombocytopenia. Tylenol can also reduce platelet counts, as can the heartburn medicine *cimetidine* (*Tagamet*).

Women with cardiovascular disease may need low-dose aspirin (81 milligrams a day), but it needs to be monitored carefully. "I advise women to take aspirin if their platelet counts are 50 to 60,000 and they are stable. They will get the same benefits from aspirin as other people with cardiovascular disease," says Dr. Bussel. "If you don't take prophylactic aspirin because you have ITP, and your platelet counts improve, you can run the risk of strokes and heart attacks. So it is something that must be used cautiously."

Other drugs for heart-related conditions can affect platelet counts, including diuretics like *chlorothiazide* and *chlorthalidone*; *digoxin* (any *digitalis* preparation); calcium channel-blockers like *Cardizem*; and antiarrhythmics such as *procainamide*.

Many commonly used antibiotics like *ampicillin*, *cephalosporin*, and *sulfamethoxazole* can also affect platelet counts. So alert your hematologist to *all* medications you're taking.

Vasculitis

Vasculitis means inflammation of blood vessels, and the different disorders that result (*vasculitides*) can affect every type of blood vessel from the major arteries to the tiny capillaries, from small *venules* to large veins.

Inflammation from vasculitis causes two types of damage. It can weaken a section of the blood vessel wall, causing it to stretch and bulge out like a tiny balloon (an *aneurysm*). In rare cases, the bulging vessel wall can become so weak that it ruptures and bleeds. In other cases, the inflamed blood vessel wall becomes narrowed, restricting blood flow (*ischemia*). A blood vessel may even close off (*occlusion*), blocking blood flow altogether. Sometimes the body compensates for hampered blood supply by rerouting blood to other blood vessels (*collateral blood supply*), but sometimes there simply isn't enough collateral flow and the affected tissue dies (*infarction*).

Vasculitis can affect one organ, such as the kidneys, or it can affect several organ systems at once (*systemic vasculitis*); symptoms can vary depending on the parts of the body affected. Vasculitis is often called the "great mimicker" because the symptoms can mimic those of other diseases.

Women are at particular risk for two types of systemic vasculitis: *Takayasu's arteritis*, which affects the aorta and its branches, and *giant cell arteritis* (*GCA*, also called *temporal arteritis*), an inflammation of the arteries that primarily supply the head. Takayasu's is nine times more common in women and typically occurs before age forty; GCA affects two to three times more women than men, usually later in life.

Other types of systemic vasculitis include *polyarteritis nodosa, Churg-Straus syndrome,* and *Wegener's granulomatosis.* Wegener's affects men and women equally at any age and can be life threatening. It most often affects the upper respiratory tract (the sinuses, nose, trachea) but can also cause problems in the ears, eyes, skin, lungs, heart, kidneys, and the nervous system.

What Causes Vasculitis?

Some forms of vasculitis are thought to be separate from autoimmune diseases, while others are a consequence of systemic inflammatory disease that can inflame and damage blood vessels, such as scleroderma or lupus.

There are autoantibodies that act against components of blood vessel walls, including the cells lining the inside of the vessel (*endothelial cells*) and the thin cell membrane that separates the vessel lining from the smooth muscle (*basement membrane*). When autoantibodies attack the vessel wall, it causes immune complexes to form inside the wall and attract inflammatory cells. (Immune complexes are latticelike structures created when antibodies bind to antigens.) Immune complexes that form in the blood of lupus patients may also attach themselves to the endothelial cells, damaging the blood vessel lining. Some evidence suggests that this may also occur in rheumatoid arthritis and in Sjögren's syndrome. Autoantibodies in diseases like lupus may also cause blood vessel damage.

The *vasculitides* that occur on their own, such as giant cell arteritis or Takayasu's arteritis, are believed to be caused by damage from autoreactive T-cells, which provokes an inflammatory reaction in the blood vessel wall. Overexpression of the inflammatory cytokine *tumor necrosis factor alpha* (*TNFα*), involved in diseases like rheumatoid arthritis and Crohn's disease, is also thought to contribute to vasculitis. Much of the pathophysiology of vasculitic diseases has not been worked out. Different immune cell types are in each, and different layers of the vessel wall are affected.

Vasculitis can also be triggered by a past or present infection (including hepatitis) that leads to formation of immune complexes, by certain cancers, or by an allergic reaction to medication (such as sulfa drugs, *sulfonamides*). In most cases the trigger is not known.

Genes also play a role. Some forms of vasculitis cluster in families and may affect certain racial groups more often. Caucasians (especially those of Scandinavian descent) are more prone to temporal arteritis and *polymyalgia rheumatica* (*PMR*); Asian women are more susceptible to Takayasu's arteritis.

Symptoms of Vasculitis

The symptoms of vasculitis can be nonspecific; inflammation can often provoke body-wide symptoms such as fever, fatigue, aches, and a general feeling of just being ill. There may be appetite loss, weight loss, and lack of energy.

Other symptoms depend on the area of the body or even the type of blood vessel that's affected, says Hal J. Mitnick, MD, a clinical professor of medicine at the New York University School of Medicine with a special expertise in vasculitis. Vasculitis affects the venous system more often than the arterial system, probably because veins are "leakier" than arteries. The damage caused by vasculitis in the smallest veins (*venules*) may allow leakage of both plasma and red blood cells, explains Dr. Mitnick. "The most common syndrome is *leukocytoclastic vasculitis*, it's predominantly an inflammation of the venules.

When red blood cells leak from the venules, it usually produces a rash you can feel that has some bruising associated with it, called *palpable purpura*. When the rash appears as flesh-colored hives that don't go away in less than twenty-four hours, it's due to inflammation that doesn't usually involve red cell leakage. This is called *urticarial vasculitis*."

Vasculitis in the blood vessels of the eyes can cause vision loss, or if the kidneys are affected (as in Wegener's), it can lead to progressive kidney failure and/or high blood pressure. Some forms of vasculitis have specific symptoms:

Giant cell arteritis (*GCA*) causes inflammation that damages large- and medium-sized arteries, often the temporal arteries along the sides of the head at the temples, just in front of the ears (hence the disorder's other name, *temporal arteritis*). It usually occurs after age fifty (the average age of a GCA patient is seventy).

Eighty percent of women with GCA have severe, throbbing headaches, usually in the temples or forehead on one or both sides of the head. The scalp over the affected blood vessels may feel tender and sore (it may even hurt to brush or comb your hair). Many women with GCA have facial or jaw soreness (especially with chewing), says Dr. Mitnick. Depression is also common. If the ophthalmic artery is blocked, it can cause vision loss. If larger arteries leading to the arms or legs are affected, women may have fatigue or aching in the limbs or *intermittent claudication*, muscle aching during exercise. Muscle aches or pain can also be due to coexisting polymyalgia rheumatica.

Polymyalgia rheumatica (*PMR*) occurs in about 30 percent of women with giant cell arteritis. PMR is often characterized by the rapid onset of muscle pains or aching in the large muscle groups, especially those around the shoulders and hips. Symptoms of PMR can be somewhat vague, and it's not uncommon for it to be initially misdiagnosed as an infection, rheumatoid arthritis, or other illness that affects muscles (or even cancer).

Takayasu's arteritis, chronic inflammation of the aorta and its branches, has two phases: A *systemic* phase that causes body-wide symptoms of inflammation as well as joint pains and nonspecific aches and pains. In the *occlusive* phase, women develop symptoms because of the closing off of the affected blood vessels, usually during repetitive activities (*claudication*). Most commonly, sharp pains occur in the arms while cutting meat, or in the calves of the legs while walking. A woman may also experience dizziness when abruptly standing up after sitting or lying down, headaches, and visual problems.

Takayasu's is often called the "pulseless disease" because it can cause a pulse that's barely felt. This occurs because blood vessels are narrowed to such an extent that the normal push of blood being pumped through the aorta from the heart cannot be felt in the wrist, neck, elbow, or lower extremities. When a stethoscope is placed over an affected blood vessel, a whooshing sound called a *bruit* (pronounced *broo-ee*) can be heard as blood pushes through narrowed blood vessels.

Although high blood pressure is common in Takayasu's (from narrowing of arteries in the kidneys), restricted blood flow in the arms or ankles can make it difficult to get an accurate blood pressure reading. Unfortunately, the disease can be present for some time before symptoms appear and some women are not diagnosed until they suffer a stroke or other complication of the occlusive phase.

Wegener's granulomatosis results from inflammation in blood vessels in a variety of tissues and can produce the same body-wide inflammatory symptoms as other forms of vasculitis. Wegener's can cause inflammation of the nose or sinuses, with a persistent runny nose (*rhinorrhea*), nasal crusts and sores, nosebleeds, nasal discharge, and facial pain. When Wegener's affects the middle ear, it can cause middle ear inflammation (*otitis media*), pain, and hearing loss. Respiratory tract symptoms include a cough, bloody phlegm, and chest pain. You may also experience hoarseness, vocal changes, wheezing, or shortness of breath, caused by inflammation of the trachea. Wegener's can also affect the kidneys.

Diagnosing Vasculitis

Because many vasculitis symptoms are nonspecific, diagnosis can be difficult. Often a biopsy of the skin or other affected areas may help in confirming a diagnosis. For example, a skin biopsy can reveal inflamed blood vessels beneath the second layer of skin (*dermis*).

Blood tests that measure inflammation are often done, such as an *erythrocyte sedimentation rate* (*ESR*). As you'll recall, the ESR measures the speed at which red blood cells settle in a vertical glass tube. When there's inflammation present, the cells settle to the bottom faster than in people who don't have inflammatory conditions. Women with vasculitis may also have a slight anemia, which can be detected with a red blood cell count.

The diagnosis of giant cell arteritis is based on the symptoms noted on page 318 and a finding of abnormal blood flow in the arms, legs, or aorta. Your physician will look for tenderness of the scalp or temples and visual abnormalities; your SED rate will be high (greater than fifty). A temporal artery biopsy involves taking a small tissue sample from a part of the temporal artery located in the hairline in front of the ear. When viewed under a microscope, the tissue from the temporal arteries reveals inflammation and unusually large macrophages, or "giant cells." A biopsy can be helpful in most cases, but the disease can "skip" areas of the artery, so a biopsy on both sides of the head may be done, says Dr. Mitnick. The use of color Doppler ultrasound to image the temporal arteries has been proposed as a useful diagnostic test, but is not always accurate.

Polymyalgia rheumatica (PMR) can mimic so many illnesses, and it can only be diagnosed after these other illnesses are excluded. During your physical exam, your doctor will look for pain, aching, and stiffness in the shoulder, pelvic, and hip regions. A high *ESR* is common among patients with PMR. Sometimes a short course of low-dose corticosteroids is given; if symptoms disappear fairly quickly, then it's likely to be PMR.

Takayasu's arteritis used to be diagnosed with **angiography**, but **magnetic resonance angiography** (MRA) has now become the primary diagnostic test. Thickening of the aortic wall can be seen on MRA. In some cases, damage to the aorta, the aortic valve, or other large blood vessel is found and surgery is needed to repair it. In angiography, a special dye (which appears opaque on x-ray) is injected into an artery and x-rays are taken of key blood vessels. In many cases, the aorta will show long areas of narrowing (*stenosis*). But these narrowed areas can also be found in many or all of the large blood vessels.

Wegener's granulomatosis is diagnosed by the results of a physical exam, together with symptoms, lab tests, x-rays, and sometimes a biopsy of affected tissue (skin, nose, lung, or kidney). These factors are also used to judge whether the disease is active or in remission. Other tests include a blood test for **antineutrophil cytoplasmic antibodies** (ANCAs), antibodies to enzymes located in the cytoplasm of white blood cells called neutrophils, a red blood cell count to test for anemia, an ESR, urinalysis to detect protein in the urine (*proteinuria*), and x-rays of the sinuses or chest may also be done.

Vasculitis that occurs in rheumatoid arthritis or lupus is often diagnosed by problems that arise in those diseases. "To a greater or lesser extent, lupus is a vasculitic illness," remarks Dr. Mitnick. "There are frequent skin manifestations, but there may also be vasculitis affecting internal organs, such as the kidneys, lungs, or brain. When a patient with *lupus nephritis* becomes hypertensive, we worry the renal arteries are affected with vasculitis. Likewise, if a lupus patient has a stroke, we wonder about vasculitis in the brain, *cerebral vasculitis*."

Treating Vasculitis

Corticosteroids, most commonly prednisone, are the usual treatment for the most common types of vasculitis. Corticosteroids relieve symptoms of both giant cell arteritis and polymyalgia rheumatica within days and slow or stop the progression of the disease. While low doses of corticosteroids are effective in treating PMR, higher doses (40 to 60 mg of oral prednisone a day) are often required initially to control temporal arteritis and Takayasu's arteritis. Unfortunately, the blindness that can occur in rare cases of temporal arteritis may not be reversible with treatment. (This is why it is so important to diagnose the disease before permanent damage takes place.)

Takayasu's may also be treated with *angioplasty* (in which a balloon-tipped catheter is threaded into blood vessels to widen narrowed arteries, such as in the kidneys). Low doses of *methotrexate, cyclophosphamide* (*Cytoxan*), or *azathioprine* (*Imuran*) may be used as "steroid-sparing" agents, so that lower doses of prednisone can be used. Cyclophosphamide can cause bladder irritation, bleeding, and cancer.

In some cases, damage from severe inflammation can require bypass procedures or aortic valve replacement, but the surgery must be done when the disease is inactive. Active GCA may last only a year or two, but continued low-dose treatment may be needed after remission.

Because Wegener's can be life threatening, it's treated with high doses of prednisone and cyclophosphamide or methotrexate. Extended treatment with corticosteroids may be needed in Wegener's; eventually the dose of prednisone is slowly decreased. Some women may have a remission, but it's difficult to predict how long it will last. Half of all Wegener's patients may have a relapse, so close monitoring is vital.

Drugs that block the inflammatory cytokine *tumor necrosis factor alpha* (*TNFα*) are also being used in clinical trials to treat different forms of vasculitis. These include *etanercept* (*Enbrel*) and *infliximab* (*Remicade*).

How Vasculitis Can Affect You Over Your Lifetime

Vasculitis in women of reproductive age does not affect pregnancy and fertility, but the medications can.

Menstruation and Fertility

As mentioned in previous chapters, prednisone can cause menstrual irregularities but can safely be used during pregnancy and breastfeeding. Because prednisone (and similar drugs) can lead to osteoporosis, women may need bone-building drugs and bone scans to monitor bone mineral density regardless of their age. However, the effects of vasculitis on pregnancy and fertility have not been studied.

Menopause and Beyond

Because vasculitis often arises in later life, when the risk of heart disease also increases, researchers are investigating connections between the two conditions. Blood vessel inflammation is known to be a component of cardiovascular disease, and people with vasculitis also have an increased risk of arteriosclerosis, or narrowing of blood vessels by fatty plaques. Blood clots can form at the site of active inflammation, and vasculitis itself can also cause heart attacks and strokes. For now, women with vasculitis would do well to take steps to reduce any of the accepted risk factors for coronary disease, such as obesity, high blood pressure, high cholesterol, and a sedentary lifestyle.

12

Assault on the Liver—
Autoimmune Hepatitis and
Primary Biliary Cirrhosis

I turned yellow when I was a senior in college. Having jaundice was the first sign that there was something really wrong with me. I had been under a lot of stress, was feeling tired and lethargic, and had no appetite. But I hadn't been sleeping or eating that well, and I had just gotten over the flu. So nothing really rang alarm bells until a friend of mine said to me, "You don't look so well—you look yellow." I looked in the mirror, and sure enough, I was. I went to the college health center and they tested me for everything possible: mono, hepatitis A, hepatitis C, Epstein-Barr virus. My tests did show I'd been exposed to Epstein-Barr virus, but there were no viruses in my blood. The only thing they found was that my liver enzymes were off the charts. But I tested negative for primary biliary cirrhosis and gallstones. So no one knew what was wrong with me. The college sent me to a couple of local doctors; one of them was even a liver doctor. And he said it was probably mono, that 4 percent of people with mono had jaundice. He told me I'd been working too hard, and to take it easy. It took two and a half months and four doctors to find out what I really had.

HANNAH, TWENTY-SEVEN

The liver is the body's main chemical processing plant. Autoimmune diseases can cause it to seriously malfunction, spilling chemicals into areas where they shouldn't be and damaging the processing equipment.

The liver's amazing processing system makes bile to help digest food; stores iron (along with vitamins and minerals); and stockpiles carbohydrates, glucose, and fat until the body needs them for energy. The liver manufactures components of blood, including clotting factors to help wound healing; and detoxifies the various chemicals we ingest, including alcohol and drugs (both legal and illegal). In fact, much of what we eat, drink, breathe, and even absorb through the skin passes through the liver to be detoxified and excreted in bile. The liver also makes cholesterol, a fat needed by all the cells in our body, and proteins that help carry fats in the bloodstream (having too much of certain types of cholesterol and other blood fats contributes to heart disease). It also produces complement, which plays a role in many autoimmune diseases.

Autoimmune hepatitis (AIH) and *primary biliary cirrhosis (PBC)* affect the small bile ducts in the liver. *Sclerosing cholangitis* affects the larger bile ducts, and is primarily seen in men. These diseases are caused by an immune attack on specific cells in the liver and bile ducts, producing inflammation and scarring (*cirrhosis*), and eventually compromising the liver's ability to function. Autoimmune hepatitis occurs four times more often in women than men; PBC strikes women six to ten times more often than men, mostly in middle age and later life.

"I often describe the liver as a tree. The *hepatocytes*, the cells of the liver, are the leaves; the bile ducts and the little ductules are the trunk and the twigs. In autoimmune hepatitis, the immune system attacks the leaves of the tree; in PBC, it attacks the twigs. And in sclerosing cholangitis, it attacks the trunk of the tree and the major branches," explains Henry C. Bodenheimer, Jr., MD, chief of the division of digestive diseases at Beth Israel Medical Center in New York City. "Think of these diseases as an arthritis of the liver or bile ducts. Just as in arthritis, where there's inflammation in the joints and destruction of the joints, there is inflammation and scarring in the liver."

In some women, the scarring becomes so extensive that the liver begins to fail and a transplant is needed. Although some women can experience a remission, autoimmune hepatitis is a disease that may require lifelong treatment.

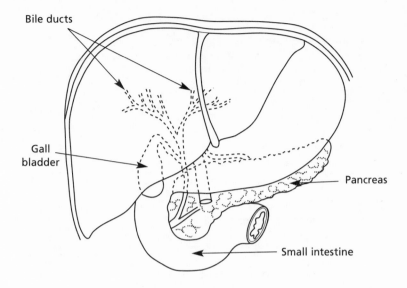

The Liver and Bile Ducts

Autoimmune Hepatitis

When you think of hepatitis, you probably think about the infectious kind—like hepatitis B or hepatitis C—but autoimmune hepatitis is not related to infectious hepatitis. It's a completely separate and distinct condition, caused by an immune system assault on the liver. Why this happens isn't known; a number of genes have been linked to vulnerability to the disease. AIH typically hits women during their twenties, and there's another peak during the sixties. Between 10 and 20 percent of cases of chronic hepatitis are due to AIH.

But it's not a disease that often makes its presence known early. The most pronounced outward sign, yellowing of the whites of the eyes and the skin (*jaundice*), appears only after the liver has sustained severe damage.

What Causes Autoimmune Hepatitis?

While there's no link between autoimmune hepatitis and any of the infectious hepatitis viruses, some women with AIH may have had a past infection with

---

Warning Signs of Autoimmune Hepatitis

- Cessation of menstruation (*amenorrhea*)
- Decreased fertility
- Fatigue, malaise
- Poor appetite
- Upper abdominal discomfort
- Swelling of the abdomen and legs
- Yellowing of the skin and whites of the eyes (*jaundice*)
- Abnormal liver tests
- Dilated capillaries under the skin (*spider angiomas*)

---

hepatitis C and gotten over it without ever knowing they had it. Between 15 and 40 percent of people infected with hepatitis C completely clear it from their system, remarks Dr. Bodenheimer.

As many as 5 percent of people with AIH may have false-positive antibody tests to the hepatitis C virus (10 percent of people with viral hepatitis may also have autoantibodies). "We can test for the presence of hepatitis C virus, and do a sensitive test called a RIBA that looks at the quality of the antibody to see if it's truly reactive against the virus, which tells us whether a woman is truly positive," says Dr. Bodenheimer.

Instead of a viral attack on liver cells, in autoimmune hepatitis the damage is done by T-cells and liver-specific autoantibodies. But the initiator of this attack is not known. Women with autoimmune hepatitis produce antinuclear antibodies (ANAs) and antibodies to smooth muscle cells, and to liver-kidney cell components. A liver biopsy will reveal T-cells and plasma cells, which manufacture the autoantibodies (see pages 328 to 329). As the inflammation and damage progress, tissues in the liver become hardened (*fibrotic*) and scarred. Progressive scarring called *cirrhosis* spreads throughout the liver, eventually choking off vital nutrients, and cells begin to die (*necrosis*). As more and more liver cells die, the liver begins to fail. Although immunosuppressant drugs can slow this process, some women eventually require a liver transplant.

Among the genes associated with autoimmune hepatitis are genes linked to rheumatoid arthritis, in particular a gene called DR4. Patients with one AIH-related gene (DR3) often have a faster progression of the disease and fewer remissions, and require a transplant more often. Women may also have other immune abnormalities or a family history of autoimmune diseases, such as thyroid disease or ulcerative colitis.

Autoimmune hepatitis may be triggered by environmental factors, such as a virus, bacteria, chemicals, or drugs. Some studies have suggested—but not proven—that AIH can develop after infection with hepatitis A, B, or C. Other suspect viruses include *Epstein-Barr virus* (*EBV*), measles virus, and *herpes simplex type 1* (*HSV-1*).

There are also drug-induced forms of hepatitis. Other cofactors may be needed, such as genes, female hormones, alcohol, and nicotine that up-regulate or down-regulate the immune system or liver enzymes that metabolize drugs, which, by being unusually elevated, may provoke an immune reaction. "It may be a case of molecular mimicry, where the immune system is mistaking cells in the liver for something else," speculates Dr. Bodenheimer. This is one of the lingering mysteries of autoimmunity.

Hannah's story continues:

I was getting ready to go home for Christmas when I saw the first liver doctor, who had said I had mono. I even asked him if it was OK to drink alcohol. He told me it was fine to have a beer or two. That amazes me now. By then, the jaundice had gone away, I started feeling better, I got my appetite back. I figured he must be right; it was mono. But while I was visiting my mother that January, the jaundice came back. I lost my appetite, and had this gurgling in my stomach, which I realized later were other symptoms of autoimmune hepatitis. My stools had also been white and my urine bright yellow, but I hadn't paid it much attention the first time. My mother said my eyes were the color of electric daffodils—that's how yellow I was when the jaundice came back. My mother made me promise I'd see a doctor.

When I got back to college, I did go back to the local hepatologist, who realized it wasn't mono. He tested me for antinuclear antibodies and smooth muscle antibodies, and said, "You have this rare disease, autoimmune hepatitis." I had a liver biopsy, and fortunately my liver wasn't damaged—there was no cirrhosis. The most uncomfortable thing about the biopsy is that even

*though the needle goes into your right side, you feel a pain in your left shoul-
der. But I was very lucky. Some people only have symptoms when their liver
is so damaged that their only hope is a liver transplant.*

Diagnosing Autoimmune Hepatitis

AIH can be present for some time before producing any symptoms at all. Typically, the disease has been present for at least six months (or longer) before a
woman is diagnosed.

"Often a woman will come in after having abnormal liver function tests.
She may be taking medications that require liver function tests, or maybe she's
just not feeling well. Fatigue is very common," says Dr. Bodenheimer. Up to
40 percent of people with AIH present with acute hepatitis, but others can
have a subclinical disease with very small elevations of liver enzymes.

Liver function tests (LFTs) are often part of routine bloodwork and include
bilirubin, various liver proteins, *cholestatic* liver enzymes (which indicate
inflammation or blockage of bile ducts), and *aminotransferases*, which are elevated when there's inflammation or injury to liver cells. These enzymes can
be elevated in a number of conditions, including viral hepatitis, alcoholic liver
disease, medication-induced liver disease, a "fatty" liver (excess fat deposits),
and liver tumors. So when liver enzymes are elevated, these other problems
must be ruled out.

AIH is usually diagnosed by doing a liver biopsy to see whether there is
inflammation and scarring. The liver is located on the right side of the body
underneath the diaphragm. Under local anesthesia, a hollow needle is gently
inserted between the right lower ribs to take a small tissue sample the size of
a pencil eraser that's analyzed by a pathologist. If autoimmune hepatitis is
present, the tissue sample will show an infiltration of T-cells and plasma cells,
as well as scarring and tissue death.

"Even though it's a small sample, a liver biopsy indicates what's going on
in the rest of the liver, as well as how severe the disease is," explains Dr.
Bodenheimer.

Women with AIH also have elevated levels of *gamma globulin*, a substance
in the blood containing antibodies and immune cells, and liver enzymes called
aminotransferases, given off when liver cells are damaged.

Almost all AIH patients have autoantibodies, but only about two-thirds have one of the autoimmune markers for the disease: *antinuclear (ANA)* or *anti-smooth muscle (SMA)* antibodies. These are detected in liver cells, using a staining process that makes them fluorescent when seen under a special microscope (a technique called *immunofluorescence*). Another antibody often seen in AIH is to *liver-kidney microsomal antigen (LKM)*, mostly found in young women and children.

There are two subcategories of AIH, depending on which antibodies are found. The most common is type 1, or classic AIH, in which there are elevated antinuclear antibodies and anti-smooth muscle antibodies. In the less common type 2, levels of LKM antibodies are elevated and the disease seems to have a more rapidly progressing course. There also seems to be a third type of AIH, where no autoantibodies are found.

There is a "scoring" system used to determine AIH if there's any uncertainty. For example, being a woman is two points; having elevated aminotransferase is another two points. Included in the list: levels (*titers*) of autoantibodies (ANAs, SMAs) are one to three points each, depending on the amount seen; increased gamma globulin (two times the normal level is three points); and having another autoimmune disease (or a first-degree relative with an autoimmune disease) is one point. A total score of 15 or greater indicates

---

Autoimmune Hepatitis Clusters

Women who have autoimmune hepatitis often develop other autoimmune diseases after several years. These diseases are varied, and may affect any part of the body, from the joints to the skin.

- Thyroid disease
- Ulcerative colitis
- Rheumatoid arthritis
- Type 1 diabetes
- Celiac sprue
- Myasthenia gravis
- Sjögren's syndrome
- Vitiligo

---

autoimmune hepatitis; probable AIH is 10 to 15 points. The scoring system can be used to determine if asymptomatic patients need treatment.

The Female Factor

Seventy to 80 percent of autoimmune hepatitis occurs in women, usually before age thirty and less often after age fifty (it's more common in older age in men), says Melissa Palmer, MD, a noted hepatologist in private practice in Plainview, New York. But research into possible hormonal aspects is scant.

It is known that processing (*metabolism*) of male and female hormones by the liver can be abnormal in people who have cirrhosis. "Both testosterone and estrogen can be altered in some people with cirrhosis. In women, estrogen metabolism may be inhibited in some way, and that could be a contributing factor in why some women with cirrhosis have abnormal menstrual cycles or, in severe cases, stop menstruating," explains Dr. Palmer. "In men, it seems to go the opposite way. Men with cirrhosis often get feminization—*gynecomastia*, enlarged breasts—and a change in hair distribution."

Primary biliary cirrhosis is a disease of middle age and older women, but there's no indication of any link to low estrogen in menopause. "Women may be diagnosed later in life, but they may have had the disease for years. If you biopsy the liver years before the disease was diagnosed, it would usually show some microscopic changes," she remarks.

Hannah's story continues:
I started on the prednisone and Imuran a week after my diagnosis. At first I didn't want to take them; I knew they were really powerful drugs and I was afraid of what they might do to my body. But I also knew that they would help get rid of the inflammation and calm down my immune system. I was put on a big dose of prednisone, 60 milligrams a day, which acted like caffeine for me—it gave me lots of energy. I didn't gain a lot of weight, but I did get the steroid moon face. On the advice of a naturopathic physician I had been seeing since before I was diagnosed, I also started taking calcium and magnesium to prevent osteoporosis from the steroids. Thanks to her, I was doing that from the beginning.

Treating Autoimmune Hepatitis

Some women have mild AIH and may not even need treatment. However, treatment is always begun if a patient

- has symptoms,
- has liver enzymes three times greater than normal, and
- has a liver biopsy that shows active inflammation.

Immunosuppressive drugs are the standard treatment for autoimmune hepatitis, usually *prednisone* or *prednisolone*, or a combination of prednisone and *azathioprine* (*Imuran*), for two years. Adding azathioprine can help keep the needed dose of corticosteroids low. Azathioprine takes several weeks to work, so it should be started as soon as possible after a diagnosis is made.

Prednisone is usually started out at a high dose (40 to 60 milligrams a day), then is tapered to a lower dose (10 mg). A maintenance dose may be lower. About 65 percent of women with AIH will have a complete remission. After that, the drugs are slowly reduced to a low dose. A remission is characterized by a drop in serum aminotransferase concentrations.

"If they have a flare-up of disease, they go back on medication, usually permanently. There are no clear-cut triggers for a relapse, but factors like viruses or stress may be important," says Dr. Palmer. "Infection with one of the hepatitis viruses may cause a flare, or they may have a worse course of hepatitis A or B. So we recommend that all patients be vaccinated against hepatitis A and B."

There are risks to long-term maintenance therapy. In younger women, who may require lifelong treatment, there's an increased risk of cancer with long-term, high-dose azathioprine. Symptoms of steroid withdrawal, such as body and joint aches, can also occur if steroid doses are reduced too abruptly. Steroid drugs also carry the risk of osteoporosis (for more, see pages 49 to 50).

For women who cannot tolerate azathioprine (or who do not have a complete remission), *6-mercaptopurine* (*6-MP*) or *cyclophosphamide* (Cytoxan) may be tried, says Dr. Palmer.

Most women with autoimmune hepatitis need lifelong treatment. However, 10 to 30 percent of women will stay in remission without medications after a minimum of four years of maintenance therapy. A liver biopsy is performed to make sure there is no inflammation before maintenance medications are stopped. Relapses occur most often the first year after medications are stopped, but can also occur many years later, so patients need to be followed closely.

Liver transplants can replace a damaged liver, but do not correct the underlying problem in autoimmune hepatitis. "If you start out with a liver that's badly damaged and you put in a new one, it resets the clock. You do have the potential for the return of the disease. But you are starting over and it may take years. Plus, you are giving the patient immunosuppressants, which may slow the process down," says Dr. Bodenheimer. "It can be a pretty aggressive disease with or without a transplant, however. What we're doing is fixing the results of the disease, but not the immune problem that caused it."

Other medications being tested in AIH include *tacrolimus* (*FK-506*), which is used in transplant patients (as is cyclosporine). Both may have potent anti-inflammatory effects. *Budesonide* (*Entocort EC*), a steroid with fewer side effects than prednisone, and *ursodeoxycholic acid* or *ursodiol* (*Actigall*), used to treat primary biliary cirrhosis, are also being tested.

How Autoimmune Hepatitis Can Affect You Over Your Lifetime

Autoimmune hepatitis can have a variety of effects during the childbearing years.

Menstruation and Fertility

The first sign of AIH in young women is often a stoppage of menstruation, *amenorrhea*. "Because of menstrual cycle irregularities, it's hard for some women to become pregnant," remarks Dr. Palmer. However, treatment with prednisone and azathioprine can normalize menstrual cycles and ovulation, so women can have successful pregnancies and deliveries. Women without cirrhosis have normal fertility.

Oral contraceptives containing estrogen may cause the growth of benign tumors (*hemangiomas, hepatic adenoma,* and *focal nodular hyperplasia*), so women with AIH are usually advised to take all-progestin birth control pills (or a long-acting injection of medroxyprogesterone, Depo-Provera). Women who have fluid in the abdomen (*ascites*) are advised to avoid progesterone because it can cause sodium and fluid retention. Oral contraceptives do not protect against sexually transmitted diseases, including hepatitis B (and in rare cases, hepatitis C). AIH is not infectious.

Pregnancy

Women may have a remission of AIH during pregnancy. "That's because of the immunosuppressive effects of pregnancy, and perhaps higher estrogen levels," says Dr. Palmer. "Some women may have a disease flare during pregnancy, but that's rare."

Although prednisone is considered safe, azathioprine is usually discontinued as soon as a woman becomes pregnant, since it has been associated with birth defects. Women planning to become pregnant are advised to discontinue azathioprine approximately six months before conceiving, says Dr. Palmer. If a woman's steroid dose was reduced because she was also taking azathioprine, she may need an increased dose. Cholestyramine and ursodeoxycholic acid are considered safe during pregnancy. If a woman has had a flare of AIH or liver-related complications (such as bleeding from varices), pregnancy should be postponed for at least a year, she adds.

Hannah's story continues:
The problem with our medical system is that you see specialists. So I have a doctor that focuses on my liver. And I have a gynecologist who focuses on that. And I have an internist I see for everything else. The gynecologist knows that I have autoimmune hepatitis, but he hasn't discussed any of the gynecologic or reproductive issues with me. My hepatologist knows I'm taking birth control pills, but he never asked which one or what dose. You have to find out so much for yourself. For instance, I noticed that in the three years I've been taking the pill, the symptoms of the prednisone have been mini-

mal. I had bad acne when I first started prednisone, and that cleared up. They're good doctors, but neither really looks at the whole person. I found out on my own about the other diseases that people can have with autoimmune hepatitis. The first liver doctor I saw didn't tell me much about the effects of prednisone on bones, maybe because of my age. This year I had a bone density scan that showed that I had lost a lot of bone despite taking calcium. So now I'm taking Fosamax once a week. I was a bit scared of it at first; you can't lie down for a half hour after taking it, or it can harm the esophagus, and you can't eat anything for two hours after taking it. Really, you do need a doctor who will give you all the information.

Menopause and Beyond

Taking oral estrogens for menopausal symptoms is not recommended for women with AIH. "I usually shy away from oral estrogens in women with liver disease, since estrogens may elevate liver enzymes and tend to promote the growth of hemangiomas. Women experiencing severe hot flashes or other symptoms and wish to use estrogen can use the estrogen patch or estrogen cream with an oral progestin. Transdermal estrogen enters the bloodstream directly, bypassing the liver on the first pass, so it has lesser effects on the liver," says Dr. Palmer.

There are several types of estrogen patches, which look like large, clear bandages. They are worn on the lower abdomen, upper thigh, or buttocks, and are changed once a week (*Climara, FemPatch*) or twice a week (*Alora, Vivelle,* or *Estraderm*). Estrogen creams (like *Premarin*) are inserted into the vagina with an applicator to prevent atrophy and drying of tissues. Very little is absorbed into the bloodstream.

There's no physical reason for sexual dysfunction in women with AIH, but, as in any chronic disease, depression and fatigue can affect libido. Note that androgen therapy may be dangerous. "Some androgens, like anabolic steroids, have been shown to lead to liver cancer. They really have not done the studies to see what kinds of effects androgens will have on someone with liver disease," remarks Dr. Palmer.

As with other autoimmune diseases, the chronic use of corticosteroids causes bone loss. "I give alendronate or one of the other bone-building drugs, and I usually follow women with bone density tests," says Dr. Palmer. "I also tell patients they need to do weightbearing exercises to protect their bones, and take calcium and vitamin D."

Women with AIH (and primary biliary cirrhosis) are advised to avoid iron, vitamin A, and niacin, which can be toxic to the liver in high doses, unless they are found to be deficient in these vitamins. "Women may not realize they are getting so much iron, for example, if they take a multivitamin. Also, some herbs may be coated with iron and this information may not be listed on the label. But too much iron can speed any kind of liver disease," cautions Dr. Palmer. "I advise women to buy a multivitamin without iron, and not to take any over-the-counter products that contain vitamin A or iron. The best thing is to take vitamins separately. The only supplements I find helpful are calcium and vitamin D." However, women in advanced stages of PBC may actually have a deficiency in vitamin A, so get vitamin A levels checked, adds Dr. Palmer. "Supplementation is recommended only if a deficiency is found and a woman experiences night blindness, a side effect of vitamin A deficiency."

Cases of autoimmune hepatitis that arise in later life can also pose a problem. Women may already have severe osteoporosis or other medical problems, and steroid drugs may make them worse. So the decision to treat aggressively is a highly individualized one in older age. "For some people, the treatment may be worse than the disease," remarks Dr. Bodenheimer.

Primary Biliary Cirrhosis

Primary biliary cirrhosis is another autoimmune disease that damages the liver, but results from an attack on bile ducts rather than liver cells.

Primary biliary cirrhosis involves an autoimmune attack on the smaller bile ducts and ductules, causing damage and leakage of bile acids into nearby tissues. (Bile, which helps break down fat during digestion, is normally stored in the gallbladder and released through the bile ducts into the small intestine when fat enters the intestine.) Bile acids are toxic and inflame liver cells,

---

Warning Signs of PBC

- Fatigue
- Itching
- Upper abdominal pain
- Dry eyes (Sjögren's syndrome)
- Jaundice
- Gastrointestinal bleeding
- Problems with taste or swallowing
- Clubbing of nails; whitening of nails

---

attracting T-cells and causing small, granular inflammatory lesions (*granulomas*) to form as the liver attempts to contain bile seepage. Copper, normally excreted in bile, also accumulates in liver cells, as does *bilirubin*, the orange-yellow pigment that gives bile its color (bilirubin is normally excreted in stool). Cells in the small bile ducts overgrow, eventually replacing the ducts with hardened scar tissue.

Immune complexes form in the blood vessels of the liver and cause increased blood pressure (*portal hypertension*) in the network of veins that carry blood to the liver from the stomach and other organs of the digestive system. The increased pressure causes bulging of the veins (*varices*) and bleeding in the stomach and esophagus.

As tissue injury progresses in the liver, inflammation and scarring spread and liver function becomes impaired. PBC is slow, chronic, and progressive, eventually causing liver failure, and is a common reason for a liver transplant.

What Causes Primary Biliary Cirrhosis?

The cause of primary biliary cirrhosis is not known. Some research suggests that the immune system may mistake liver cells for bacteria commonly present in the gut, such as *Escherichia coli* (*E. coli*), Epstein-Barr virus, and *cytomegalovirus*. These are among the infectious agents associated with bile duct injury. Some drugs have also been associated with PBC, but there's little evidence of any cause and effect.

The autoantibodies seen in PBC are not specific to the bile ducts, but attack the tiny energy-producing components of cells called *mitochondria*.

PBC strikes women six to ten times more often than men, and mostly affects those aged thirty-five to sixty-five, but can also occur in young women and in the elderly, says Dr. Bodenheimer. There's a genetic component, with a higher prevalence among first-degree relatives with the disease, and among women with family members who have other autoimmune diseases.

About 70 percent of women with PBC have another autoimmune disease. Between 50 and 75 percent of women with PBC may have Sjögren's syndrome. Scleroderma is also common. About 6 percent of women with PBC also have rheumatoid arthritis, and another 6 percent have thyroid disease. Other autoimmune diseases seen in women with PBC include pernicious anemia, autoimmune thrombocytopenia, celiac disease, and polymyositis. Women with PBC may also be at higher risk for liver and other cancers, including lymphoma and cancers of the breasts, ovaries, and thyroid.

Symptoms of PBC

As with autoimmune hepatitis, fatigue may be one of the earliest symptoms of primary biliary cirrhosis, occurring in as many as 78 percent of patients. You may find that you're unable to exert yourself physically, especially with exercise.

Another common symptom is itching (seen in over 60 percent of women), which may worsen at bedtime. The dry mouth of Sjögren's syndrome can alter taste and hamper swallowing and even vocal cord function. Dry eyes are also common, and there may be enlargement of the parotid glands in women who also have Sjögren's.

Women may also complain of upper abdominal pain on the right side. There may be weight loss and diarrhea with pale, bulky stools. Some women may have brownish hyperpigmentation of the skin. Signs of later disease and liver failure include fluid in the abdomen, gastric bleeding, and jaundice (caused by accumulation of bilirubin in the skin and other tissues).

PBC is also associated with bone loss (see page 341); in some cases, poor absorption of vitamin D (a fat-soluble vitamin) may contribute. "But we really don't know that this occurs," remarks Dr. Bodenheimer. The degree of osteoporosis can be severe, with spinal fractures and compression, resulting in back pain and muscle spasms. Older women may experience spontaneous fractures of the ribs and bone pain.

Up to 60 percent of people with PBC have no symptoms at all (some may even have normal liver enzymes). As with AIH, routine blood tests may reveal abnormalities in liver function that alert a woman's doctor to a problem. In PBC, the red flag is an elevation in the enzyme *alkaline phosphatase* to more than twice the normal level. Cholesterol may also be mildly elevated, due to backflow of bile fats into the blood and increased cholesterol production by liver cells. However, some women may have normal liver enzymes and even in advanced disease may show no outward signs.

However, two physical signs are the hallmarks of PBC: One is yellow, fatty nodules in the skin, caused by abnormal cholesterol metabolism. When these nodules appear around the eyes, they are called *xanthalasmas*, and when they arise in folds or creases of the skin (such as on the hands, elbows, or knees) they are termed *xanthomas*. People with PBC may also display severe scratch marks and breaks in the skin, caused by scratching to relieve intense itching (*excoriations*); these scratch marks can often bleed.

Diagnosing PBC

It's often difficult to tell PBC from autoimmune hepatitis, because both cause the death of liver cells (*necrosis*). However, a liver biopsy will reveal damage to bile ducts, granulomas, fibrosis, and an infiltration of inflammatory cells. A liver biopsy can also reveal the extent of damage to the bile ducts and the liver.

Ninety to 95 percent of PBC patients will have *antimitochondrial antibodies (AMAs)* detected in blood or liver cells using *immunofluorescence*. The amount of AMAs does not indicate how severe the disease is or predict how rapidly it will progress. Unlike antinuclear antibodies, which often decline after treatment for other autoimmune diseases, AMAs do not respond to treatment.

Women with primary biliary cirrhosis also have elevated levels of alkaline phosphatase, an enzyme found in bile that increases when there's an obstruction in the flow of bile (*cholestasis*). Cholesterol may also be elevated (and can top 1,000 milligrams per deciliter of blood [mg/dl] in late-stage disease).

PBC Clusters

Autoimmune thyroid disease occurs in 20 percent of women with primary biliary cirrhosis. Many of the same diseases that cluster with autoimmune hepatitis also occur with PBC. They include the following:

- Thyroid disease
- Sjögren's syndrome
- Rheumatoid arthritis
- Scleroderma
- Raynaud's phenomenon
- Lupus
- Celiac disease
- Pernicious anemia
- Vitiligo

More than 80 percent of women with PBC have other autoimmune disorders (see list), which must be treated separately. Because of the overlap with autoimmune hepatitis, some patients are given a trial of prednisone to help separate the two; PBC does not respond to corticosteroids, but AIH does.

Treating PBC

Ursodeoxycholic acid, or ursodiol (Actigall) is the most common treatment for PBC. It improves symptoms of PBC, prolongs survival, and postpones the need for a liver transplant. Ursodiol lowers levels of alkaline phosphatase, bilirubin, and other liver enzymes, and is also prescribed to dissolve certain kinds of gallstones. Side effects include abdominal pain, arthritis, back pain, bronchitis, flulike symptoms, headache, and fatigue. Ursodiol can interact with cholesterol-lowering medications, aluminum-based antacids (such as *Rolaids*), and estrogens (see page 340).

Clinical trials have been conducted of high-dose ursodiol, and ursodiol in combination with corticosteroids. Ongoing trials of the drug with the topical steroid budesonide (which is highly absorbed into the liver) show benefits with fewer side effects than for other steroids.

"The therapies we have do not cure the disease, and many patients will need a liver transplant," says Dr. Bodenheimer. "When there's narrowing of the bile ducts, they can be stretched with a balloon, in a catheter procedure similar to angioplasty."

A **liver transplant** improves the course of PBC. It doesn't cure the underlying problem, and PBC can recur after a transplant. One-year survival is 85 to 90 percent; after that, women with PBC can have the same lifespan as healthy individuals.

Symptom relief. The itching associated with PBC is treated with *cholestyramine resin* (*Questran, Questran Light*) taken three times a day. Questran is a bile-acid binder that comes in powder form and must be mixed with water or other liquids. The main side effect is constipation. It can also interact with estrogens and progestins, as well as thyroid medications such as *Synthroid*. Questran can also interfere with the normal digestion and absorption of fats and fat-soluble vitamins. The effects of Questran during pregnancy have not been well studied, so women need to take it under a doctor's supervision.

How PBC Can Affect You Over Your Lifetime

Ursodiol can interfere with the estrogens in oral contraceptives, so women may need to use a second form of birth control or another method of contraception.

While no evidence exists to indicate that ursodiol can harm an unborn baby, it is not recommended during pregnancy. It's not known whether the drug passes into breast milk, so caution is advised for those women who are breastfeeding.

Menopause and Beyond

Ursodiol can also interfere with the effectiveness of oral estrogen in hormone replacement therapy (HRT), such as *conjugated equine estrogens* (*Premarin*). Again, women are advised to use estrogen patches or cream (see page 334).

Osteoporosis is a serious concern for postmenopausal women in general, but women with PBC may have a greatly accelerated course. Older women with PBC can have vertebral fractures, spinal compression, loss of height, and sudden rib fractures. So women with PBC may need to be put on drugs such as alendronate to slow bone loss.

The Risk of Cancer

Liver cancer can develop in anyone with cirrhosis, but the incidence is low in both PBC and autoimmune hepatitis. "The risk of liver cancer in women with autoimmune liver disease is increased compared to the general population, but not as much as in people with the viral hepatitis," remarks Dr. Palmer. "We really don't know why. In hepatitis C there's a 25 percent chance of developing liver cancer, but in autoimmune hepatitis and PBC it's much, much lower, perhaps around 2 to 6 percent in PBC. Preventing the development of cirrhosis will also prevent liver cancer."

13

Mysterious Fellow Travelers— Fibromyalgia, Chronic Fatigue, Endometriosis, and Interstitial Cystitis

I was diagnosed with juvenile rheumatoid arthritis when I was in eighth grade. But I've been fortunate in that I only seem to get bad flares every few years. I was always able to stay active in some way; I've even run marathons. When I have a flare, the pain and fatigue are very bad . . . it's hard to do my job . . . I can't write or type, I can't open a car door, or even turn the key in the ignition . . . but I would take different drugs and it would get better. Even with those problems, I had started to think of my RA as kind of predictable. But then I started to develop pain in other areas of my body. Not in the joints, but in the muscles around them . . . and at very specific points like my shoulders, elbow, or knees. And I got this overwhelming aching fatigue, like I had the flu . . . I couldn't seem to think straight . . . I just wanted to sleep all the time, but I never really felt rested. This was unlike any of the RA flares I'd ever had, and none of the drugs I normally took seemed to help it. My rheumatologist kept saying it was my RA getting worse, but the blood tests did not show any signs of a flare and my joints were not affected. My doctor finally diagnosed me with fibromyalgia.

CATE, THIRTY

Fibromyalgia

Fibromyalgia is not an autoimmune disease. But it occurs so often with autoimmune diseases, and has such a major impact on so many women's lives, that we felt it was important to include it in this book. Symptoms of fibromyalgia can overlap with autoimmune connective tissue diseases, and it's often difficult to tell whether it's a disease flare or something else. So you need to know enough about fibromyalgia to be able to recognize the signs and alert your physician.

Fibromyalgia isn't a new problem. In the late nineteenth century it was called *neurasthenia*, a vague ailment attributed to "weakness or exhaustion of the nervous system" that sent women to their beds with aches and pains, unexplained fatigue, and depression (and a bottle of *Lydia Pinkham's Vegetable Compound*, a cure-all of 20 percent alcohol). But it wasn't until 1975 when two Canadian researchers studying rheumatoid arthritis patients described the distinct symptoms—including sleep disorders, diffuse musculoskeletal

---

Warning Signs of Fibromyalgia

- Pain or sensitivity when applying pressure to "tender points" around the body
- Widespread body pain lasting more than three months
- Muscle pain and malaise after physical activity
- Low energy and fatigue
- Irritable bowel (cramps, bloating, alternating diarrhea and constipation)
- Chronic sleep problems
- Chronic headaches
- Inability to concentrate, memory impairment
- Depression, anxiety
- Temporomandibular joint (jaw) pain (TMJ)
- Vulvar pain
- Dizziness or lightheadedness
- Allergies or multiple chemical sensitivities
- Irritable bladder symptoms

---

pain, and tenderness at specific points around the body—that characterize fibromyalgia.

It was first called *fibrositis*, meaning "muscle inflammation," but studies later showed there was no inflammation in the muscles of patients with the disorder. Today, the constellation of symptoms known as *fibromyalgia syndrome (FMS)* is recognized as a distinct medical disorder involving pain amplification or hypersensitivity. The American College of Rheumatology (ACR) established diagnostic criteria for FMS in 1990.

Fibromyalgia typically strikes women between the ages of twenty and forty, possibly caused by abnormalities in the processing of pain signals by the central nervous system. Studies suggest it may be triggered by injuries, infections, or autoimmune diseases.

Between 2 and 4 percent of women in the general population may be affected by this disorder, and up to 25 percent of women with autoimmune diseases, including rheumatoid arthritis, lupus, and Crohn's disease meet the ACR criteria for fibromyalgia (see page 350). Fibromyalgia symptoms also overlap with other autoimmune "fellow travelers" such as chronic fatigue syndrome (CFS), irritable bowel syndrome (IBS), and interstitial cystitis (IC).

What Causes Fibromyalgia?

The causes of fibromyalgia are unknown, but experts believe that some stressor or trauma—be it a physical injury, immune overstimulation (as in autoimmune disease), hormonal alterations (such as being hypothyroid), infections, extreme emotional stress, or a combination of factors—triggers disturbances in the central nervous system of susceptible women, leading to oversensitivity to even low levels of pain. It's been likened to having the "volume turned up" to pain and other stimuli.

Fibromyalgia can run in families, with women primarily affected by pain amplification. "We don't have a single candidate gene, and it's probably a combination of genetic factors, but the evidence is that there's a predisposition to this disorder," remarks Laurence A. Bradley, PhD, professor of medicine in the division of clinical immunology and rheumatology at the University of Alabama at Birmingham. "There may be multiple disruptions in the function of structures in the central nervous system involved in pain transmission and modulation, along with dysregulation of neurotransmitters involved in pain processing and stress hormones."

Brain activity in processing pain seems to be different in people with FMS. "We identified resting state abnormalities in cerebral blood flow in two brain structures involved in processing pain in patients with fibromyalgia, compared to healthy people. And in nonpatients who report pain, we also saw low levels of blood flow in one of those structures," says Dr. Bradley. Many people with fibromyalgia appear to have abnormalities in the *autonomic nervous system* (which governs breathing, heart rate, and blood pressure, among other things), causing symptoms like *orthostatic hypotension* (dizziness when going from a sitting to standing position).

Brain chemicals that may be affected in FMS include *serotonin* (which helps regulate mood, sleep, and appetite) and *norepinephrine* (a stress hormone). Studies have also found levels of *substance P*, a chemical that helps transmit pain signals, to be up to three times higher in the spinal fluid of fibromyalgia patients than levels in healthy individuals.

One recent study at the Cedars-Sinai Medical Center in Los Angeles also found increased levels of inflammatory cytokines stimulated by substance P in blood samples from 56 people with fibromyalgia, compared to healthy people. One cytokine, *interleukin-8* (*IL-8*) promotes pain, and another, *interleukin-6* (*IL-6*), induces hypersensitivity to painful stimuli, fatigue, and depression. (IL-6 is also elevated in people with lupus and rheumatoid arthritis.) The researchers theorize that these cytokines may play a role in modulating symptoms of fibromyalgia.

"The evidence is not very consistent, but there is some question as to whether there may be abnormalities in some of the cytokines that promote inflammation in people with fibromyalgia. However, there is no reliable evidence so far that there is an immune system problem in fibromyalgia, and certainly not an autoimmune problem," says Dr. Bradley, who is among those studying the disorder. "Nevertheless, there are individuals with autoimmune diseases such as rheumatoid arthritis who develop fibromyalgia as a secondary condition."

Psychological factors also come into play. The lifetime incidence of mood disorders like depression and anxiety in people with fibromyalgia ranges from 40 to 70 percent, but that may be an overestimate. "When we compare peo-

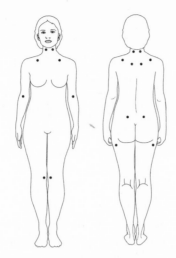

Tender Point Locations in Fibromyalgia
Source: American College of Rheumatology

ple being treated for fibromyalgia with nonpatients, nonpatients tend to have lower scores on questionnaires that measure depression or other kinds of psychological distress, and they often feel they're more able to use their internal resources to cope with their pain than the people who are treated in the clinic," comments Dr. Bradley.

Symptoms of Fibromyalgia

Chronic, diffuse pain and tenderness around the body is the major symptom of fibromyalgia. But the hallmark of FMS is pain when pressure is applied to specific "tender points" located around the neck, shoulder, chest, hip, and lower back.

While many women with fibromyalgia also have painful connective tissue diseases like lupus or rheumatoid arthritis, in many cases no physical joint, bone, or tissue damage or inflammation can be found. Fibromyalgia pain often waxes and wanes, shifts from one area of the body to another, and is often accompanied by numbness or tingling. Some women complain that they "ache all over," while others report pain only in certain regions of the body, like the lower back and hip. In fact, many women may initially be diagnosed with lower back problems or an overuse injury like tennis elbow (*lateral epicondylitis*) or heel pain (*plantar fascitis*).

Other problems common in fibromyalgia include migraine and tension headaches, dry eyes, jaw pain (*temporomandibular joint syndrome, TMJ*), mitral valve prolapse, noncardiac chest pain, heartburn, painful periods, urinary frequency and urgency (irritable bladder), and chronic pelvic pain. Women with FMS may also have other, more regional pain-related syndromes, such as irritable bowel syndrome, interstitial cystitis, endometriosis, and vulvar pain syndromes (*vulvodynia, vulvar vestibulitis*).

"Many of these symptoms and syndromes cluster together. For example, it's much more likely for someone with chronic pain to have irritable bowel syndrome or TMJ syndrome than someone who doesn't have chronic pain," observes Daniel J. Clauw, MD, professor of medicine in the division of rheumatology and director of the Center for the Advancement of Clinical Research at the University of Michigan, Ann Arbor. A majority of women with fibromyalgia report severe fatigue; at least half of those who meet the criteria for FMS will also meet diagnostic criteria for chronic fatigue syndrome, says Dr. Clauw. "While the defining symptom of CFS is fatigue, you also have to have four of eight minor criteria, including joint pain, muscle aches, headaches, and sore throat, which are all pain-based symptoms."

In FMS, fatigue and pain are worse after physical activity, and women may also experience major problems with concentration and memory. Other symptoms can include weight gain (or loss); intolerance to heat, cold, and loud noises; and problems with vision or hearing. Women may also complain of "allergic" symptoms, ranging from drug reactions and multiple chemical sensitivities to respiratory symptoms like runny nose and nasal congestion.

Symptoms of fibromyalgia may come on after viral infections, such as Epstein-Barr virus (infectious mononucleosis), Lyme disease, parvovirus, or Q fever, all of which have a pain component. "Two to 3 percent of people who develop these infections will never completely recover and end up with fibromyalgia or chronic fatigue syndrome," says Dr. Clauw. "There's also a subset of people who develop hypothyroidism and have chronic widespread pain as a result. And even after their thyroid hormone is replaced and they are made euthyroid, they never regain their baseline state of health and have something indistinguishable from fibromyalgia."

Certain medications, like the cholesterol-lowering drugs called *statins*, can provoke chronic widespread pain, which persists even after the drug is stopped. Symptoms mimicking fibromyalgia can also occur when women are being tapered off high-dose corticosteroids. However, regular pain medicines (like aspirin, ibuprofen, or acetaminophen) don't help the pain of fibromyalgia, and that's often what brings a woman to her doctor's office.

The symptoms of fibromyalgia and autoimmune disorders overlap, including joint and muscle pain, fatigue, and morning stiffness, as well as a feeling that the hands or feet are swollen. Some women may have symptoms similar to Raynaud's phenomenon, but their entire hand turns pale or red, instead of just the fingers. Facial flushing and a mottled red rash on the legs (*livedo reticularis*) are also common in fibromyalgia, and women may initially be misdiagnosed with lupus. FMS often coexists with autoimmune diseases.

How can you tell the difference between symptoms of fibromyalgia and symptoms of your RA or lupus? For one thing, fibromyalgia always has the characteristic tender points "and no one ever sees swollen joints due to fibromyalgia," emphasizes Michelle Petri, MD, MPH, professor of medicine and director of the Lupus Clinic at Johns Hopkins.

"In fibromyalgia there isn't truly joint pain as much as there is muscle pain, but since muscles overlie some joints, patients will often have difficulty differentiating them," says Dr. Petri. "We can show women where the tender points are and how to apply pressure, and we can teach them to differentiate between muscle pain and true joint pain and swelling, so they can tell the difference between fibromyalgia and chronic pain from a lupus flare."

Diagnosing FMS

If you or your doctor suspects you have fibromyalgia, you'll undergo a thorough physical examination to exclude neurological, orthopedic, and rheumatological causes for your pain. Your physician will then apply pressure to the nine pairs of tender points to see whether the palpation provokes pain. The amount of pressure needed is usually around nine pounds, or enough force to blanch the fingernail of the finger applying the pressure. In some cases, the pain from one tender point will radiate to another spot.

To meet the criteria for fibromyalgia set by the ACR, you need a history of chronic widespread pain involving all four quadrants of the body, as well as areas overlying the bones of the skull, backbone, ribs, and chest (the *axial skeleton*), and pain on pressure at eleven of eighteen tender points.

But if you have fibromyalgia you won't just have pain at tender points— you'll be more sensitive to pain all over your body. To some degree everyone has tenderness at the tender points (like the shoulder blades or elbows). When there's more overall tenderness, there tends to be more positive tender points. Women also have more tender points than men, and older age, lack of fitness, and depression or anxiety will also increase sensitivity at those points.

"A person with diffuse pain that has been present for a number of years is more likely to have fibromyalgia, especially if the pain is accompanied by fatigue, memory difficulties, sleep disturbances, and irritable bowel symptoms," notes Dr. Clauw.

More acute, short-term pain may be due to an injury or disease flare, and may need a more extensive workup. Physical signs of inflammation like swollen joints (*synovitis*) or muscle weakness are not signs of fibromyalgia. But inflammatory and noninflammatory mechanisms can both cause fibromyalgia symptoms, so having a response to anti-inflammatory medications doesn't automatically rule out FMS. "Since one in three lupus patients also has fibromyalgia, often doctors try to explain symptoms by saying it's due to the lupus, and try to treat it with prednisone. In fact, some of the problems will be fibromyalgia related, and a woman may be given prednisone that she didn't need," adds Dr. Petri. Lupus patients don't usually have the overall pain sensitivity seen in fibromyalgia.

Tests You May Need and What They Mean

Laboratory testing in a fibromyalgia workup will include a complete blood count; blood tests for liver, kidney, and thyroid function, and a sedimentation rate or level of C-reactive protein to detect inflammation. Unless your pain has come on suddenly or there's evidence that you may have an autoimmune disease, testing for markers such as rheumatoid factor or antinuclear antibodies (ANAs) is usually not done.

If you have dizziness when going from a prone to standing position, your **blood pressure** will be measured as you do this to see if you have a sudden drop in pressure (orthostatic hypotension), a common symptom in fibromyalgia. If you're having pain and stiffness in weightbearing joints, **x-rays** or other imaging may be done to look for evidence of arthritis, either rheumatoid arthritis or osteoarthritis (the wear-and-tear kind that breaks down cartilage).

Cate's story continues:
My husband was fine through my RA flares, but he doesn't understand this. It really has put a strain on our relationship. He keeps saying, "Why do you need to sleep so much? Why can't you do things? Why are you upset so easily? Can't you take something for the pain?" It's very frustrating. I know if my RA got bad, there are drugs I could take to help it. But nothing really seems to make fibromyalgia better . . . I've had antidepressants . . . I've taken bigger doses of pain medications. The only thing that really seems to help is exercise. So I just force myself to go out and walk or run. It's hard, and I can't exercise as much as I used to, and that gets me down sometimes, much more so than having RA. But I refuse to give in to this. Since I've had RA for so long, I understand what's going on in my body. But fibromyalgia? This, I just don't understand.

Treating Fibromyalgia

Treatment for fibromyalgia usually involves a combination of medication and exercise, along with behavior modification techniques, like stress reduction, and other coping strategies.

"Regular analgesics don't work very well in pain amplification syndromes. Things like acetaminophen and nonsteroidal anti-inflammatory drugs have virtually no effect in pain amplification syndromes. Opioids also do not seem to work well," comments Dr. Clauw. "The best drugs for these syndromes are those that act on the central nervous system, like tricyclic antidepressants. Some randomized controlled trials indicate that medications that act on the neurotransmitters serotonin and norepinephrine are among the most effective." Aerobic exercise acts as a natural painkiller and an antidepressant, he adds.

Antidepressant medications can help reduce pain signals from nerves and aid sleep. "While the major treatment of fibromyalgia is really physical exercise, for those patients who have sleep disturbances we often use a low dose of a tricyclic antidepressant, or the antiseizure medication *gabapentin* (*Neurontin*), which helps both chronic pain and sleep problems," says Dr. Petri. "We also use *selective serotonin reuptake inhibitors* (*SSRIs*) for patients who have clinical depression."

The tricyclic antidepressant used most often is *amitriptyline* (*Elavil*). Low doses of tricyclics have also been shown to help women who suffer migraine and tension headaches, noncardiac chest pain, irritable bowel syndrome, insomnia, and a variety of chronic pain syndromes. Women with insomnia who can't tolerate tricyclics are often helped by *trazodone* (*Desyrel*) or *zolpidem* (*Ambien*) taken at bedtime.

The SSRIs and mixed antidepressants (which affect both serotonin and norepinephrine, neurotransmitters that modulate sleep and immune system function) most frequently prescribed for fibromyalgia patients include *fluoxetine* (*Prozac*), *nefazodone* (*Serzone*), and *paroxetine* (*Paxil*). Antianxiety medications like *alprazolam* (*Xanax*), *diazepam* (*Valium*), and *clonazepam* (*Klonopin*) are occasionally used. The muscle relaxant *cyclobenzaprine* (*Flexeril*) can also be helpful.

Atypical antidepressants, such as *bupropion* (*Wellbutrin*) and nefazodone (Serzone), which affect the neurotransmitters norepinephrine and dopamine, have been shown to help FMS patients whose major complaints are fatigue or cognitive problems.

Women who have orthostatic hypotension or palpitations may benefit from increasing fluid intake, along with sodium and potassium; low doses of betablockers are also helpful in women with these signs of autonomic nerve dysfunction.

Nondrug Therapies

Exercise, both aerobic exercise and stretching exercises, may be the best prescription for FMS pain. Exercise not only helps to combat deconditioning

Chronic Fatigue Syndrome

Many autoimmune diseases can cause fatigue that is chronic. However, *chronic fatigue syndrome (CFS)* is a separate disorder. It is not believed to be autoimmune, but it may occur with autoimmune diseases. CFS is believed to involve interactions between the immune and central nervous systems, but the cause is unknown.

CFS can come on suddenly, often after a viral infection, with extreme fatigue and a cognitive "fog" that can last for months or even years. Infections that have been linked to CFS include colds, bronchitis, hepatitis, and infectious mononucleosis (Epstein-Barr virus).

Symptoms of CFS may linger or come and go frequently for more than six months. They include fatigue and weakness, muscle and joint aches, headaches, inability to concentrate, allergic symptoms, and tender lymph nodes. For most people, CFS symptoms plateau early in the course of illness and wax and wane thereafter, with some people completely recovering.

CFS is diagnosed two to four times more often in women than in men. The federal Centers for Disease Control and Prevention estimate that as many as 500,000 people in the United States have a CFS-like condition. The criteria for a diagnosis of CFS include:

- Unexplained fatigue of at least six months' duration that is not alleviated by rest and is associated with a marked reduction in activity levels
- Having four of seven possible symptoms: memory impairment; tender lymph nodes; muscle pain; pain in multiple joints; new-onset headaches; unrefreshing sleep; malaise lasting more than twenty-four hours after exertion

There's no specific treatment for CFS. But nonsteroidal anti-inflammatory drugs (NSAIDs), such as ibuprofen, may help ease body aches or fever, and nonsedating antihistamines may help relieve allergic symptoms, such as runny nose. Learning how to manage fatigue and plan activities can help improve day-to-day functioning.

The same kinds of treatments that help women with fibromyalgia also work with CFS. Cognitive behavioral therapy and graduated exercise programs can greatly help many women, and low-dose tricyclic antidepressants help with sleep and pain. While other antidepressants, including the selective serotonin reuptake inhibitors, can also improve symptoms of CFS, they can cause fatigue in therapeutic doses, so your doctor may have to increase the dosage slowly. Some women with CFS benefit from benzodiazepines, used to treat anxiety and sleep problems. You may need to try more than one drug before finding one that works for you.

---

from inactivity that can lead to disability, but can also help relieve pain by triggering production of the body's own painkilling chemicals, *endorphins*. In fact, a recent three-year study at Helsinki University Central Hospital in Finland found exercise to be more effective in alleviating pain symptoms of fibromyalgia than medications. Numerous studies have also found that exercise relieves depression as well as, or even better than, medications. A physical therapist who works with fibromyalgia patients can help design an exercise program for you, provide therapies for easing pain and stiffness, and offer pointers for minimizing stress during daily activities.

Physical therapy and other techniques to ease pain include cortisone injections at tender points, injections of local anesthetic (such as *procaine*) at tender points that produce pain that radiates to other areas (called *trigger points*), massage, moist heat, *myofascial release therapy* (in which pressure is applied to trigger points to "release" tightened muscles), chiropractic (a technique of spinal manipulation), and acupuncture (the application of hair-thin needles to specific points along the body called meridians, triggering the release of endorphins and stimulating nerve endings). There have been only a few studies of these therapies in fibromyalgia, but some of the data support their use.

Dietary changes might even be helpful. A small preliminary study at the Center for Integrative Medicine at Thomas Jefferson University Hospital in Philadelphia suggests that symptoms can be reduced by eliminating potential food allergens, including wheat, dairy, and citrus. "However, given the fact that fibromyalgia is a neural pain amplification syndrome, it's unlikely that nutritional factors play a really prominent role," remarks Dr. Clauw.

Cognitive behavioral therapy (CBT) teaches coping skills and behavioral changes to help you manage an often-frustrating illness. "Every randomized, controlled trial of cognitive behavioral therapy in any chronic illness has shown it to be effective," says Dr. Clauw. For women with fibromyalgia, a pain-based CBT program can be especially effective. In CBT, you'll learn relaxation techniques (such as deep breathing and positive visual imagery), how to reframe negative thoughts and behaviors that intensify pain responses, how to effectively solve problems, and how to pace activities to accommodate whatever limitations you may have. The ultimate goal is to provide you with tools to take control over your fibromyalgia . . . and your life.

> *I have probably had endometriosis since I was sixteen, when I started having severe pain with my periods. It has taken a tremendous toll on me. I developed severe osteoporosis from the hormonal treatments, and over the years I have had a half-dozen surgeries for the endometriosis, as well as a hysterectomy. After that I took hormones for a few years because I had severe hot flashes. But it caused my endometriosis to kick in again, so I had to stop them. I was diagnosed with Hashimoto's thyroiditis in 1991, and I have also developed horrific joint pain. I also have terrible allergies. Although we really can't say yet whether endometriosis is autoimmune, this is obviously a disease caused by immune problems. Many of the women in our database have irritable bowel syndrome, and half have at least one family member with type 1 diabetes.*
>
> Mary Lou Ballweg, thirty-eight, founder and president,
> Endometriosis Association

Endometriosis

Endometriosis is a painful, chronic condition that affects up to five and a half million women in the U.S. and Canada. The problem arises when *endometrial* tissue, which normally lines the uterus, is found outside the uterus, where it grows in response to estrogen. These implants cause pain and inflammation, irritating the pelvic cavity, the reproductive organs, and/or the bowel. As the inflammation heals, scar tissue can form weblike growths called *adhesions*, which can also cause pain.

There's evidence to suggest there may be an autoimmune *component* in endometriosis. Endometrial implants are tolerated as self-antigens, but act

---

Warning Signs of Endometriosis

- Unusually painful menstrual periods
- Chronic pelvic pain
- Painful sex
- Infertility
- Fatigue
- Diarrhea, painful bowel movements, and other gastrointestinal symptoms at the time of the menstrual period.

---

as irritants to promote inflammation, and levels of inflammatory cytokines found in many autoimmune diseases are elevated in women with endometriosis.

A recent study also found that autoimmune diseases are more common in women with endometriosis. The study, presented at the 8th World Congress on Endometriosis in February 2002, found that 12 percent of women with endometriosis also had an autoimmune disorder, such as lupus or multiple sclerosis; 2 percent of women in the general population have either disease. Researchers from the National Institutes of Health and the Endometriosis Association polled 3,680 women aged fourteen to eighty-nine with surgically diagnosed endometriosis and asked whether they had ever been diagnosed with an autoimmune disorder, an endocrine disorder, fibromyalgia, chronic fatigue syndrome, and allergies or asthma. More than 28 percent reported having either FMS or chronic fatigue, more than 12 percent of the women said they had asthma (20 percent of the women with autoimmune diseases reported having asthma), and 63 percent of the women suffered allergies. "This suggests an association of endometriosis with autoimmune diseases," the researchers concluded.

What Causes Endometriosis?

Despite decades of research, the exact cause of endometriosis remains unclear. The earliest theory linked endometriosis to "retrograde menstruation," the purported backward flow of menstrual discharge through the fallopian tubes into the pelvic cavity, but it's now known that most women actually experience some backflow. Evidence is mounting that women with the disease have some type of immune dysregulation, which fails to destroy the rogue tissue.

Normally, the scavenger cells of the immune system (*macrophages*) get rid of foreign cells and bacteria, but in endometriosis these "big eaters" don't clean up all the stray endometrial cells and cell fragments. The macrophages gobble the errant endometrial cells and present the remains of their dinner to T-cells, which recognize the tissue as self and don't attack. There's also reduced activity of NATURAL KILLER (NK) T-CELLS, which don't need to be sensitized to react against viruses or tumors. So inflammation and irritation caused by the implants continue, possibly leading to production of cytokines that foster the growth of endometrial implants.

Researchers at the Institute for the Study and Treatment of Endometriosis in Oak Brook, Illinois, and the Medical College of Ohio told the 2002 World Congress that the inflammatory cytokine tumor necrosis factor alpha (TNFα, found in many autoimmune diseases), is elevated in women with endometriosis, preventing normal programmed cell death and allowing endometrial implants to proliferate. A review of studies on TNFα in endometriosis by the University of Kansas Medical Center published in *Fertility and Sterility* in September 2001 found "overwhelming evidence" that immunologic factors play a role in endometriosis.

Previous research has found elevations of other inflammatory cytokines, including *interleukin-6 (IL-6)*, *interleuken-8 (IL-8)*, and *Rantes*. "The theory has been that abnormal amounts of these cytokines and other chemicals produced by immune cells, along with retrograde flow, may overwhelm the immune system's ability to eliminate migratory endometrial cells," says David L. Olive, MD, director of reproductive endocrinology and infertility at the University of Wisconsin, Madison. "There are subtle immunologic disorders that occur with endometriosis. Are they the primary disorder or are they the result of endometriosis? We simply don't know."

Endometriosis *is* considered a chronic pain syndrome. Cytokines produced in reaction to endometrial implants may cause malaise, fatigue, fever, and other inflammatory symptoms. Pain from implants may be caused by chemicals such as *prostaglandins* (which are also produced by the uterine lining and cause menstrual cramps). "It's unclear why endometriosis causes pain in some women, and not in others. It may be specific to the site of the implants, the amount of prostaglandins secreted by the implants, or the implants may be secreting something that irritates nerves or causes inflammation," adds Dr. Olive.

Autoimmune diseases are characterized by the presence of autoantibodies, and researchers have looked for such antibodies in blood and secretions from women with endometriosis. Scientists have found *antiendometrial antibodies*, which may be triggered by the presence of the endometrial implants and contribute to symptoms. But their exact role is not understood. Many women have autoantibodies without disease; one antibody linked to lupus—*antinuclear antibodies (ANAs)*—has been found in 12 percent of women with endometriosis.

However, there's no definitive evidence that endometriosis actually has an autoimmune component, stresses D. Ware Branch, MD, professor of obstetrics and gynecology at the University of Utah at Salt Lake City. "It's an attractive hypothesis, but the proof is not there yet. And until someone translates the research into solid basic evidence, and then into a better treatment, this remains a research question."

Symptoms of Endometriosis

The most common symptom of endometriosis is severe pain before and during menstrual periods caused, in part, by prostaglandins produced by the endometrial implants.

However, some women may have no symptoms at all and are diagnosed only when they're unable to become pregnant, sometimes due to scars or adhesions that block the release of eggs from the ovaries or their passage into the fallopian tubes, inflammation, or other factors.

Common sites for endometrial implants include the outer surface of the uterus and supporting ligaments, the space between the uterus and the rectum (called the *cul-de-sac*), the ovaries, and the membrane that lines the pelvic cavity. As the implanted tissue grows under the influence of estrogen, it can invade nearby organs, including the intestines and the bladder, causing painful bowel movements, irritable bowel symptoms, diarrhea and/or constipation, and intestinal upsets during menstruation.

A 1998 survey by the Endometriosis Association found that more than 87 percent of patients felt lethargic and fatigued, a majority was unable to carry out normal activities one to two days a month, and 57 percent had allergies. Sixty-five percent of the 4,000 women surveyed experienced painful intercourse. In addition, 44 percent of the women reported low resistance to infection, around 30 percent low-grade fever, and others reported severe problems with yeast infections (*candidiasis*) and yeast allergies. Up to 65 percent of women with endometriosis experience their first symptoms before the age of 20.

Diagnosing Endometriosis

While endometriosis can produce nodules or cysts on the ovary that can be felt during a pelvic exam, laparoscopy is the gold standard for a diagnosis.

Diagnostic laparoscopy uses a thin, lighted telescope to look inside the pelvis and inspect the reproductive organs. It's done under general anesthesia, using small incisions in the abdomen to insert the fiber-optic scope to view the pelvic organs, and surgical instruments for a biopsy.

The amount of endometriosis seen on laparoscopy is assigned a numerical score; treatment decisions are usually based on the stage of the disease. The disease staging system divides endometriosis into minimal (Stage 1), mild (Stage 2), moderate (Stage 3), and severe (Stage 4). However, the staging system may be unreliable since symptoms may not correlate with the stages. For example, someone with stage 1 disease can have severe pain. In some cases, implants can be vaporized (burned away), excised (cut out), or ablated (destroyed) during diagnostic laparoscopy using a laser or electrocautery instruments.

MetrioTest is a new test that combines an endometrial biopsy with a blood test to detect endometriosis in women suffering pelvic pain. It's done in a doctor's office and takes around fifteen minutes. The test looks for the presence of immunological markers in endometrial tissue and in the blood, predicting endometriosis with around 90 percent accuracy. The test is available in Canada and is expected to be marketed in the United States in the future.

Treating Endometriosis

Medical treatment is aimed at suppressing the female hormones that fuel the growth of endometrial implants, using various hormones to prevent or lessen menstruation. It's not a cure; recurrence rates range from 30 to 60 percent. Surgery can eradicate endometrial implants and remove adhesions that cause pain, but cannot cure the disease.

Hormonal Therapy

Oral contraceptives are usually the initial treatment for endometriosis. Various formulations and strengths of estrogen and progesterone act together to prevent ovulation; the progestins in the pill suppress growth of endometrial tissue, reduce production of prostaglandins, and lessen pain. Oral contraceptives may be effective for short-term relief in 50 to 80 percent of women.

Danazol (Danocrine, Cyclomen) is a derivative of testosterone, which reduces the amount of estrogen produced by your body to menopausal levels. A six-month regimen of danazol reduces the size and extent of endometrial implants by up to 50 percent; a majority of women experience pain relief, and as many as 70 to 100 percent of women go into remission. Danazol has *androgenic* side effects, including acne, growth of facial hair, water retention, and weight gain. It can also raise cholesterol. A vaginal preparation to minimize side effects is being researched.

GnRH agonists mimic the natural gonadotropin releasing hormone produced by the body that regulates estrogen production, but are much more potent. These drugs fool the body into thinking you're in menopause, reducing the symptoms of endometriosis. GnRH agonists come in several forms, including *leuprolide* (*Lupron*), given as injections; *nafarelin acetate* (*Synarel*) and *buserelin acetate* (*Suprefact*) in nasal spray form; or *goserelin acetate* (*Zoladex*), an implant placed under the skin of the abdomen. They relieve pain in most women and produce up to a 90 percent regression of implants. The artificial menopause they create has all the symptoms of natural menopause: hot flashes, vaginal dryness, decreased sex drive, mood swings, and fatigue. GnRH agonists also cause accelerated bone loss (around twice the normal rate of the first year of menopause) increasing the risk of osteoporosis. If prolonged treatment is needed, drugs are given to prevent bone resorption, including *alendronate* (*Fosamax*) and *risedronate* (*Actonel*).

Newer **GnRH antagonists** are being developed that work faster than GnRH *agonists*, directly blocking secretion of gonadotropins by the pituitary gland. Other hormonal treatments for endometriosis include progestogens, such as *Depo-Provera*, which inhibit the growth of endometrial tissue.

Clinical trials were conducted with Enbrel and with the immune inhibitor *pentoxifylline* (*Trental*) to see if they improve fertility rates; the results were not statistically significant.

Surgery is usually done when hormonal therapy fails or women don't wish to take hormones. Endometriosis surgery is usually done laparoscopically, making small incisions to admit tiny surgical instruments, lasers, or electro-cautery devices that remove or destroy implants.

Laparoscopic surgery is done as a day surgery under general anesthesia. Laparoscopic surgery causes far less pain than open abdominal surgery and recovery is faster; most women return to work within a week. For severe, invasive implants in and around the bowel or bladder, open abdominal surgery (*laparotomy*) may be needed.

How Endometriosis Can Affect You Over Your Lifetime

Endometriosis takes its biggest toll during a woman's reproductive years, sometimes causing pain during her teens.

Menstruation and Fertility

Endometriosis can cause extremely painful menstrual periods, and according to surveys by the Endometriosis Association, more than 40 percent of women with endometriosis report fertility problems. Surgery to remove adhesions or blockages that interfere with the release and uptake of an egg can improve fertility. But some women aren't helped by surgery, and turn to in-vitro fertilization. However, hormones needed for these procedures may stimulate endometrial implants, so experts urge women to proceed cautiously.

Women with endometriosis also have a high rate of tubal (*ectopic*) pregnancies and an increased risk of miscarriage. Some studies suggest that autoantibodies may interfere with the implantation of the fetus. One study presented at the 2002 World Congress on Endometriosis found that a combination of low-dose aspirin and prednisone improved pregnancy and implantation rates in women undergoing in-vitro fertilization who were found to have autoantibodies.

Menopause and Beyond

For some women, pregnancy brings temporary relief from endometriosis, and menopause usually ends symptoms in women who have moderate disease. Estrogen replacement therapy (ERT) can occasionally reactivate endometriosis (even in women who have had a hysterectomy).

The course of endometriosis in later life has not been well-studied. But studies suggest that women with endometriosis have an increased risk of ovarian and breast cancer, as well as melanoma.

Interstitial Cystitis

Interstitial cystitis (IC) is another chronic condition scientists suspect may have an autoimmune component. IC is a chronic bladder disorder that causes nerve endings to be irritated by elements in urine, resulting in bladder pain on filling, so it holds less urine. The cause is not known. It was once thought to be inflammatory, but bladder biopsies show very little inflammation.

One theory is that the cells lining the bladder are somehow "leaky" in women with IC, allowing substances in urine to penetrate the bladder wall, irritating muscle tissue and nerve endings, resulting in symptoms of urinary urgency and pain.

Other research suggests IC may be an autoimmune problem, with autoantibodies attacking bladder tissue. Around 25 percent of women with IC are found to have increased levels of antinuclear antibodies (ANAs). Autoantibodies to mitochondria, the energy-generating components of cells, found in women with scleroderma, have also been found in around 2.5 percent of IC patients. It's not known exactly what role autoantibodies may play. Women found to have these antibodies may have a separate form of the disease.

Mast cells, which play a role in allergies and in inflammation, have turned up in bladder biopsies of some women with IC, and 40 percent of IC patients also have allergies.

There's also a connection with chronic pain disorders. A study by Temple University found that 25 percent of women with IC have irritable bowel syndrome, almost 20 percent have migraines, 13 percent had endometriosis, and 10 percent had vulvodynia. The Temple study found that other IC patients have been diagnosed with (or have occasional symptoms of) fibromyalgia, ulcerative colitis, chronic fatigue, lupus, and asthma. Experts say there are probably multiple causes for IC, which affects as many as 500,000 women.

The most common symptom is an urgent need to urinate, sometimes as many as sixty times over a twenty-four-hour period. Women also experience a burning or cramping pain before and after urinating. Over half of women with IC have pain during or after intercourse, possibly due to spasms in pelvic muscles caused by irritation. IC is diagnosed by cystoscopy. The procedure is done under general anesthesia: the bladder is filled with water (distended) and drained, and then a flexible, lighted fiber-optic scope is inserted into the urethra to examine the lining of the bladder to look for tiny hemorrhages, ulcers (*Hunner's ulcers*), or cracks in the mucosa. The distention of the bladder with water (*hydrodistention*) may have therapeutic effects.

Treatments include the drug *dimethyl sulfoxide* (*DMSO*), infused into the bladder by a catheter weekly (or every other week) for four to six weeks. A newer drug, *pentosan polysulfate sodium* (*Elmiron*), is given orally. It seems to help coat the bladder lining, protecting it from irritants. Other treatments include the tricyclic antidepressant *amitriptyline* (*Elavil*), which lessens nerve pain and seems to increase bladder capacity, and the antihistamine *hydroxyzine* (*Atarax*). Since both can cause drowsiness, they're usually taken at bedtime.

Dietary changes—avoiding bladder irritants like alcohol, citrus fruits and juices, spicy foods, coffee, vinegar, and high-oxalate foods like spinach and rhubarb—may help some women.

There are no cures for interstitial cystitis. But, as with other chronic pain syndromes, women are urged to learn stress management techniques to help cope with the disorder.

14

Navigating the Medical Maze

I was incredibly lucky—it only took me a couple of months to get a diagnosis. I now have an excellent liver doctor. But his focus is on the liver, not on the fact that I have an autoimmune disease. He doesn't discuss my diseases with me in that context. He discusses my medications and my liver function tests, and he makes sure that I'm doing OK. I get my bloodwork done at my GP's office. And even then I don't see the doctor. Once I found the American Autoimmune Diseases Association, I was able to learn a lot about autoimmunity and my own disease. And I was able to connect with other women who have these diseases, and it's really wonderful. We exchange E-mails and we call each other. That support is really important. But I do wish there were doctors who dealt with autoimmunity, so you could get a more complete picture of what's going on. You learn things bit by bit, and so much is left for you to figure out on your own.

HANNAH

Hannah *is* lucky. The typical woman with an autoimmune disease may spend several years, see a half-dozen doctors, and spend upward of $50,000 before there's a correct diagnosis. Some women have a tough time just getting their symptoms taken seriously. A survey by the American Autoimmune Related Diseases Association (AARDA) found that over 45 percent of patients were labeled hypochondriacs in the early stages of their illness. All too many women are told their symptoms are "all in their head" and are referred to a psychiatrist instead of a rheumatologist or endocrinologist, remarks Virginia Ladd, founder and president of AARDA.

Autoimmune diseases consume more than $86 billion annually in health care dollars, and are the fourth leading cause of illness in American women, after heart disease, lung cancer, and breast cancer. Yet there are few centers that "triage" women to the proper care and help them form a care team, says Ladd; and no specialty in autoimmunology exists, so it may not be easy to find the proper doctor to manage your care.

> *There needs to be an autoimmune specialty. We can have wacko symptoms that often make no sense. And each specialist is only looking at his one specialty. We need to have doctors who get the big picture. In my medical odyssey there were actually only two doctors who did not suspect what I had. The specialists, the ophthalmologist, the neurologist, the rheumatologist, and the hematologist all suspected it was antiphospholipid syndrome. But my primary care physician and the first ER doctor I saw discounted it. I do think that part of it is that outside of big cities, in rural areas particularly, doctors may be insular and they are not comfortable with collaborative diagnoses in the way that doctors at major medical centers are. So I would tell women to get to a major medical center in a big city.*
>
> MARGARET

Who Should Be Your Doctor?

If you think you have an autoimmune disease, or need better care for an existing problem (or problems), you need to find the right specialist to obtain the proper diagnosis, treatment, and followup. As a starting point, AARDA suggests identifying the type of medical specialist who deals with your major symptom, then looking for physicians who have board certification in that particular area. They should be certified by one of the twenty-three specialty boards of the American Board of Medical Specialties. To check on a doctor's certification status, call **(800)** 776-2378. Following are some general guidelines for choosing a specialist.

Rheumatoid arthritis, lupus, Sjögren's syndrome, and other connective tissue diseases are usually managed by a rheumatologist. This is a specialty that encompasses diseases of the joints, bones, and muscles, and related diseases. A rheumatologist may have dual board certifications in internal medicine and rheumatology from the American Board of Internal Medicine, and will often belong to the American College of Rheumatology (ACR).

As your treatment progresses, other professionals often help, including nurses, physical or occupational therapists, orthopedic surgeons, psychologists, and social workers. Physical therapists are certified by the American Board of Physical Medicine and Rehabilitation. If you should need joint replacement, you'll need an orthopedic surgeon certified by the American Board of Orthopaedic Surgery; they can often be found through the American Association of Orthopaedic Surgeons (AAOS).

Endocrine disorders, including thyroid disease and type 1 diabetes, require the care of an endocrinologist. This specialist can also deal with issues of osteoporosis that arise from corticosteroid treatments.

Women with diabetes ideally should look for a physician who specializes in managing diabetes—an endocrinologist who's a diabetologist, says Cornell's Dr. Carol Levy. Your care team might include a certified diabetes educator (who may be a registered nurse or registered dietitian) to help you learn to manage glucose self-testing and insulin injections and structure a healthy eating plan that fits your likes, dislikes, and lifestyle. "Many internists will not have access to these people, so I recommend looking for a hospital that has a diabetes program or clinic," she advises. "This is a lifelong condition that needs lifelong management, so it's important to have an endocrinologist who can follow you. Your condition can change over time; you can develop complications or other autoimmune endocrine diseases, or new treatments may come out that will benefit you. So, ideally, the best person to manage your care is an endocrinologist."

A diabetologist is an endocrinologist who specializes in diabetes and is board certified in Diabetes and Metabolism by the American Board of Internal Medicine; other board certifications include those with Special Qualifications in Endocrinology and/or Reproductive Endocrinology.

For neurological diseases, such as multiple sclerosis and myasthenia gravis, a neurologist is the best physician to diagnose and manage your condition.

He or she should be board certified by the American Board of Neurological Surgery.

Gastrointestinal diseases, including Crohn's disease, ulcerative colitis, and celiac disease, should be managed by a gastroenterologist. Autoimmune hepatitis and primary biliary cirrhosis are managed by gastroenterologists who specialize in liver disease called *hepatologists*. Your gastroenterologist should be a Diplomate of the American Board of Gastroenterology. For surgery, you'll need a physician board certified in Colon and Rectal Surgery by the American Board of Colon and Rectal Surgery. The professional group is the American Society of Colon and Rectal Surgeons.

Specialists in blood disorders, called *hematologists*, can manage not only platelet disorders like immune thrombocytopenia, but also antiphospholipid syndrome. However, if APS occurs with another autoimmune connective tissue disease, such as lupus, your rheumatologist can often manage APS. A hematologist is board certified in that specialty by the American Board of Internal Medicine, and will usually be a member of the American Society of Hematology.

A dermatologist is best qualified to manage autoimmune skin disorders, including psoriasis, alopecia areata, and vitiligo. They can have general certification in Dermatology, with special qualifications in Dermatological Immunology/Diagnostic and Laboratory Immunology (for biopsies) from the American Academy of Dermatology.

A reproductive endocrinologist or gynecologist who specializes in infertility is ideally suited for diagnosing premature ovarian failure and helping you get pregnant. The American Board of Obstetrics and Gynecology offers general certification in Obstetrics and Gynecology, with special Qualifications in Reproductive Endocrinology. A good OB/GYN will often be a fellow of the American College of Obstetricians and Gynecologists (ACOG). Infertility specialists are usually members of the American Society for Reproductive Medicine (ASRM).

Asthma and allergies can coexist with some autoimmune diseases. Specialists in this area are certified by the American Board of Allergy and Immunology. They typically belong to either the American College of Asthma, Allergy and Immunology (ACAAI) or the American Association of Allergy, Asthma and Immunology (AAAAI).

In general, large teaching hospitals affiliated with medical schools are more likely to have an array of specialists to consult. You can also find an appropriate specialist by visiting the websites of the various professional organizations. Support groups for various disorders often keep lists of specialists and can be a valuable resource in finding the right doctor. (See Appendix A.)

Being followed by the right kind of specialist can make a *big* difference to your care. A study reported at the 2002 ACR Annual Scientific Meeting looked at the treatment of patients with RA belonging to a large health insurance plan in Pittsburgh and found 67 percent of those being followed by a rheumatologist were prescribed disease-modifying antirheumatic drugs (DMARDs), compared to only 27 percent of those seen by a nonrheumatologist. And RA patients seen by nonrheumatologists were more likely to be given narcotics for their pain, rather than drugs that also target inflammation.

Interview your prospective physician. Ask how many patients he or she has treated with your particular problem. The more patients the doctor sees with your disease, the more skilled he or she is likely to be in treating it. However, personal "fit" is important too. Even if you have found "the" expert in the field, the personal empathy may not be there. You'll be revealing some of the most intimate details of your life to this person, so if you don't feel comfortable talking to him or her, keep looking until you find the right fit. Too many of us choose a doctor who will have a major impact on our quality of life after just one visit. Even though he or she may be an expert on your disease, you're the expert on your own experiences with your illness.

When I was diagnosed with autoimmune hepatitis and my family started talking about it, we realized there was a family history of autoimmune disease. My mother has Hashimoto's thyroiditis, and my grandfather was also hypothyroid. My grandmother had type 1 diabetes. So there was definitely a history, but we'd never talked about it as autoimmunity. It turns out my dad's brother also had hypothyroidism. So we have it on both sides of the family. But no one had liver disease, at least that I know of.

HANNAH

I never even asked questions until recent years, and found out we had an extensive family history of thyroid disease that stretched into my second and

*third cousins. I've persuaded my brother to be tested, since his daughter has
a thyroid problem. And it wasn't just thyroid—my father had Crohn's disease and Hashimoto's, my second cousin had celiac disease, and another
cousin has lupus. And honestly, I might never have known.*

LYNNE

What You Can Do to Take Charge

Taking charge of your care means getting as much information as you can,
keeping track of symptoms and medications, and coming prepared to every
doctor visit.

Make a Family Tree

Ask questions about other family members and make a family medical tree.
It's not simply an exercise in genealogy. In some cases, testing may be advised
for close family members, especially in cases of type 1 diabetes and thyroid
disease. You may need additional testing for autoimmune diseases that cluster with your particular problem.

"When someone presents with type 1 diabetes we automatically look for
thyroid autoimmunity because the concurrence is so high. If positive, then
we look for thyroid autoimmunity in the parents— if the child has it, then
the mother often has it as well," comments Dr. Noel Maclaren of Cornell.
"Thyroid autoimmunity is somehow predisposing to type 1 diabetes. Addison's disease, adrenal gland insufficiency, is found more commonly in patients
with type 1 diabetes; about 1 in 200 to 250 patients with type 1 diabetes will
also develop adrenal insufficiency. This can be a very serious problem in a diabetic, because it can be life threatening and is often missed in a diabetic
patient. Doctors don't always have the thought that this patient is developing
this second problem."

Vitiligo is a skin marker for propensity to autoimmunity, especially thyroid problems, adrenal insufficiency, and type 1 diabetes, Dr. Maclaren
believes. "Half the patients we see with vitiligo also have autoimmune thyroid disease, so they all ought to be screened for it."

In some cases, if a disease has a strong genetic component, genetic counseling may be needed. You also need to ask questions about the chances of passing along an autoimmune disease to your child. Physicians should be board certified in Medical or Clinical Genetics by the American Board of Medical Genetics. A genetic counselor (who could be a social worker or other health professional) is usually trained in a graduate program.

Keep Track of Details

Just as physicians keep an up-to-date file on each patient, so should you keep a medical file for yourself. This can be a notebook or a file folder, and it should contain a record of doctor visits, copies or records of lab reports and other diagnostic tests, and a list of medications you're taking (the dose, when and how each drug is taken, and so on).

You should have a section in your diary for symptoms. Because knowledge of autoimmune clusters is just beginning to reach physicians who are not specialists in rheumatology or endocrinology, you need to keep track of symptoms, even those that don't appear to be related to your specific diagnosis. An unusual symptom may be the very first clue that you have a second (or third) autoimmune disease.

At each doctor visit, bring a list of symptoms you're experiencing; review that list with your doctor and give him or her a copy to keep in your file. As you've learned from reading this book, when you have an autoimmune disease you can often experience a number of symptoms that may seem unrelated. So let your doctor know about any new symptom. And don't worry that your doctor will think you're a chronic complainer, or that you'll just end up with another prescription. Be honest. You only hurt yourself if you don't speak up.

Autoimmune diseases are not simple. And many times, especially during the first physician visits, you may get a lot of information to process in a short amount of time. Bring your medical diary or a pad and paper, or even a small tape recorder.

Make sure you understand unfamiliar terms, the tests you may need, and treatment options. And before you leave, go over what was discussed so you're clear about the details.

You need someone who not only knows about your disease, but who's alert to the other complications and other diseases. When you have a symptom, they have to think it may not just be your disease acting up. You have to be very alert, you have to know your body, and you have to speak up when there's something bothering you. We may not always be good at articulating exactly what's wrong, but there are also too many things that doctors will say are "all in your head."

LAURA, FORTY-SIX

After I was first diagnosed with Crohn's, I had to have surgery. They removed a foot of my small intestine, my appendix, and some of my colon. But the gastroenterologist I was seeing in the hospital didn't really explain what any of the followup was going to entail and basically discharged me without any medication or anything. And about a month after I got out of the hospital, I started having trouble again. I tried to call him, but he never returned any of my phone calls. About two years later I started developing some symptoms, and they finally put me on medication. But that was a gap of two years, which allowed my disease to get worse again. Now I know to ask questions and find out as much as I can.

JANINE

A Team Effort

The time is long past when patients blindly accepted a doctor's pronouncements. And that's a positive thing. You need to ask questions from the outset. Don't allow any physician to dismiss your symptoms as stress. Make sure you get a thorough clinical examination.

As you've seen, tests *vary* for different autoimmune diseases, and often there's no single test that can diagnose your condition. You may be faced with the prospect of undergoing a battery of tests, and you need to ask what each is for and whether there are any alternatives. Will a diagnostic procedure be done on an outpatient or inpatient basis? Will there be any pain or discomfort? Will you need anesthesia? If you suffer from claustrophobia and need an MRI (which means spending thirty minutes inside a magnetic tube) ask about medications to make you more comfortable during the procedure. Ask how much a procedure costs, and whether it will be covered by your health insurance. Who will get the test results, and what will they tell us about your condition? Although diagnostic criteria can define a disease, your particular array of symptoms may be uncertain.

Get a second, third, or fourth opinion if need be. Because autoimmunity is just now being recognized as an underlying cause of many diseases, and because symptoms can be vague, many doctors don't initially think to test for autoimmune diseases.

Ask questions about treatment options. What are the advantages and disadvantages? How long will the treatment last? You can only benefit by working together with your doctor.

> *I was seriously depressed from the prednisone, though I didn't know it at the time. Prednisone increases anger, anxiety, and depression—none of which any doctor ever told me. And the methotrexate was even worse. When I had a period I thought I was hemorrhaging, and twice I almost went to the hospital just thinking, "This is it. This is the end." Again, no one spoke to me about any of this. I'd look it up in a medical guide and find out what the hell was going on for myself. And I would wake up each morning in this rage, and have to tell myself, "OK, wait a minute. This is not me. I'm not angry. I don't have any reason to be angry other than life, and what was going on with my disease, but there's nothing to be angry at. Just chill out. Calm down. It's the medication, it's not me." Which I needed to do . . . I was risking personal relationships all over the place. I have wonderful friends and a wonderful husband, but there's only so far you can go before they say, "Would you please stop?" And I wish someone had spoken to me about the possible effects of the medication on my thinking, my emotions.*
>
> KATHLEEN TURNER

Find Out All You Can About Your Medications

As Kathleen Turner found out the hard way, medications can have unexpected side effects. And in all likelihood you're going to be taking several medications, all of which have side effects. So you need to know how they can affect you, and how they may interact with other drugs you may be taking (including over-the-counter drugs, supplements, and herbs).

Write down the name of the drug, what it's used for (an immunosuppressant or a pain reliever, for example), the dose you need to take and how often, if it needs to be taken with (or without) food, and any potential side effects.

It's probably wise to buy a consumer copy of the *Physician's Desk Reference*, or check your library's copy of the *PDR*, to obtain complete information on medications that have been prescribed for you.

If you're seeing more than one doctor, make sure they all know what medications you're taking, including over-the-counter drugs and herbal preparations. Sit down once a year to review those medications to make sure you still need the same drug and the same dose.

Save the package inserts in your medical folder at home. Even commonly used drugs may, in very rare cases, cause severe, possibly fatal reactions. There's usually a section that says "Contact your doctor immediately if. . . ." This contains key information about potential side effects and interactions. Your risk of serious side effects may be small, but you need to know the warning signs. If you don't get the insert, ask for it, or get a computer printout of drug instructions and precautions. If you have *any* reaction to a drug, call your doctor immediately.

Don't be surprised if your questions about how medications affect women prompt a response of "We don't know—there haven't been any studies on that." In writing this book and talking to preeminent experts around the country, many of them conceded that knowledge is lacking about the effects of female and male sex hormones, and even the effects on pregnancy or menopause of medications that have been used for long periods of time. Clinical trials of medications sponsored by the National Institutes of Health have only been required to include women since 1989 (women had been excluded because of concerns about potential birth defects and the notion that female hormones could confuse trial results). And reporting of those clinical trials to include sex differences in the responses and side effects of medications has only been mandated by the Food and Drug Administration since 1999.

The cost of medications can be staggering. The newest drugs to treat autoimmune diseases can cost hundreds of thousands of dollars; the multiple sclerosis drug Avonex can cost upward of $60,000 a year. Many insurers will not cover the cost of new drugs, but pharmaceutical companies can often help you get into a program to obtain these drugs at low or no cost. Many states have drug discount plans as well. These sources are listed in Appendix A.

There's a lot you need to learn on your own. I had to learn how to adjust my insulin intake to match my natural appetite, which is something most doctors don't encourage diabetics to do. They want to get everyone on the same schedule, which makes it easier for them to explain. I had to find endocrinologists and doctors who understood, who would spend the time with me to work this out. No one told me to increase the amount of blood testing when I started on estrogen for my hot flashes. I knew about gestational diabetes and I thought there could be a reaction that could increase the need for insulin. But when my gynecologist prescribed estrogen, she never mentioned it and she knew I was a diabetic. I just started testing more on my own. I almost did that automatically. There's a lot that you have to find out for yourself.

MARY KAY

I was extremely lucky to find a gynecologist who worked closely with the MS center. She wanted me to take estrogen because she thought it would help my disease, even though there hadn't been clinical studies at the time. She just knew MS got better during pregnancy. So the choice of a gynecologist can be critical.

ANA

Find a Gynecologist Familiar with Autoimmune Disease

As Mary Kay and Ana discovered, having a gynecologist who's knowledgeable and up to date on your particular autoimmune disease is extremely important, since you'll need expert guidance and followup should you choose to have a child or take estrogen (or its alternatives).

For example, says Cornell diabetologist Dr. Carol Levy regarding decisions about taking oral contraceptives or hormone replacement, "Up until a few years ago there was this misconception among doctors that women couldn't go on birth control pills because it would cause fluctuations in blood sugar levels. That misconception has been passed along to patients, and it often makes them fearful. Oral contraceptives can make glucose fluctuations more predictable, but we need to be able to work with the gynecologist."

Information may not be offered, or your questions about hormones may (again) be answered with "We don't know" or "That's a question you need to take up with your gynecologist." "Rheumatologists aren't discussing it, and the gynecologist may not know anything about autoimmune disease," remarks Lila E. Nachtigall, MD, of the NYU School of Medicine, who has been researching estrogen for more than thirty years. "The question of hormones, be it birth control pills or hormone replacement, is part of the whole patient picture. So a woman needs to get answers somewhere. For our part, we find it extremely helpful when a woman keeps track of her symptoms, because it can help us individualize care."

Keep a symptom diary during the menstrual cycle, pregnancy, or menopause, and bring it with you to doctor visits and ask questions. *Don't* ignore regular pelvic exams and Pap smears, and periodically have pelvic floor muscle function assessed, especially in diseases that affect muscle and nerve function. Many women who become disabled as a result of their disease often have difficulty finding a gynecologist who's not only knowledgeable, but also has adequate equipment (like specially designed examining tables that can adjust to women who must use wheelchairs). Incontinence and sexual problems can be side effects of multiple sclerosis or myasthenia gravis, and other diseases, and require special and empathetic attention. The specialist treating your disease can often help with a referral to a gynecologist. Sources of information include the American College of Obstetricians and Gynecologists (ACOG). Your specialist can often make a referral to an OB/GYN.

I decided to combine drug therapy with the natural treatments. I had been seeing a naturopathic doctor before I was diagnosed with autoimmune hepatitis, and she had recommended milk thistle for my liver. Milk thistle is an herb that contains Silybum marianum, which has been shown to help regenerate liver cells. It doesn't cure the hepatitis. She also told me to avoid fatty foods and alcohol, and had also recommended acupuncture before I was diagnosed. That made me feel better, psychologically at least. Thanks to that naturopath, I was also taking calcium from the beginning. When I moved to New York I started seeing a liver specialist, who told me there was no harm in my taking milk thistle, but it was probably a waste of my money. I've continued to take it, and I think it's helped.

HANNAH

What About Alternative and Complementary Therapies?

In writing this book, we made a decision not to delve into the myriad complementary therapies being used by women with autoimmune diseases. That's a subject for another book. Fortunately, there is a reliable source for women affected with many of the autoimmune diseases: *The Arthritis Foundation's Guide to Alternative Therapies* (see Appendix B). There are many helpful books on herbal remedies, as well.

But there are many cautions. While many women find complementary therapies extremely helpful, it's important to remember that "natural" doesn't always mean safe, and that supplements are largely unregulated. There's no guarantee that you'll get what you pay for. We urge you to investigate everything carefully, consult the physician managing your care, and don't be afraid to discuss herbs and other things you've tried. (After all, glucosamine was once on the fringes, and now it's an accepted therapy for osteoarthritis.) Some drugs may make your condition worse or cause interactions with medications you're taking (such as evening primrose oil and anticoagulants); many herbs should not be taken before surgery; and some herbs (like kava) may even be toxic to the liver.

This is one area where you need to do your homework. Realize that many remedies have a powerful placebo effect—if you believe something is going to help you, chances are it will.

It sounds weird, but if you have to have one of these diseases, this is a great time. They have made leaps and bounds in research. There is some real hope for MS and other diseases, and you need to hang on to that hope. They've made more progress in the last few years than they have in the last twenty-five years. Because of AIDS, they've learned a great deal about the immune system and the central nervous system that will benefit people with autoimmune disease. We also have the Internet, which is a godsend. You get a lot of support and information. There are bulletin boards and chat rooms. And there's tons of information. Even if you have a handicap, so much more is accessible than before, and I thank God I was born now rather than twenty-five, thirty years ago. I would tell women, don't shut yourself in, get out and be part of the world you live in. The more you isolate yourself, the scarier the world becomes. That can be quite a rut, and it's easy to slip into that when you have a chronic disease. The Internet is also a great place to make contact with people, and women should get in touch with support groups, because they can give you so much. Whatever you do, don't isolate yourself.

MARIANA

With a Little Help from Some Friends

As Mary Kay puts it, you almost have to make a profession out of your own health care. But you can't go it alone, and any chronic disease can have its rough spots. Support groups can be lifesavers. It may be hard to walk into that group meeting for the first time, but once you get over that hurdle, a group can be a source of information, friendship, and emotional support.

Millions of people are finding those resources on the Internet. You can do a surprising amount of research right from your own home. You can find information that can help clarify symptoms, uncover resources for finding a good diagnostician, and share your experiences with others. If you don't have your own computer, many libraries provide access to the Internet through their computers. Contact your hospital's community education or outreach program to find out about support groups.

A comprehensive listing of resources and self-help groups appears in Appendix A, and a list of recommended readings is included in Appendix B.

I'm obviously a success story, but what I really want women to know is not to give up, not to think that this is going to be the only controlling factor of

their lives from now on. Because that's not necessary at all . . . They find
their way to fight it, whether it's through exercise or medication. I think
exercise is totally essential. I can't imagine doing without it. I would put
that right on par with medication, frankly. But you need to take action.
There's so much fear of being crippled, or permanently damaged, or not being
able to pursue the work you love and being dependent on loved ones. You
need to keep moving and be as strong as you can be; you can't feel helpless.
They told me I would never recover, but here I am.

KATHLEEN TURNER

Afterword

Where the Future May Take Us

When I first learned I had an autoimmune disease, I had just completed my MD and was moving along on my PhD training in the laboratory. Just like the stories contained in this book, the diagnosis took a long time in coming, probably a good six months. Ironically, I was studying autoimmunity in mice at the time, and as the old adage goes, if you study it long enough you will finally get it.

It was a senior and very seasoned laboratory technician who noticed I was turning yellow. Indeed, I ate lots of carrots every day (my excuse) and was pale from long hours in the lab instead of the summer sun. The consensus lab diagnosis, a dangerous concept in and of itself, was that I must have been coming down with hepatitis from some patient encounter over the past year. After much prodding I dutifully went to student health service (a highly risky venture). It took many trips to rule out the common causes of yellowed skin, but eventually I was diagnosed as having severe hypothyroidism. My yellow skin represented a very long-standing disease.

I was relieved to know what was wrong, but my PhD advisor was very stressed. He personally called the physician in charge of health service to let her know that she needed to reevaluate her diagnosis; he was certain I had *hyper*thyroidism (overactive thyroid). My nickname in the lab was "fireball" and it was hard for everyone to believe that the corrective therapy might actually supercharge the already energetic Faustman. My story had a happy ending. If there is one autoimmune disease that is almost entirely corrected by a little pill, it is hyperthyroidism. (And yes, I did get my PhD done on time.)

But for millions of women, diagnosis and treatment do not come as easily. One of my long-term acquaintances, who herself worked in the field of autoimmunity for twenty-five years, had three major surgical interventions, all mistakes. Her dentist later correctly diagnosed her as having multiple sclerosis. You can be fully educated and be in the care of smart doctors, and those smart doctors can miss these diseases time and time again.

If you have autoimmune disease or know someone close to you who has one of these dreadful diseases, consider becoming a lay advocate. You can have a significant impact at influencing funding for research. You have unique motivation that distinguishes you from the scientists who do the research work; you do not care *who* discovers the cure, you only want the cure and with as great a speed as possible.

I think as scientists we must do significantly better at coming up with cures for these diseases. In my lifetime, I want to hear someone say: "I had type 1 diabetes ten years ago." Over the next decade, I think it is highly feasible that we may be able to actually cure some of these diseases.

Because there are so many different aspects to autoimmunity, we will be attacking these diseases on a number of fronts. As this book outlines, there will be new ways to diagnose these diseases before they occur. This may be by a simple blood sample. There may be ways to stop certain forms of autoimmunity prior to severe end organ damage and there is hope, yes hope, that even once these diseases occur, there may be ways beyond treatment of symptoms to actually reverse the disease.

In this book you've learned about inflammatory cytokines and the damage they can cause. We have already developed medicines to disable some of these cytokines, but the task is now to uncover and interfere with the pathways that lead to their release. The anti-cytokine therapies in their many forms are on the pharmacy shelves, but just remember they do not stop the disease, they only treat the symptoms.

We must also target the cells that cause destruction in autoimmunity. It was long thought that once the disease was fully established, identifying markers of only "bad" cells would not exist. On the research side, at least in spontaneous mouse models, these "bad" cells can be uniquely identified.

Finally, we need a greater understanding of the antigens that provoke autoimmunity to begin. This research is moving forward, albeit more slowly. It was long thought there would only be one antigen per disease, but perhaps the more typical picture is that there are many antigens that trigger disease.

The challenge will be to make the agents that target these pathways nontoxic (or at least less toxic). Corticosteroids are an example of a wonderful medicine that has devastating effects. The cost of a cure should not be another disease or disability.

Indeed, there are medications in the pipeline and in research laboratories that appear for the first time to not only be specific for the "bad" cells but also to selectively eliminate the "bad" cells. The remarkable data in autoimmune diseases shows that the disease is permanently eliminated by a short course of these drugs and the end organ, in this case the insulin secreting islet cells, regrow in adult animals. This sort of research opens up new opportunities for all afflicted with autoimmunity but also opens up the paths for identifying the adult stem cells with unrecognized potential for many diseases, including the aging process that we all hope to experience.

Why talk about all of this work if it is still years away from clinical use? I believe it helps the public and physicians to appreciate the importance of further research into stopping—not just suppressing—the symptomatology of these diseases. And it provides hope. Which leads me to my final thought: Do not be discouraged.

Denise L. Faustman, MD, PhD
Associate Professor of Medicine, Harvard Medical School; Director, Immunobiology Laboratory, Massachusetts General Hospital

Appendix A

Where to Go for Help—
Information and Support Groups

Alopecia Areata
  Alopecia Areata National Registry
  Madeline Duvic, MD
  Lead Investigator
  M. D. Anderson Cancer Center
  University of Texas
  Department of Dermatology
  Box 434 1515 Holcombe Boulevard
  Houston, TX
  (713) 792-5999
  Fax: (713) 794-1491
  E-mail: alopeciaregistry@mdanderson.org

  Affiliated Centers:
  University of Colorado Health Sciences Center, Denver
  University of California, San Francisco
  University of Minnesota, Minneapolis
  Columbia University College of Physicians & Surgeons, New York

  National Alopecia Areata Foundation
  714 C Street
  San Rafael, CA
  (415) 456-4644
  www.naaf.org

Antiphospholipid Syndrome
  Antiphospholipid Syndrome National Registry Coordinating Center
  University of North Carolina, Chapel Hill
  Department of Rheumatology and Immunology, CB #7280
  Thurston Building, Room 3330
  Chapel Hill, NC 27599-7280
  (919) 966-0572
  E-mail: apscore@med.unc.edu

Seven centers are participating in this registry of patients and repository for tissue samples:
Hospital for Special Surgery
Weill Cornell University Medical Center, New York
Johns Hopkins University Medical Center, Baltimore, MD
Duke University Medical Center, Durham, NC
Morehouse School of Medicine, Atlanta, GA
Ball Memorial Hospital, Indiana University–Muncie
University of Texas Health Sciences Center, San Antonio
University of Utah Health Sciences Center, Salt Lake City

The Registry for the Antiphospholipid Syndrome
Clinical Pharmacology Research Program
Oklahoma Medical Research Foundation
825 Northeast 13th Street
Oklahoma City, OK 73104
(866) SLRAPLS (toll-free number)
www.slrapls.org
Note: This registry accepts patients from all locations around the United States.

Arthritis

American College of Rheumatology
60 Executive Park South, Suite 150
Atlanta, GA 30329
(800) 346-4753
www.rheumatology.org

The Arthritis Foundation
1330 West Peachtree Street
Atlanta, GA 30309
(800) 283-7800
www.arthritis.org

Autoimmune Disease Centers

The Arthritis Center
Silvio O. Conte Medical Research Center
Boston University Medical Center
715 Albany Street, K-501
Boston, MA 02118
(617) 638-5180
Fax: (617) 638-5239

Barbara Volcker Center for Women & Rheumatic Diseases
The Hospital for Special Surgery
535 East 70th Street
New York, NY 10021
(212) 606-1461
Fax: (212) 774-2374
E-mail: volckerctr@hss.edu

Center for Arthritis and Autoimmunity
Hospital for Joint Diseases Orthopaedic Institute
303–305 2nd Avenue, Suite 16
New York, NY 10003
(212) 598-6516

Johns Hopkins Autoimmune Disease Research Center
Ross Building, Room 659
School of Medicine, Pathology Department
720 Rutland Avenue
Baltimore, MD 21205

Autoimmune Diseases/General Information

American Autoimmune Related Diseases Association, Inc.
Michigan National Building
22100 Gratiot Avenue
Eastpointe, MI 48021-2227
(586) 776-3900
Fax: (586) 776-3903
www.aarda.org

National Institute of Allergy and Infectious Diseases
Building 31, RM7A-50
31 Center Drive
MSC 2520
Bethesda, MD 20892
(800) 874-2572
www.niaid.nih.gov

National Institute of Arthritis and Musculoskeletal and Skin Diseases
National Institutes of Health
Building 31, Room 4C05
Bethesda, MD 20892
(301) 496-8188
www.niams.nih.gov

Autoimmune (Immune) Thrombocytopenia Purpura

ITP Society of the Children's Blood Foundation
333 East 38th Street, Room 830
New York, NY 10016
(800) ITP-7010
www.ultranet.com/~itpsoc

National Heart, Lung, and Blood Institute
Information Center
P.O. Box 30105
Bethesda, MD 20824
(301) 251-1222
www.nhlbi.nih.gov

Platelet Disorder Support Association
P.O. Box 61533
Potomac, MD 20859
87-PLATELET (877-528-3538) or (301) 294-5967
Fax: (301) 294-3125
E-mail: pdsa@pdsa.org
www.pdsa.org

Celiac Disease

American Celiac Society
Dietary Support Coalition
58 Musano Court
West Orange, NJ 07052
(973) 325-8837
Fax: (973) 669-8808
E-mail: bentleac@umdnj.edu

Celiac Disease Foundation
3251 Ventura Boulevard, Suite #1
Studio City, CA 91604-1838
(818) 990-2354
www.celiac.org

Celiac Sprue Association/USA Inc.
P.O. Box 31700
Omaha, NE 68131-0700
(402) 558-0600
Fax: (402) 558-1347
www.csaceliacs.org

Gluten Intolerance Group of North America
15110 10th Avenue SW, Suite A
Seattle, WA 98166-1820
(206) 246-6652
www.gluten.net

National Center for Nutrition and Dietetics
American Dietetic Association
216 West Jackson Boulevard, Suite 800
Chicago, IL 60606-6995
(800) 366-1655
www.eatright.org/ncnd.html

Chronic Fatigue Syndrome

The CFIDS Association of America
P.O. Box 220398
Charlotte, NC 28222-0398
(800) 442-3437
Resource line: (704) 365-2343
Fax: (704) 365-9755
www.cfids.org

Crohn's Disease and Ulcerative Colitis

Crohn's & Colitis Foundation of America, Inc.
386 Park Avenue South, 17th Floor
New York, NY 10016-8804
(800) 932-2423 or (212) 685-3440
www.ccfa.org

National Digestive Diseases Information Clearinghouse
2 Information Way
Bethesda, MD 20892-3570
E-mail: niddic@info.niddk.nih.gov
www.niddk.nih.gov/health/digest/niddic.htm

Pediatric Crohn's & Colitis Association, Inc.
P.O. Box 188
Newton, MA 02468
(617) 489-5854
www.pcca.hypermart.net

United Ostomy Association, Inc.
19772 MacArthur Boulevard, Suite 200
Irvine, CA 92612-2405
(800) 826-0826 or (949) 660-8624
www.uoa.org

Diabetes

American Diabetes Association
1211 Connecticut Avenue NW
Washington, DC 20036-2701
(800) 342-2383 or (202) 331-8303
www.diabetes.org

Juvenile Diabetes Research Foundation International
120 Wall Street
New York, NY 10005-4001
(800) 533-CURE or (212) 785-9500
Fax: (212) 785-9595
www.jdf.org

To find a local chapter: www.jdf.org/chapters/homepage.php

National Institute of Diabetes & Digestive & Kidney Diseases
National Institutes of Health
(301) 496-3583
www.niddk.nih.gov

Disability Resources

The National Information Center for Children and Youth with Disabilities (NICHCY)
P.O. Box 1492
Washington, DC 20013
(800) 695-0285
www.nichcy.org

U.S. Department of Education and Office of Special Services Clearinghouse on
    Disability
330 C Street SW
Washington, DC 20202
(202) 732-1723

Endometriosis

The Endometriosis Association (EA)
International Headquarters
8585 North 76th Place
Milwaukee, WI 53223
(800) 992-3636 or (414) 355-2200
Fax: (414) 355-6065
www.endometriosisassn.org

Fibromyalgia

Fibromyalgia Alliance of America
P.O. Box 21990
Columbus, OH 43221-0990
(614) 457-4222
E-mail: masaathoff@aol.com
www.stanford.edu/~dement/fibromyalgia.html

Fibromyalgia Network
P.O. Box 31750
Tucson, AZ 85751
(800) 853-2929
www.fmnetnews.com

National Fibromyalgia Research Association, Inc.
P.O. Box 500
Salem, OR 97308
(503) 588-1411
www.nfra.net

Immunology

American Academy of Allergy, Asthma & Immunology
611 East Wells Street
Milwaukee, WI 53202
(414) 272-6071
(800) 822-2762 (Patient information and physician referral line)
E-mail: info@aaaai.org
www.aaaai.org

Multiple Sclerosis

American Academy of Neurology (AAN)
1080 Montreal Avenue
St. Paul, MN 55116
(800) 879-1960
www.aan.com

National Institute of Neurological Disorders and Stroke (NINDS)
NIH Neurological Institute
P.O. Box 5801
Bethesda, MD 20824
(800) 352-9424
www.ninds.nih.gov

National Multiple Sclerosis Society
733 Third Avenue
New York, NY 10017
(800) 344-4867
www.nmss.org

MS Medication Information and Support
Avonex Alliance & MS Resource Center
Biogen Services
(800) 456-2255
www.avonex.com

Betaseron Resource Center
MS Pathways Resource
Berlex Laboratories
(800) 788-1467
www.betaseron.com

Team Copaxone & Shared Solutions
Teva Marion Partners
(800) 887-8100
www.copaxone.com

Myasthenia Gravis

Myasthenia Gravis Foundation of America
5841 Cedar Lake Road, Suite 204
Minneapolis, MN 55416
(800) 541-5454 or (952) 545-9438
Fax: (952) 545-6073
www.myasthenia.org

Myositis (Polymyositis, Dermatomyositis)
Myositis Association of America
755 Cantrell Avenue, Suite C
Harrisonburg, VA 22801
(540) 433-7686
Fax: (540) 432-0206
www.myositis.org

Pemphigus
International Pemphigus Foundation
Atrium Plaza, Suite 203
828 San Pablo Avenue
Albany, CA 94706
(510) 527-4970
www.pemphigus.org

Psoriasis
National Psoriasis Foundation
6600 SW 92nd Avenue, Suite 300
Portland, OR 97223
(800) 723-9166 or (503) 244-7004
Fax: (503) 245-0626
www.psoriasis.org

Rare Diseases
National Organization for Rare Disorders
55 Kenosia Avenue
P.O. Box 1968
Danbury, CT 06813-1968
(203) 744-0100 or (800) 999-6673
Fax: (203) 798-2291
E-mail: orphan@rarediseases.org
www.rarediseases.org

Office of Rare Diseases
National Institutes of Health
6100 Executive Boulevard
Room 3A07, MSC 7518
Bethesda, MD 20892-7518
(800) 999-6673 or (301) 402-4336
Fax: (301) 480-9655
http://rarediseases.info.nih.gov

Scleroderma

International Scleroderma Network
www.sclero.org/isn/a-to-z.html

National Scleroderma Federation
Peabody Office Building
One Newberry Street
Peabody, MA 01960
(800) 422-1113 or (508) 535-6600
Fax: (508) 535-6696

Scleroderma Family & DNA Registry
Marilyn Perry, Registry Coordinator
Wayne State University School of Medicine
University of Texas Health Science Center at Houston
6431 Fannin Street, MSB 5.270
Houston, TX 77030
(800) 736-6864
Fax: (713) 500-0723
E-mail: sclerodermaregistery@uth.tmc.edu

Scleroderma Foundation
12 Kent Way, Suite 201
Byfield, MA 01922
(978) 463-5843
Info line: (800) 722-HOPE (4673)
Fax: (978) 463-5809
www.scleroderma.org

Sjögren's Syndrome

Sjögren's Syndrome Foundation, Inc.
8120 Woodmont Avenue, Suite 530
Bethesda, MD 20814
(301) 718-0300
Info line: (800) 475-6473
Fax: (301) 718-0322
www.sjogrens.org

Systemic Lupus Erythematosus (SLE)

Lupus Foundation of America
1300 Piccard Drive, Suite 200
Rockville, MD 20850
(800) 74-LUPUS or (800) 558-0121
www.lupus.org

LupusLine (telephone counseling for people with lupus by people with lupus, offered in
coordination with S.L.E. Foundation, Inc.)
Department of Social Work
The Hospital for Special Surgery
535 East 70th Street
New York, NY 10021
(212) 606-1952

S.L.E. Foundation, Inc.
149 Madison Avenue, Suite 205
New York, NY 10016
(800) 74-LUPUS or (212) 685-4118
Fax: (212) 545-1843
E-mail: lupus@lupusNY.org
A chapter of the Lupus Foundation of America

Thyroid Disease
American Foundation of Thyroid Patients
18534 North Lyford
Katy, TX 77449
(281) 855-6608
www.thyroidfoundation.org

The American Thyroid Association, Inc.
Townhouse Office Park
55 Old Nyack Turnpike, Suite 611
Nanuet, NY 10954
www.thyroid.org

The Thyroid Society
7515 South Main Street, Suite 545
Houston, TX 77030
(800) THYROID
www.the-thyroid-society.org

Appendix B

Recommended Reading

Arthritis

The Arthritis Sourcebook, Earl J. Brewer, MD, and Kathy Cochran Angel, 1998, Lowell House, Chicago.

The Arthritis Bible: A Comprehensive Guide to Alternative Therapies and Conventional Treatments for Arthritic Diseases, Leonid Gordon and Craig Weatherby, 1999, Healing Arts Press, Rochester, VT.

The Arthritis Foundation's Guide to Alternative Therapies, Judith Horstman, 1998, Arthritis Foundation, Atlanta.

The Duke University Book of Arthritis, David S. Pisetsky, MD, PhD, and Susan Flamholtz Trien, 1992, Fawcett Columbine, New York.

The Rheumatoid Arthritis Handbook, Stephen Paget, MD, Michael Lockshin, MD, and Susanne Loebl, 2002, John Wiley & Sons, New York.

Autoimmune Hepatitis

Dr. Melissa Palmer's Guide to Hepatitis and Liver Disease: What You Need to Know, Melissa Palmer, MD, 2000, Avery, New York.

Autoimmunity

At War Within: The Double-Edged Sword of Immunity, William R. Clark, PhD, 1995, Oxford University Press, Inc., New York.

Thriving with Your Autoimmune Disorder: A Woman's Mind-Body Guide, Simone Ravicz, PhD, 2000, New Harbinger, Oakland.

Crohn's Disease and Ulcerative Colitis

Controlling Crohn's Disease the Natural Way, Virginia M. Harper and Tom Monte, 2002, Kensington Publishing Corp., New York.

Crohn's Disease & Ulcerative Colitis: Everything You Need to Know, Fred Saibil and Frederic G. Saibil, 1997, Firefly, New York.

The First Year: Crohn's Disease and Ulcerative Colitis Handbook: An Essential Guide for the Newly Diagnosed, Jill Sklar and Michael Sklar, 2002, Marlowe & Co., New York.

The New Eating Right for a Bad Gut: The Complete Nutritional Guide to Ileitis, Colitis, Crohn's Disease, and Inflammatory Bowel Disease, James Scala, PhD, 2001, Plume/Penguin Putnam, New York.

Diabetes

The American Diabetes Association Complete Guide to Diabetes, Second Edition, 2001, American Diabetes Association, Bantam Books, New York.

The Joslin Guide to Diabetes, Richard S. Beaser, MD, with Joan V. C. Hill, RD, CDE, 1995, Fireside Books, New York.

Lupus

The Lupus Book (Revised Edition), Dan Wallace, 1999, Oxford University Press, New York.

Lupus: Everything You Need to Know, Robert Lahita, MD, and Robert Phillips, 1998, Avery Publishing Group, New York.

New Hope for People with Lupus: Your Friendly, Authoritative Guide to the Latest in Traditional and Complementary Solutions, Theresa Foy Digeronimo, Stephen Paget, MD, and Sara J. Henry, 2002, Prima Publishing, New York.

Multiple Sclerosis

Living with MS: A Guide for Patient, Caregiver, and Family, David L. Carroll and Jon Dudley Dorman, MD, 1993, Harper Perennial, New York.

Me and My Shadow: Living With Multiple Sclerosis, Carole MacKie, Ronnie Wood, and Sue Brattle, 1999, Aurum, Ltd., London.

Multiple Sclerosis: The Facts You Need, Paul O'Connor, 1999, Firefly, New York.

Women Living With Multiple Sclerosis, Judith Lynn Nichols, 1999, Hunter House, Alameda, CA.

Scleroderma

The Scleroderma Book: A Guide for Patients and Families, Maureen Mayes, 1999, Oxford University Press, New York.

Sjögren's Syndrome

The New Sjögren's Syndrome Handbook, Steven Carsons and Elaine K. Harris, 1998, Oxford University Press, New York.

Thyroid Disease

Graves' Disease: A Practical Guide, Elaine A. Moore, Lisa Moore, and Kelly R. Hale, 2001, McFarland & Co., New York.

Living Well With Hypothyroidism: What Your Doctor Doesn't Tell You . . . What You Need to Know, Mary J. Shomon, 2000, Harper Resource, New York.

Index